Applied Technologies in Pulmonary Medicine

Applied Technologies in Pulmonary Medicine

Editor

Antonio M. Esquinas Murcia

56 figures, 9 in color and 29 tables, 2011

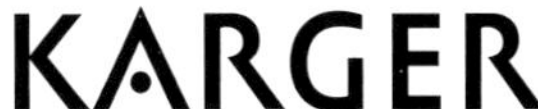

Basel · Freiburg · Paris · London · New York · Bangalore · Bangkok · Shanghai · Singapore · Tokyo · Sydney

'To Rosario, my wife, inspiration and love for all.'
Antonio M. Esquinas

Antonio M. Esquinas
Intensive Care Unit
Hospital Morales Meseguer
Murcia, Spain

Library of Congress Cataloging-in-Publication Data

Applied technologies in pulmonary medicine / editor, Antonio M. Esquinas.
p. ; cm.
Includes bibliographical references and indexes.
ISBN 978-3-8055-9584-1 (hard cover: alk. paper) — ISBN 978-3-8055-9585-8 (e-ISBN)
1. Respiratory therapy — Technological innovations. 2. Respirators (Medical equipment)
I. Esquinas, Antonio M.
[DNLM: 1. Pulmonary Medicine — Instrumentation. 2. Pulmonary Medicine – methods. 3. Biomedical Technology.
4. Respiratory Physiological Phenomena. 5. Respiratory Tract Diseases. 6. Technology, Medical — instrumentation. WF 100]
RC735.I5A67 2011
615.8'36 — dc22

2010036628

Bibliographic Indices. This publication is listed in bibliographic services.

Disclaimer. The statements, opinions and data contained in this publication are solely those of the individual authors and contributors and not of the publisher and the editor(s). The appearance of advertisements in the book is not a warranty, endorsement, or approval of the products or services advertised or of their effectiveness, quality or safety. The publisher and the editor(s) disclaim responsibility for any injury to persons or property resulting from any ideas, methods, instructions or products referred to in the content or advertisements.

Drug Dosage. The authors and the publisher have exerted every effort to ensure that drug selection and dosage set forth in this text are in accord with current recommendations and practice at the time of publication. However, in view of ongoing research, changes in government regulations, and the constant flow of information relating to drug therapy and drug reactions, the reader is urged to check the package insert for each drug for any change in indications and dosage and for added warnings and precautions. This is particularly important when the recommended agent is a new and/or infrequently employed drug.

All rights reserved. No part of this publication may be translated into other languages, reproduced or utilized in any form or by any means electronic or mechanical, including photocopying, recording, microcopying, or by any information storage and retrieval system, without permission in writing from the publisher.

© Copyright 2011 by S. Karger AG, P.O. Box, CH–4009 Basel (Switzerland)
www.karger.com
Printed in Switzerland on acid-free and non-aging paper (ISO 9706) by Reinhardt Druck, Basel
ISBN 978–3–8055–9584–1
e–ISBN 978–3–8055–9585–8

Contents

Applied Technologies in Specific Clinical Situations

Technology in Sleep Pulmonary Disorders

Technology in Cardiopulmonary Resuscitation

Technology in Inhalation Therapy

Technology in Diagnosis and Pulmonary Problems

Technology in Anesthesiology

Technology in Transplants

Technology and Monitoring

Technology and Equipment in Transport

Respiratory Technology in Abdominal Syndromes

Critical Care Problems

Applied Technologies in Pulmonary Diagnosis

Infections – Ventilator-Associated Pneumonia

Oncology and Pulmonary Complications

Prognosis and Readmission

Pulmonary Rehabilitation and Technology

Pulmonary Medicine in Pediatrics and Neonatology Critical Care

Respiratory Health Problems and Environment

Preface

Technological innovations in the treatment of respiratory diseases involve a critical vision of all aspects from basic physics, pathophysiology, diagnosis and treatments, to clinical experience.

Applied Technologies in Pulmonary Medicine is an updated selection of the most current original articles published on new technological advances in the diagnosis and treatment of respiratory problems. The analytical methodology is a very original aspect of this book in comparison to other textbooks on respiratory medicine, where invited authors critically present their results and the clinical implications of their findings.

The analysis includes basic areas such as pulmonary and critical care medicine, mechanical ventilation, ventilator modes (extracorporeal membrane oxygenation, time-adaptive modes, proportional assist ventilation, automatic control mechanical ventilation, etc.), new pharmacological treatments during mechanical ventilation (weaning options and post-extubation failure), the basics of pathophysiology, treatment and how to prevent ventilator-associated pneumonia (new antibiotics, viral infections and healthcare-associated pneumonia). We have also included original advances in technologies that are applied in anesthesiology and postoperative critical care (minimally invasive thoracic surgery, open-heart surgery, intraoperative and pulmonary resections) and in the preservation of organs.

Further topics that the readers will find in this book include the outcome of patients with lung cancer admitted to the ICU, new results on pulmonary rehabilitation and technologies, evidence-based guidelines and the basics on discharge from the ICU, how to optimize the problems in pediatric and neonatal critical care telemonitoring and assistance in chronic respiratory failure and capnography innovations, the newest options for diagnosis of pulmonary diseases (polysomnography, ultrasound), technology in emergency medicine such as cardiopulmonary resuscitation, and new options in inhalation therapies (macromolecules such as insulin).

Recently, two new major topics have gained the interest of all specialists engaged in the field of pulmonary medicine and related technologies: firstly the diagnosis of health respiratory problems and the environment, and secondly new concepts of organizational issues in global disaster management and the role of mechanical ventilation, guidelines and options.

The major topics in *Applied Technologies in Pulmonary Medicine* and their clinical implications have involved hard and meticulous work. It presents a novel approach to help clinicians easily understand the technologies provided in the numerous papers. We hope that the reader and younger researchers will acquire practical ideas when carrying out their laboratory and clinical trials on a daily basis.

I would like to thank all the authors as well as the following collaborators: Penny Andrews, BSN, RN, Baltimore, Md., USA; Melissa Brown, RRT-NPS, San Diego, Calif., USA; Andrea Calkovska, MD, PhD, Martin, Slovakia; Ettore Capoluongo, MD, Rome, Italy; Bart L. De Keulenaer, MD, FJFICM, East Fremantle, W.A., Australia; Emmanuel Douzinas, MD, Athens, Greece; Lothar Engelmann, MD, Leipzig, Germany; J. Pat Herlihy, MD, Houston, Tex., USA; Pavlos M. Myrianthefs, MD, PhD, Kifissia/Athens, Greece; Naomi Kondo Nakagawa, BSc, PhD, São Paulo, Brazil; Catherine S. Sassoon, MD, Long Beach, Calif., USA; Ilias I. Siempos, MD, Athens, Greece; Giovanni Vento, MD, Rome, Italy, and M.Terese Verklan, PhD, CCNS, RNC, Houston, Tex., USA. Their efforts to reach these objectives are greatly appreciated. I personally believe that the knowledge and '*application of technologies in pulmonary medicine*' will become a continuous dynamic process of ideas and experiences of trial and error, where the final conclusions can be drawn once they become routine.

Antonio M. Esquinas
Murcia, Spain

Esquinas AM (ed): Applied Technologies in Pulmonary Medicine. Basel, Karger, 2011, pp 1–5

Proportional Assist Ventilation and Neurally Adjusted Ventilatory Assist

Jennifer Beck[a] · Christer Sinderby[b]

[a]Department of Pediatrics, University of Toronto, and [b]Keenan Research Centre, Li Ka Shing Knowledge Institute and Department of Critical Care Medicine, St. Michael's Hospital, Toronto, Ont., Canada

Abbreviations

EAdi Electrical activity of the diaphragm
NAVA Neurally adjusted ventilatory assist
PAV Proportional assist ventilation

Historically, patients in need of mechanical ventilation were often heavily sedated or paralyzed and placed on time-cycled modes of ventilation. There is now clear evidence showing that reduced sedation and spontaneous breathing improve patient outcome in terms of days on ventilation and mortality [1]. Under these conditions (less sedation and more spontaneous breathing), unless the patient 'entrains' themselves to the rate of the breath delivery, time-cycled modes may not be the most appropriate, especially in light of the recent work demonstrating that patient-ventilator asynchrony increases the duration of mechanical ventilation and mortality [2].

Two new modes of mechanical ventilation are now available on the market that can synchronize not only the timing, but also the level of assist to the patient's own effort, PAV and NAVA. This article describes the concepts related to PAV and NAVA, their similarities and their differences, and the recent physiological studies. For a more detailed review of this topic, the reader is referred to Sinderby and Beck [3].

Patient-Ventilator Interaction

Ideally, a mechanical ventilator should behave as a respiratory prosthesis, providing air in tandem with the patient's breathing in terms of timing and the magnitude of the inspiration. The prevalence of patient-ventilator asynchrony has recently been revealed [2] and it is now readily accepted that during conventional ventilation, such as pressure support ventilation, poor patient-ventilator asynchrony does occur [4, 5]. Patient-ventilator asynchrony ranges at its worst from completely missed patient efforts (so-called wasted efforts) and auto-triggering in the absence of spontaneous efforts, to delays in ventilator triggering and cycling-off. Modes with fixed levels of assist (such as assist control, pressure control, and pressure support ventilation)

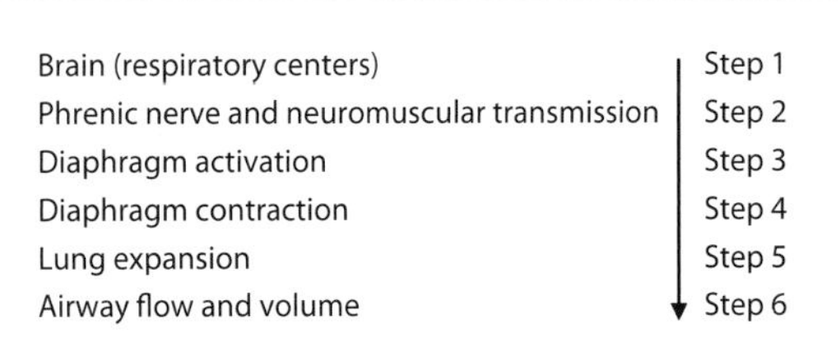

Fig. 1. Simplified chain of events involved with spontaneous breathing, beginning with central respiratory drive (Step 1), to the final ventilatory output at the airway (Step 6).

may also be asynchronous since the ventilator cannot respond to changes in patient demand on a breath-by-breath basis. Patient-ventilator asynchrony has now been shown to affect patient outcome in terms of prolonged weaning [6], poorer sleep quality [7], longer duration of mechanical ventilation and tracheotomy [2], and in infants, higher incidence of pneumothorax [8].

From Brain to Breath: Spontaneous Breathing

A simplified schematic of the chain of events that occur during spontaneous breathing is presented in figure 1. The signal for spontaneous breathing originates in the respiratory centers (Step 1) and in the case of the diaphragm – the most important muscle of respiration – travels down the phrenic nerves, then passes through the neuromuscular junction (Step 2) to activate the diaphragm electrically (Step 3). It is only after this step of electrical activation of the diaphragm, that cross-bridge cycling is initiated and the muscle contracts (Step 4). Contraction of the diaphragm results in lung expansion (Step 5), resulting in flow and volume at the airway (Step 6). Depending on the type and severity of the disease, the final output of airflow and volume at the airway may not represent the true neural respiratory output.

Proportional Assist Ventilation

In PAV [9], the ventilator generates airway pressure in proportion to instantaneous flow and volume (Step 6). The flow assist, which is a percentage of the airway resistance, dictates how much airway pressure is delivered per unit of flow. The volume assist, which is a percent of the pulmonary elastance, dictates how much pressure is delivered per unit of volume. The degree of assist can range to provide unloading between 0 and 100%. During PAV, knowledge about respiratory system mechanics and endotracheal tube resistance are required. This is especially important in preterm neonates as there is a large breath-to-breath variability in resistance and compliance of the respiratory system. Recently, 'PAV+', with updated measurements of resistance and elastance and implementation of load-adjustable gain factors, has the potential to account for this.

With regard to physiological studies [for a review, see 3], PAV has been shown to improve patient comfort, improve patient-ventilator interaction, improve sleep quality, and allows greater variability in breathing pattern (i.e. more physiological) in comparison with pressure support. In both adults and neonates, PAV has been demonstrated to unload the respiratory muscles, with lower mean airway pressures than pressure support ventilation – with similar clinical short-term outcomes (gas exchange and hemodynamics). Recently, PAV with load-adjustable gain factors has been shown to be feasible in critically ill patients, and to require fewer interventions with respect to sedation and ventilator settings [10] compared to pressure support.

Neurally Adjusted Ventilatory Assist

NAVA uses the EAdi (Step 3) – a signal representative of the output from the respiratory centers – to control both the timing and the magnitude of delivered pressure [11]. The EAdi is obtained by an array of miniaturized sensors placed on a conventional nasogastric (or orogastric) feeding tube. The electrode array is positioned in the esophagus at the level of the gastroesophageal junction, where the spontaneous activity of the crural diaphragm is sensed. Standardized signal processing algorithms automatically take into account diaphragm displacement, motion artifacts, filtering of the electrocardiogram, and cross-talk from other active muscles [12]. The processed signal, known as the EAdi waveform, can be characterized by its amplitude on inspiration (phasic EAdi) and expiration (tonic EAdi) as well as its timing (neural inspiratory time, neural expiratory time, neural respiratory rate). When compared to the airway pressure waveform in other modes of ventilation, the EAdi provides information about patient-ventilator synchrony. In the absence of the EAdi signal (and the catheter position has been deemed appropriate), it is an indication of central apnea, or suppression of spontaneous breathing activity. Hence, the EAdi signal has monitoring capabilities as well as controlling the ventilator.

In infant and adult patients, NAVA has been shown to significantly improve patient-ventilator interaction compared to conventional modes of assist [4, 5, 13], in terms of both improved timing and proportionality. Neural triggering and cycling-off on non-invasive (helmet) ventilation in healthy adults has demonstrated that this improved synchrony improves comfort [14].

During NAVA, the assist levels are adjusted by changing the proportionality between the EAdi and delivered pressure (the so-called 'NAVA level'). Stepwise increases in the NAVA level cause a gradual reduction in respiratory drive, and therefore the expected increase in pressure is not necessarily achieved. Due to this physiological downregulation of the EAdi signal, airway pressure and tidal volume 'plateau' at adequate levels of unloading [15].

Since the EAdi controller signal for NAVA is pneumatically independent, application of NAVA with excessively leaky non-invasive interfaces does not affect patient-ventilator synchrony.

Discussion

The similarities and differences between PAV and NAVA can only be discussed theoretically as there are no studies in the literature comparing these two modes of ventilation. The lack of a single device providing both modes of ventilation is likely the responsible factor.

In principle, NAVA and PAV are similar in that they are both modes of assisted ventilation where the applied airway pressure is servo-controlled continuously throughout spontaneous inspiration, changing in proportion to the patient's breathing effort and allowing the patient to control the extent and timing of lung inflation. During both NAVA and PAV, the amplification 'gain' between patient effort and delivered pressure can be adjusted, in order to achieve more or less unloading of the respiratory muscles. This is very different from modes of ventilation that are volume- or pressure-targeted, where fixed levels of assist are delivered independent of patient effort.

Both PAV and NAVA require that the patient is spontaneously breathing. However, it should be noted that NAVA uses the neural output signal (EAdi), whereas PAV has no monitoring capabilities for quantifying respiratory drive. This means that, similar to other patient-triggered modes of ventilation, a back-up mode of ventilation is required in the case of central apnea. As well, upper pressure limits should be adjusted accordingly, in the case of large and central respiratory drive. The fact that PAV and NAVA require some degree of spontaneous breathing may actually be a clinical advantage, in that the respiratory muscles are encouraged to be used during partial ventilator assist. Inactivity of respiratory muscles during mechanical ventilation (due to too high levels of sedation or too high levels of assist) has a negative impact on diaphragm muscle fiber integrity and prolongs the duration of mechanical ventilation [16].

Unlike pressure support ventilation, increasing levels of assist with PAV and NAVA have little effect on respiratory rate and tidal volume when unloading is sufficient. In modes of ventilation that allow the patient the freedom to control the rate and depth of inspiration, it seems that there is a desired minute ventilation, rate and volume. When unloading is adequate to satisfy the patient's demand, if the assist is increased during PAV or NAVA, patient effort decreases and therefore, so does the amount of assist.

The major differences between these two modes lie in how the disease processes affect the controller signals. During NAVA, the EAdi (the neural respiratory drive to the diaphragm from the respiratory centers, Step 3 in figure 1) is the controller signal. PAV uses airway flow and volume (Step 6), which is a surrogate measurement of respiratory drive, and further down the chain of events involved with spontaneous breathing.

In the presence of a leak – for example in infants with leaks around the endotracheal tube, or during non-invasive ventilation – the flow and volume signal in Step 6 will be misinterpreted as patient flow and volume. For triggering and delivering proportional assist during PAV, the leak may auto-cycle the ventilator and may call for increased flow delivery during inspiration. In sharp contrast, NAVA, using a neural trigger, is not affected by leaks for obtaining synchrony. Depending on the size of the leak, an increase in the NAVA level however may be required to unload the respiratory muscle sufficiently.

The major difference between NAVA and PAV might be observed in the case of dynamic hyperinflation, where shortening of the respiratory muscles affects the force output for a given neural activation. In fact, any disease process affecting the contractile properties of the diaphragm (Step 4) will in theory cause an 'uncoupling' between neural respiratory drive (Steps 1–3) and patient flow and volume (Step 6). In the case of dynamic hyperinflation, if the respiratory drive stays the same (i.e. same EAdi), the flow and volume will be lower, and the controller signal for PAV may reduce the airway pressure delivery.

Conclusion

PAV and NAVA are both modes of partial ventilator assist delivering assist in proportion to patient effort. During NAVA, the diaphragm electrical activity – a true signal of neural respiratory output – is the controller signal for delivered ventilation. During PAV, a surrogate measurement of respiratory drive is used to control the ventilator. The inherent benefits of these two modes lie in the fact that these modes require spontaneous breathing and offer synchronized delivery of assist.

Recommendations

- Implement spontaneous mode of ventilation as soon as possible/tolerable.
- Ensure that respiratory drive is not suppressed by too high levels of sedation or too high levels of assist, i.e. ensure that patients are spontaneously breathing.
- Optimize patient-ventilator synchrony.

References

1 Girard TD, Kress JP, Fuchs BD, et al: Efficacy and safety of a paired sedation and ventilator weaning protocol for mechanically ventilated patients in intensive care (Awakening and Breathing Controlled trial): a randomised controlled trial. Lancet 2008;371:126–134.

2 Thille AW, Rodriguez P, Cabello B, et al: Patient-ventilator asynchrony during assisted mechanical ventilation. Intensive Care Med 2006;32:1515–1522.

3 Sinderby C, Beck J: Proportional assist ventilation and neurally adjusted ventilatory assist – better approaches to patient-ventilator synchrony? Clin Chest Med 2008;29:329–342.

4 Colombo D, Cammarota G, Bergamaschi V, et al: Physiologic response to varying levels of pressure support and neurally adjusted ventilatory assist in patients with acute respiratory failure. Intensive Care Med 2008;34:2010–2018.

5 Spahija J, De Marchie M, Albert M, et al: Patient-ventilator interaction during pressure support ventilation and neurally adjusted ventilatory assist. Crit Care Med 2010;38:518–526.

6 Chao DC, Scheinhorn DJ, Stearn-Hassenpflug M: Patient-ventilator trigger asynchrony in prolonged mechanical ventilation. Chest 1997:112:1592–1599.

7 Bosma K, Ferreyra G, Ambrogio C, et al: Patient-ventilator interaction and sleep in mechanically ventilated patients: pressure support versus proportional assist ventilation. Crit Care Med 2007;35: 1048–1054.

8 Greenough A, Wood S, Morley CJ, Davis JA: Pancuronium prevents pneumothoraces in ventilated premature babies who actively expire against positive pressure inflation. Lancet 1984;1:1–3.

9 Younes M: Proportional assist ventilation, a new approach to ventilatory support. Theory. Am Rev Respir Dis 1992; 145:114–120.

10 Xirouchaki N, Kondili E, Vaporidi K, et al: Proportional assist ventilation with load-adjustable gain factors in critically ill patients: comparison with pressure support. Intensive Care Med 2008;34: 2026–2034.

11 Sinderby C, Navalesi P, Beck J, et al: Neural control of mechanical ventilation in respiratory failure. Nat Med 1999;5: 1433–1436.

12 Aldrich T, Sinderby C, McKenzie D, et al: Electrophysiologic techniques for the assessment of respiratory muscle function; in ATS/ERS Statement on Respiratory Muscle Testing. Am J Respir Crit Care Med 2002;166:518–624.

13 Beck J, Reilly M, Grasselli G, et al: Patient-ventilator interaction during neurally adjusted ventilatory assist in low birth weight infants. Pediatr Res 2009;65:663–668.

14 Moerer O, Beck J, Brander L, et al: Subject-ventilator synchrony during neural versus pneumatically triggered noninvasive helmet ventilation. Intensive Care Med 2008;34:1615–1623.

15 Brander L, Leong-Poi H, Beck J, et al: Titration and implementation of neurally adjusted ventilatory assist in critically ill patients. Chest 2009;135:695–703.

16 Levine S, Nguyen T, Taylor N, et al: Rapid disuse atrophy of diaphragm fibers in mechanically ventilated humans. N Engl J Med 2008;358:1327–1335.

Jennifer Beck, PhD
Keenan Research Centre, Li Ka Shing Knowledge Institute
St. Michael's Hospital, 30 Bond Street, Queen Wing 4-072
Toronto, ON M5B1W8 (Canada)
Tel. +1 416 880 3664, E-Mail beckj@smh.toronto.on.ca

Esquinas AM (ed): Applied Technologies in Pulmonary Medicine. Basel, Karger, 2011, pp 6–9

Time-Adaptive Mode: A New Ventilation Form for the Treatment of Respiratory Insufficiency

D. Dellweg · T. Barchfeld · J. Kerl · D. Koehler

Pneumonology 1, Kloster Grafschaft, Schmallenberg, Germany

Abbreviations

AC Assist control
NIV Non-invasive ventilation
S Spontaneous
ST Spontaneous-timed
TA Timed automated

NIV has gained substantial importance and is considered standard medical care for hypercapnic respiratory failure of different etiologies [1]. It also has a proven benefit for certain forms of hypoxemic respiratory failure [2]. The main rationale of NIV is the unloading effect on the respiratory muscles during ventilation [3]. This results in reduction of dyspnea, increased mobility and better quality of life for the patient. NIV is usually applied using a S, ST or AC mode. In either mode, patients have to trigger the ventilator unless the programmed backup rate (ST mode) exceeds the patient's respiratory rate. The work that is necessary to trigger the ventilator can be substantial and might be as high as 39% of the total work of breathing [4]. Controlled NIV is feasible [5] and might decrease the respiratory workload, eliminating the need to trigger the ventilator. Controlled NIV however is not frequently used and might potentially increase patient-ventilator asynchrony or mismatch. Non-invasive ventilators produce a linear or curvilinear flow profile during inspiration that might not match the patient's own inspiratory flow profile. This may cause discomfort and increase patient-ventilator asynchrony.

In view of these problems, Weinmann GmbH (Hamburg, Germany) introduced a new mode of NIV (TA incorporated into the Ventilogic© ventilator) that automatically captures the patient's own flow profile and adjusts ventilation with preselected pressure levels in a controlled fashion [6].

Description of the TA Algorithm

Inspiratory and expiratory pressures must be selected on the ventilator-interactive display prior to ventilation. The operator has also to select the type of underlying airway disease (R = restrictive, O = obstructive, N = normal) and set upper and lower limits to the respiratory rate by selecting a target rate and a range of allowance. The patient must be connected (via mask) to the ventilator prior to activation of the mode.

Once activated, TA-mode ventilation begins with an analysis phase. During this phase, a continuous pressure of 4 hPa is delivered by the ventilator turbine to guarantee effective carbon dioxide washout through the whisper valve of the mask interface. During this phase, the ventilator analyzes

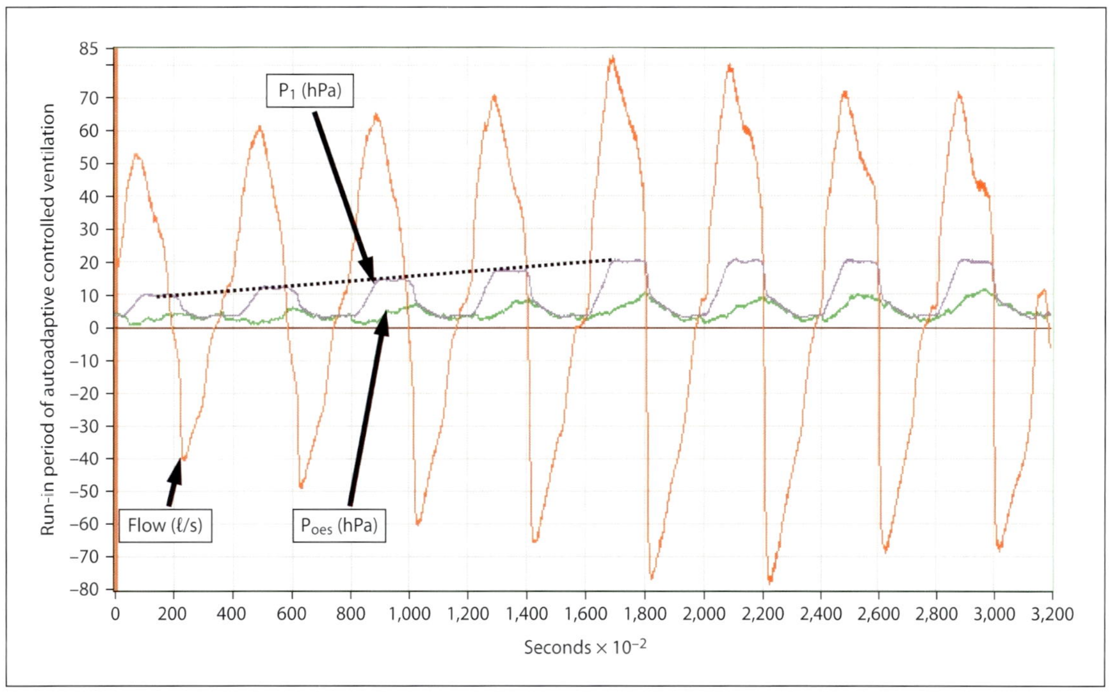

Fig. 1. Pressure and flow tracings during the run-in period of autoadaptive controlled ventilation (TA mode). According to the measured flow profile of spontaneous breathing, the ventilator slowly increases inspiratory pressure (P_I) during the run-in period, resulting in increased inspiratory flow (Flow) and raised esophageal pressure (P_{oes}), a marker of respiratory muscle unloading.

the patient's own flow profile by integration of flow and time. Once the ventilator senses a stable profile (time and flow measurements within a predefined range of allowance), the ventilator will increase inspiratory pressure over five consecutive breaths in steps of 60–70–80–90–100% of preset value (fig. 1). During the inspiratory phase, inspiratory pressure will be adjusted over inspiratory time in order to obtain a flow profile matching the patient's own pattern. One has to note that the preselected inspiratory pressure will only be achieved during peak inspiratory flow, and that the pressure level during inspiration will be adjusted to mimic the previously detected flow profile.

The inspiratory pressure curve is calculated according to the following motion equation:

$$P(t) = R \times \text{flow} + 1/C \times \text{volume}$$

P(t) represents the pressure integral, flow and volume arise from averaged flow pattern data from the analysis phase. The selection R = restrictive, O = obstructive and N = normal allocates distinct constant numbers for resistance (R given in hPa/(l/s)) and compliance (C given in ml/hPa) into the equation. The system software calculates P(t) according to the individual preselected maximal inspiratory pressures.

Inspiratory time refers to the average inspiratory time recorded during the analysis phase. We selected a broad range of the respiratory rate to allow each individual to achieve his or her natural respiratory rate. The target rate range selection can be used to prevent an inept and non-physiological breathing pattern.

Inspiratory to expiratory time ratio (I:E ratio) is determined by the subject's I:E ratio measured

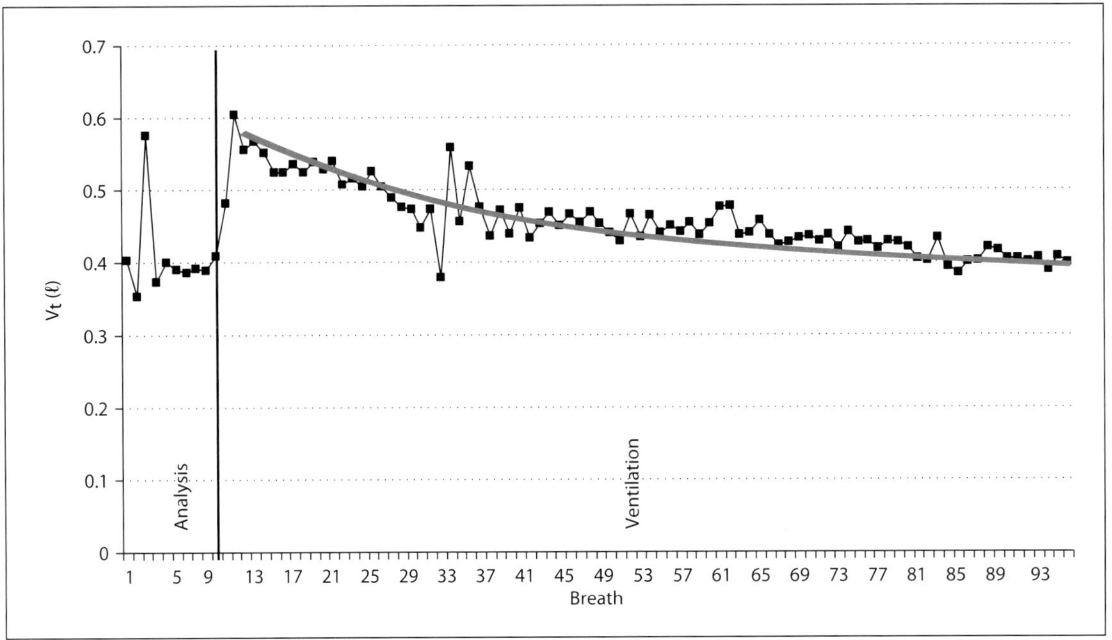

Fig. 2. Onset of ventilation (red line) increases tidal volume (V_t) initially, since patient effort is supported by gas delivery from the ventilator. While the latter is constant, patient effort decreases as indicated by the subsequent decrease in V_t.

during the analysis phase. At the end of the run-in period, ventilator gas delivery will increase (V_t) as long as the patient has not decreased his or her respiratory effort. Patient effort will then consecutively decrease as a sign of respiratory muscle rest and decreasing oxygen cost of breathing (fig. 2).

TA mode does not allow for additional triggered breaths, however if the ventilator senses subject-ventilator asynchrony, and it will reanalyze the patient's flow pattern. Asynchrony is defined by inspiratory and/or expiratory fighting in four consecutive breaths. Inspiratory fighting is defined by a flow reduction of at least 20 l/min below the mean inspiratory flow inside the middle 60% of the inspiratory time (between T_I 20 and T_I 80). Expiratory fighting is defined by the presence of flow rise of 10 l/min above leak-compensation inside the middle 40% of the expiratory time (between T_E 30 and T_E 70).

Clinical Implication of TA-Mode NIV

TA-mode ventilation has been compared to S-mode ventilation in healthy individuals and achieved a higher degree of respiratory muscle unloading (see fig. 3) [7]. It therefore represents a promising mode to better unload the respiratory muscles in patients who require NIV. Clinical studies in patients are being currently conducted but have not been published to date. From our experience, TA-mode ventilation is well tolerated and effective in the majority of patients.

Patients with a markedly irregular breathing pattern during sleep might experience recurrent phases of breathing pattern reanalysis if fighting criteria are fulfilled. This might cause sleep disturbances and can compromise compliance and practicability of this type of ventilation. According to our personal experience, the latter applies only

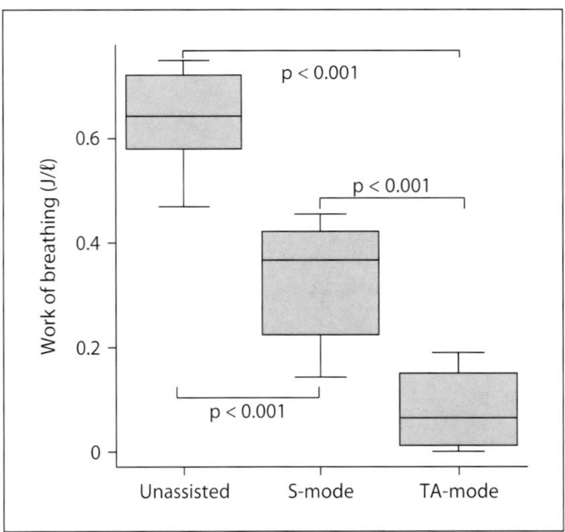

Fig. 3. Work of breathing during unassisted breathing, S-mode and TA-mode NIV.

to a minority of patients (<5%). In general, patients have to understand the functioning of the TA mode and should be instructed to breathe their usual quiet and normal breathing pattern during the analysis period. Patients however can manually select reanalysis, if they are not satisfied with the ventilator-generated breathing pattern.

TA-mode ventilation is promising and an innovative new mode of ventilation with improved unloading of respiratory muscles. Clinical studies in respiratory failure of different etiologies however are required to prove clinical feasibility and evaluate the clinical benefit.

Conclusion

TA-mode ventilation offers the opportunity of additional respiratory muscle unloading because it reduces the work required to trigger the ventilator. The mode is well tolerated by the majority of patients, however asynchrony with frequent phases of re-analysis might compromise the quality of ventilation and user compliance in some patients.

References

1 Ozsancak A, D'Ambrosio C, Hill NS: Nocturnal noninvasive ventilation. Chest 2008;133:1275–1286.

2 Ferrer M, Esquinas A, Leon M, Gonzalez G, Alarcon A, Torres A: Noninvasive ventilation in severe hypoxemic respiratory failure: a randomized clinical trial. Am J Respir Crit Care Med 2003;168: 1438–1444.

3 Girault C, Chevron V, Richard JC, et al: Physiological effects and optimisation of nasal assist-control ventilation for patients with chronic obstructive pulmonary disease in respiratory failure. Thorax 1997;52:690–696.

4 Vitacca M, Barbano L, D'Anna S, Porta R, Bianchi L, Ambrosino N: Comparison of five bilevel pressure ventilators in patients with chronic ventilatory failure: a physiologic study. Chest 2002;122: 2105–2114.

5 Dellweg D, Schonhofer B, Haidl PM, et al: Short-term effect of controlled instead of assisted noninvasive ventilation in chronic respiratory failure due to chronic obstructive pulmonary disease. Respir Care 2007;52:1734–1740.

6 Kohler D, Dellweg D, Barchfeld T, Klauke M, Tiemann B: Time-adaptive mode, a new ventilation form for the treatment of respiratory insufficiency – a self-learning system (in German). Pneumologie 2008;62:527–532.

7 Dellweg D, Barchfeld T, Klauke M, Eiger G: Respiratory muscle unloading during auto-adaptive non-invasive ventilation. Respir Med 2009;103:1706–1712.

Dr. med. Dominic Dellweg
Pneumonology 1, Kloster Grafschaft
Annostrasse 1, DE–57392 Schmallenberg (Germany)
Tel. +49 2972 791 00, Fax +49 2972 791 2526
E-Mail d.dellweg@fkkg.de

Esquinas AM (ed): Applied Technologies in Pulmonary Medicine. Basel, Karger, 2011, pp 10–14

Influence of Ventilation Strategies on Hemodynamics in Hypovolemic Shock

Holger Herff

Department of Anesthesiology and Critical Care Medicine, Innsbruck Medical University, Innsbruck, Austria

Abbreviations

CPR Cardiopulmonary resuscitation
ITD Inspiratory threshold device
ITPR Intrathoracic pressure controller
NEEP Negative end-expiratory pressure
PEEP Positive end-expiratory pressure

Influence of Intrathoracic Pressure on Blood Flow – Physiological Background

High positive ventilation pressures being induced by high PEEP levels or recruitment maneuvers are standard tools to improve oxygenation in emergency and critical care patients, especially in acute lung injury [1, 2]. However, positive pressure ventilation with PEEP increases intrathoracic pressure which is subsequently transmitted to intrathoracic vessels. Thus, venous return into the thorax is decreased which has a significant negative impact on cardiac preload, cardiac output and subsequently on blood pressure [3]. PEEP levels >15 cm H_2O increase pulmonary arterial resistance directly which may additionally result in right ventricular failure [4]. Normovolemic patients tolerate PEEP well and hypervolemic central blood volume has the potential to reduce effects of high PEEP levels on blood flow, as long as the right ventricle does not fail [5]. Vice versa, negative PEEP effects are more pronounced if the central volume state is hypovolemic [6]. Thus, central hypovolemic patients are at high risk of cardiovascular collapse even at moderate PEEP levels. Right atrial pressures <10 cm H_2O in intubated patients seem to be critical if PEEP levels are increasing [5]. It is noteworthy that while PEEP may be used in cardiogenic shock to reduce central volume and subsequently left ventricular preload [7], in cardiac arrest increased central volume improves blood flow during CPR [6, 8, 9]. Although cardiac arrest often may be the final form of cardiogenic shock, the mechanisms determining blood flow in cardiac arrest and during CPR are similar to those in hypovolemic shock. Since heart function is bridged by chest compressions during CPR, blood flow mainly depends on the quality of chest compressions and central volume status and thus central (relative) hypervolemia may increase blood flow whereas hypovolemia may reduce it. In consequence, ventilation strategies improving blood flow in cardiac arrest [10, 11] are similar to those in hypovolemic shock [12, 13].

Conventional Therapeutic Consequences – Reducing Mean Airway Pressures

In a recent study, a strong correlation between mean intrapulmonary pressure and blood flow and cardiac output was demonstrated in a simulated hemorrhagic shock animal model [14]. Thus, ventilation strategies that may decrease mean intrathoracic pressure either by reducing PEEP, lower tidal volumes, or lower respiratory rates may increase venous return to the heart and subsequently cardiac output. The easiest step to achieve reduced mean airway pressures is to reduce PEEP. Such a reduction of PEEP from 10 to 5 or 0 cm H_2O PEEP in severe hemorrhagic shock increased short-term survival in pigs substantially [15]. Another method may be to reduce tidal volumes; despite retaining PEEP and lung minute volume constant by doubling respiratory rate in an animal model, survival rate was improved by 40–60% for as much as 20 min longer due to reduced tidal volumes. In this experiment, mean airway pressure was reduced substantially by the lower inflated tidal volumes despite higher respiratory rates. Further, mean airway pressure correlated strongly with blood pressure and cardiac output [14]. Thus, despite remaining minute ventilation and subsequently blood gases constant and maintaining PEEP levels, the influence of ventilation on blood pressure could have been decreased by reducing tidal volumes and subsequently mean intrapulmonary pressure. Mean intrapulmonary pressure as an important force that interferes with venous return explains apparently discrepancies to previous studies reporting higher respiratory rates being detrimental to blood flow in acute shock states [12, 13]. In these studies, tidal volumes were constant and thus higher respiratory rates resulted in higher mean intrapulmonary pressures, whereas reduced respiratory rates with constant tidal volumes automatically resulted in lower mean intrapulmonary pressures which due to our data improve blood flow and survival chances of experimental animals [14]. However, we have to be aware that a strategy of high respiratory rates and low tidal volumes may fail in obstructive patients such as asthmatics. Due to short expiratory times, incomplete expiration might lead to intrinsic PEEP levels that may again have detrimental effects on blood flow [14].

Experimental Therapeutic Consequences – Reducing Mean Airway Pressures Sub-Zero

Another more aggressive strategy to reduce mean airway pressure further is to apply NEEP. In a pig model of severe hemorrhagic shock, intermittent negative pressure was applied by suctioning gas out of the airways during the expiratory phase [16]. Ventilation was applied using normal tidal volumes and respiratory rates. As a result, all NEEP animals survived the 120-min observational period whereas only half of the 0 PEEP and none of the 5 PEEP animals survived. Reducing the baseline pressure by reducing EEP to negative levels is the most effective way to reduce mean airway pressure. Thus, it is not surprising that NEEP ventilation significantly increases blood flow in hemorrhagic shock [16].

While this strategy needed a special technical apparatus to apply NEEP in ventilated animals this could be achieved with less technical effort in spontaneously breathing individuals. A special valve, ITD, was originally designed to be used during CPR [8, 17]. The ITD closes the airway up to a preset pressure during the chest decompression phase of CPR [8]. The forces of the recoiling chest that would suction air into the patient's lungs if the ventilation tube remains open, result in a subatmospheric pressure in the patient's lungs if this tube is closed by the ITD [8]. The recoiling forces can be further enhanced during CPR if in addition to the forces generated by passive recoiling of the chest wall, active decompression is applied to the chest [18]. These negative airway pressures substantially increase venous return to the heart resulting in a central hypervolemic state, thus 'priming the pump' for the next chest compression. This strategy resulted in better blood flow in CPR models and increased survival rates in clinical studies [17, 19].

In non-CPR states, e.g. during hemorrhagic hypovolemic shock, such a negative airway pressure cannot be generated by force on the chest. However, the forces generated by the diaphragm can be used in spontaneously breathing patients to generate subatmospheric intrapulmonary pressures. Special valves for shock (ITPR) had been developed comparable to the CPR-ITD. Within general lower cracking pressures <10 cm H_2O, the ITPR may allow patients to ventilate freely against some tolerable resistance which generates negative intrapulmonary pressures [20]. The ITPR can be set on facemasks that then have to be sealed to patients' faces tightly. These devices improved substantially blood flow in shock states in spontaneously breathing animals that were being intubated due to anesthesia for animal protection. Thus, short-term survival rates were substantially increased in hemorrhagic shock models [21, 22]. In a recent study the ITPR further improved blood flow and short-term survival in a pig model of acute heat stroke [23]. Although heat shock may have a different etiology compared to hemorrhagic shock, subatmospheric intrapulmonary pressure seems to improve hemodynamics in other forms of hypovolemic shock, too.

Testing the ITPR in healthy adult volunteers increased cardiac output up to 20%; further, heart rate increased as well as stroke volume indicating better venous return to the heart that forces the (healthy) heart to increased work [24, 25]. In further recent studies in human volunteers using the ITPR, hypotension was artificially induced by central hypovolemia due to progressive lower body negative pressure. This was achieved by a special garment applying –7 cm H_2O on the lower body half. In such a simulated central hypovolemic state, spontaneous ventilation through an ITPR resulted in significantly improved cardiac output and more stable cardiocirculatory conditions [26, 27]. Thus, despite still lacking experience in humans in severe hemorrhagic shock, spontaneously breathing through an ITPR seems to be a promising concept to improve blood flow in human hypovolemic shock.

Negative Side Effects of Decreasing Intrapulmonary Pressures and Limitations

PEEP is used to improve oxygenation in ventilated patients since it has the potential to remain the alveoli open state [1]. Further, since many shock patients may suffer from thoracic trauma as well lung-protective ventilation, strategies including PEEP are efficient against pulmonary failure [28]. Thus, concepts that omit PEEP or induce NEEP may gain some bargain in the immediate shock state while in the aftermath patients may be lost due to increased rates of pulmonary failure [29]. Thus, concepts that postulate to omit well-established clinical concepts such as PEEP have to be well deliberated and need more clinical evidence in controlled prospective studies.

Especially high negative intrapulmonary pressures may result in pulmonary atelectasis and thus right-to-left shunts that may endanger patients of hypoxia. In a study performed in 2001, we used an ITD model with a cracking pressure of 35 cm H_2O in a CPR model [30]. Without active ventilation the airway was completely obstructed which resulted in resorption atelectasis; although the oxygen concentration in the alveoli was 100% before the experiment, the animals were severely hypoxic after 2 min. In contrast, if the airway remained open the SaO_2 was still >95% after 5 min experimental time [30]. Thus, if these valves are used in intubated patients during CPR, the best way to avoid complete resorption atelectasis is intermittent active positive pressure ventilation for recruitment of atelectatic pulmonary areas [31]. In spontaneously breathing patients, airway obstruction may be especially dangerous due to rapidly developing negative pressure pulmonary edema [32]. Further, to avoid resorption atelectasis, subatmospheric pressures in spontaneously breathing patients generated by special valves as the ITPR have to be so low that the valves open during every inspiratory effort. Last, breathing through an ITPR in shock increases work of power for breathing; while healthy volunteers did not have any problems to compensate, this may be different in multiple trauma patients [33].

Conclusion

Reducing mean airway pressure may be a strategy to improve venous return to the heart and subsequently blood flow in hypovolemic shock states. One method may be to omit PEEP or to decrease tidal volumes. Experimental approaches to reduce intrapulmonary pressures to subatmospheric levels, either in spontaneously breathing patients or in the expiratory phase during artificially ventilation, are not evidenced yet and need further research.

References

1 Barbas C, de Matos G, Pincelli M, da Rosa Borges E, Antunes T, de Barros J, Okamoto V, Borges J, Amato M, de Carvalho C: Mechanical ventilation in acute respiratory failure: recruitment and high positive end-expiratory pressure are necessary. Curr Opin Crit Care 2005;11: 18–28.

2 Borges J, Okamoto V, Matos G, Caramez M, Arantes P, Barros F, Souza C, Victorino J, Kacmarek R, Barbas C, Carvalho C, Amato M: Reversibility of lung collapse and hypoxemia in early acute respiratory distress syndrome. Am J Respir Crit Care Med 2006;174:268–278.

3 Gernoth C, Wagner G, Pelosi P, Luecke T: Respiratory and haemodynamic changes during decremental open lung positive end-expiratory pressure titration in patients with acute respiratory distress syndrome. Crit Care 2009;13:R59.

4 Biondi JW, Schulman DS, Soufer R, Matthay RA, Hines RL, Kay HR, Barash PG: The effect of incremental positive end-expiratory pressure on right ventricular hemodynamics and ejection fraction. Anesth Analg 1988;67:144–151.

5 Jellinek H, Krafft P, Fitzgerald R, Schwarz S, Pinsky M: Right atrial pressure predicts hemodynamic response to apneic positive airway pressure. Crit Care Med 2000;28:672–678.

6 Ido Y, Goto H, Lavin M, Robinson J, Mangold J, Arakawa K: Effects of positive end-expiratory pressure on carotid blood flow during closed-chest cardiopulmonary resuscitation in dogs. Anesth Analg 1982;61:557–560.

7 Hoffmann B, Welte T: Non-invasive positive pressure ventilation in cardiogenic pulmonary edema (in German). Med Klin (Munich) 1999;94:58–61.

8 Lurie K, Coffeen P, Shultz J, McKnite S, Detloff B, Mulligan K: Improving active compression-decompression cardiopulmonary resuscitation with an inspiratory impedance valve. Circulation 1995;91:1629–1632.

9 Lurie K, Mulligan K, McKnite S, Detloff B, Lindstrom P, Lindner K: Optimizing standard cardiopulmonary resuscitation with an inspiratory impedance threshold valve. Chest 1998;113:1084–1090.

10 Aufderheide T, Lurie K: Death by hyperventilation: a common and life-threatening problem during cardiopulmonary resuscitation. Crit Care Med 2004;32(suppl):S345–S351.

11 Aufderheide T, Sigurdsson G, Pirrallo R, Yannopoulos D, McKnite S, von Briesen C, Sparks C, Conrad C, Provo T, Lurie K: Hyperventilation-induced hypotension during cardiopulmonary resuscitation. Circulation 2004;109:1960–1965.

12 Pepe P, Lurie K, Wigginton J, Raedler C, Idris A: Detrimental hemodynamic effects of assisted ventilation in hemorrhagic states. Crit Care Med 2004;32(suppl):S414–S420.

13 Pepe P, Raedler C, Lurie K, Wigginton J: Emergency ventilatory management in hemorrhagic states: elemental or detrimental? J Trauma 2003;54:1048–1055.

14 Herff H, Paal P, von Goedecke A, Lindner KH, Severing AC, Wenzel V: Influence of ventilation strategies on survival in severe controlled hemorrhagic shock. Crit Care Med 2008;36:2613–2620.

15 Krismer AC, Wenzel V, Lindner KH, Haslinger CW, Oroszy S, Stadlbauer KH, Konigsrainer A, Boville B, Hormann C: Influence of positive end-expiratory pressure ventilation on survival during severe hemorrhagic shock. Ann Emerg Med 2005;46:337–342.

16 Krismer AC, Wenzel V, Lindner KH, von Goedecke A, Junger M, Stadlbauer KH, Konigsrainer A, Strohmenger HU, Sawires M, Jahn B, Hormann C: Influence of negative expiratory pressure ventilation on hemodynamic variables during severe hemorrhagic shock. Crit Care Med 2006;34:2175–2181.

17 Plaisance P, Lurie K, Payen D: Inspiratory impedance during active compression-decompression cardiopulmonary resuscitation: a randomized evaluation in patients in cardiac arrest. Circulation 2000;101:989–994.

18 Plaisance P, Lurie K, Vicaut E, Adnet F, Petit J, Epain D, Ecollan P, Gruat R, Cavagna P, Biens J, Payen D: A comparison of standard cardiopulmonary resuscitation and active compression-decompression resuscitation for out-of-hospital cardiac arrest. French Active Compression-Decompression Cardiopulmonary Resuscitation Study Group. N Engl J Med 1999;341:569–575.

19 Wolcke B, Mauer D, Schoefmann M, Teichmann H, Provo T, Lindner K, Dick W, Aeppli D, Lurie K: Comparison of standard cardiopulmonary resuscitation versus the combination of active compression-decompression cardiopulmonary resuscitation and an inspiratory impedance threshold device for out-of-hospital cardiac arrest. Circulation 2003;108:2201–2205.

20 Lurie K, Zielinski T, McKnite S, Idris A, Yannopoulos D, Raedler C, Sigurdsson G, Benditt D, Voelckel W: Treatment of hypotension in pigs with an inspiratory impedance threshold device: a feasibility study. Crit Care Med 2004;32:1555–1562.

21 Yannopoulos D, Metzger A, McKnite S, Nadkarni V, Aufderheide T, Idris A, Dries D, Benditt D, Lurie K: Intrathoracic pressure regulation improves vital organ perfusion pressures in normovolemic and hypovolemic pigs. Resuscitation 2006;70:445–453.

22 Yannopoulos D, McKnite S, Metzger A, Lurie K: Intrathoracic pressure regulation improves 24-hour survival in a porcine model of hypovolemic shock. Anesth Analg 2007;104:157–162.

23 Voelckel W, Yannopoulos D, Zielinski T, McKnite S, Lurie K: Inspiratory impedance threshold device effects on hypotension in heat-stroked swine. Aviat Space Environ Med 2008;79:743–748.

24 Convertino V, Ratliff D, Ryan K, Doerr D, Ludwig D, Muniz G, Britton D, Clah S, Fernald K, Ruiz A, Lurie K, Idris A: Hemodynamics associated with breathing through an inspiratory impedance threshold device in human volunteers. Crit Care Med 2004;32(suppl):S381–S386.

25 Convertino V, Ratliff D, Crissey J, Doerr D, Idris A, Lurie K: Effects of inspiratory impedance on hemodynamic responses to a squat-stand test in human volunteers: implications for treatment of orthostatic hypotension. Eur J Appl Physiol 2005;94:392–399.

26 Convertino V, Ryan K, Rickards C, Cooke W, Idris A, Metzger A, Holcomb J, Adams B, Lurie K: Inspiratory resistance maintains arterial pressure during central hypovolemia: implications for treatment of patients with severe hemorrhage. Crit Care Med 2007;35:1145–1152.

27 Ryan K, Cooke W, Rickards C, Lurie K, Convertino V: Breathing through an inspiratory threshold device improves stroke volume during central hypovolemia in humans. J Appl Physiol 2008;104:1402–1409.

28 Laudi S, Donaubauer B, Busch T, Kerner T, Bercker S, Bail H, Feldheiser A, Haas N, Kaisers U: Low incidence of multiple organ failure after major trauma. Injury 2007;38:1052–1058.

29 Schwartz D, Maroo A, Malhotra A, Kesselman H: Negative pressure pulmonary hemorrhage. Chest 1999;115:1194–1197.

30 Herff H, Raedler C, Zander R, Wenzel V, Schmittinger CA, Brenner E, Rieger M, Lindner KH: Use of an inspiratory impedance threshold valve during chest compressions without assisted ventilation may result in hypoxaemia. Resuscitation 2007;72:466–476.

31 Dorph E, Wik L, Strømme T, Eriksen M, Steen P: Oxygen delivery and return of spontaneous circulation with ventilation: compression ratio 2:30 versus chest compressions only CPR in pigs. Resuscitation 2004;60:309–318.

32 Fremont R, Kallet R, Matthay M, Ware L: Postobstructive pulmonary edema: a case for hydrostatic mechanisms. Chest 2007;131:1742–1746.

33 Idris A, Convertino V, Ratliff D, Doerr D, Lurie K, Gabrielli A, Banner M: Imposed power of breathing associated with use of an impedance threshold device. Respir Care 2007;52:177–183.

Dr. Holger Herff
Department of Anesthesiology and Critical Care Medicine
Innsbruck Medical University, Anichstrasse 35
AT–6020 Innsbruck (Austria)
Tel. +43 512 504 80375, Fax +43 512 504 6780375, E-Mail holger.herff@i-med.ac.at

Esquinas AM (ed): Applied Technologies in Pulmonary Medicine. Basel, Karger, 2011, pp 15–18

Gas Exchange during Perfluorocarbon Liquid Immersion

Mark W. Davies[a–c] · Kimble R. Dunster[a,d]

[a]Grantley Stable Neonatal Unit, [b]Perinatal Research Centre, and [c]Department of Paediatrics and Child Health, Royal Brisbane and Women's Hospital, The University of Queensland, and [d]Medical Engineering Research Facility, Queensland University of Technology, Brisbane, Qld., Australia

Abbreviations

PFC Perfluorocarbon
CPAP Continuous positive airway pressure

Given that there is potential for transcutaneous respiration in the extremely premature newborn infant, it has been proposed that immersion of these infants in PFC liquid will allow augmentation of gas exchange. This is possible because PFC liquid has an excellent oxygen- and carbon-dioxide-carrying capacity. Immersion in PFC may allow a spontaneously breathing infant to also achieve lung gas exchange with the combination of skin and lung gas exchange being sufficient to support life. Alternatively, immersion with some skin gas exchange may allow other forms of mechanical ventilation (with or without PFC) to be used but in a far less injurious way.

Analysis Main Topics Related to Title

Immersion in PFC and the Potential for Skin Gas Exchange

The potential for gas exchange through the skin when immersed in PFC liquid is feasible given two key principles: (1) extremely preterm infants have very thin, poorly keratinized skin across which, it is well known, gas exchange can occur, and (2) PFC liquid is an excellent carrier of both oxygen and carbon dioxide.

Immersion in PFC liquid provides other potential advantages: (1) water is not soluble in, or miscible with, PFC, so water will not evaporate from the skin possibly slowing skin keratinization (thus prolonging skin respiration); (2) it may allow tidal breathing of PFC liquid in a spontaneously breathing infant providing non-injurious lung gas exchange, and (3) temperature regulation and control in the immersed infant [1].

Experimental Studies

Only two papers have explored the concept of nursing whole subjects immersed in PFC liquid. Hiroma et al. [1] nursed adult rats in PFC liquid to investigate the temperature control possibilities of their 'liquid incubator'. They found that the temperature of rats two-thirds submerged in FC-43 was readily controlled and manipulated by changing the temperature of the FC-43.

In a small experimental pilot study, Davies et al. [2] explored the possibility of using whole-body immersion in PFC to provide some degree

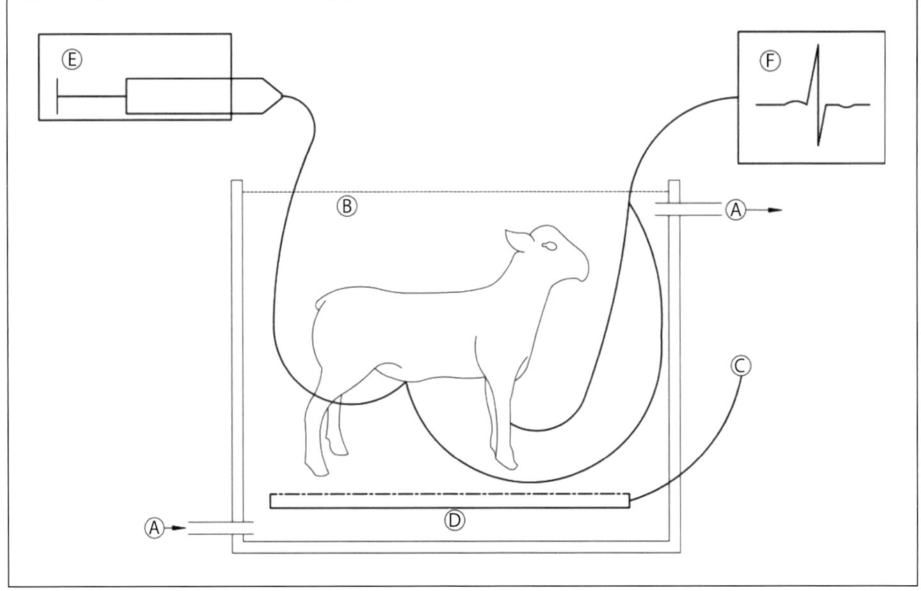

Fig. 1. A lamb immersed in PFC liquid (B) circulated – via inlet and outlet pipes (A) – with an external pump and heater. 100% oxygen (C) flows through a 'bubble curtain' (D). Fluids and drugs are given by syringe pumps (E) into the umbilical vessels. Vital signs (incl. arterial pressure and oxygen saturations) are monitored (F).

of skin gas exchange combined with tidal liquid breathing in preterm lambs (fig. 1). They did not achieve any meaningful gas exchange. They did demonstrate that the central circulation remains relatively intact immediately after birth, and whilst significant initial heat loss occurs before immersion, the fetus can be adequately warmed and temperature maintained with immersion in warm PFC liquid.

Discussion

Extremely preterm newborn infants are often critically ill from birth. Mortality in this group of infants is high and a large part of that mortality is primarily due to lung immaturity and acute lung disease. Even when the baby's death is not directly due to lung disease it is often a major contributor to it. Extremely preterm newborn infants also have a significant risk of brain injury from intracerebral bleeding (intraventricular hemorrhage) and ischemia (porencephaly and periventricular leukomalacia). Any lung disease, and its required respiratory support, along with accompanying hemodynamic disturbance will contribute to this increased risk of brain injury. Survivors are also at risk of neonatal chronic lung disease which will lead to prolonged need for respiratory support and oxygen as well as a considerably longer stay in hospital. They also have significant post-discharge respiratory morbidity and mortality.

The extremely preterm newborn infant has very immature lungs and will almost certainly need respiratory support. The incidence of severe hyaline membrane disease is very high, but even in the absence of lung disease they may require respiratory support because of their pulmonary immaturity and extremely compliant chest wall.

Any respiratory support given has the potential to cause lung injury, especially mechanical ventilation and its associated ventilator-induced lung injury. This lung injury can make the acute and chronic lung disease worse. Many forms of less injurious respiratory support have been postulated and used including nasal CPAP, high-frequency ventilation, triggered and synchronized ventilation, volume-targeted ventilation and liquid ventilation. Despite this, babies born at the margins of viability continue to have a high mortality and significant neurodevelopmental and respiratory morbidity.

If an alternative means of gas exchange could be provided then we might be able to ventilate in a less injurious way. The provision of gas exchange requires adequate gas exchange surfaces and sufficient oxygen and carbon dioxide gradients with a functioning circulation. Alternative means of gas exchange include: (1) *extracorporeal* – whilst this has the potential to provide all the gas exchange requirements it has so far not been possible in preterm infants and will likely result in intolerable fluctuations in hemodynamics and an even greater risk of brain injury; (2) *gut/peritoneum* – gas exchange is possible over the gut and peritoneum and better oxygenation has been demonstrated with intra-abdominal PFC liquid in rabbits [3, 4], and (3) *skin* – the transfer of oxygen and carbon dioxide is possible across the skin of the newborn human and the more immature the infant, the greater the degree of gas transfer [5–7].

Davies et al. [2] have proposed, and tested in a small experimental pilot study, that immersion in PFC will provide some degree of skin gas exchange. The gas exchange provided by this means would hopefully supplement that available through the lungs. Thus the degree of respiratory support that will be needed will be less because of that occurring through the skin and therefore should be able to be provided with a much lower risk of lung injury. The lung gas exchange could be provided in a number of ways: with normal spontaneous breathing on CPAP, tidal PFC breathing or any form of mechanical ventilation.

Immersion in PFC with Spontaneous Liquid Breathing

If it is possible to support a spontaneously breathing preterm infant immersed in PFC and achieve both lung gas exchange through tidal flow of PFC in and out of the lungs and skin gas exchange from direct contact with the PFC, then an extremely simple form of advanced life support would be available for the extremely preterm infant.

A number of hurdles would have to be overcome before this technique would be remotely possible, and a number of conditions would need to be optimized for its success. These include: (a) prompt delivery and immersion in PFC; (b) ensuring adequate lung expansion – may require lung recruitment maneuvers prior to immersion in PFC (with or without endotracheal intubation); (c) ensuring adequate respiratory effort; (d) ensuring an adequate circulation (may require circulatory support, e.g. adrenaline infusion), and (e) the problem of the baby floating on the top of the very dense PFC.

Immersion in PFC as an Adjunct to Conventional Forms of Respiratory Support

It may not be possible to achieve adequate gas exchange through the lungs with spontaneous tidal liquid breathing. However, the degree of skin gas exchange achieved may be sufficient to augment that provided by more conventional means. Because some of the gas exchange is provided via the skin, less will be needed through the lungs. In the infant ventilated with conventional mechanical ventilation this will allow the use of lower pressures and smaller tidal volumes and decrease baro- and volutrauma and its sequelae.

Other Uses of Immersion in PFC

Apart from providing the capacity for skin gas exchange, immersion may have other advantages. Because there is no skin-air interface the skin will not dry out and keratinization will be delayed. Any skin gas exchange can therefore be maintained. Immersion in PFC may provide a better barrier to skin colonization with potentially infecting organisms. Bacteria are not able to be carried in PFC liquid and cannot be supported by it. Control of the temperature of the PFC liquid will allow the maintenance of a normal temperature and a thermo-neutral environment thus minimizing metabolic demand, oxygen consumption and carbon dioxide production. Manipulation of the temperature of the PFC liquid will also allow an infant's temperature to be manipulated, for example for therapeutic hypothermia in infants with hypoxic ischemic encephalopathy.

Conclusion

Although the initial studies in PFC immersion have been unsuccessful in augmenting gas exchange, the large potential for its use remains. A large amount of research is needed to progress this from an embryological technique to clinical use.

References

1 Hiroma T, Baba A, Tamura M, Nakamura T: Liquid incubator with perfluorochemicals for extremely premature infants. Biol Neonate 2006;90:162–167.

2 Davies MW, Dunster KR, Wilson K: Gas exchange during perfluorocarbon liquid immersion: life-support for the ex utero fetus. Med Hypotheses 2008;71:91–98.

3 Chiba T, Harrison MR, Ohkubo T, Rollins MD, Albanese CT, Jennings RW: Transabdominal oxygenation using perfluorocarbons. J Pediatr Surg 1999;34:895–901.

4 Miyaguchi N, Nagahiro I, Kotani K, Nakanishi H, Mori H, Osaragi T, Shimizu N: Transintestinal systemic oxygenation using perfluorocarbon. Surg Today 2006;36:262–266.

5 Evans NJ, Rutter N: Percutaneous respiration in the newborn infant. J Pediatr 1986;108:282–286.

6 Cartlidge PHT, Rutter N: Percutaneous oxygen delivery to the preterm infant. Lancet 1988;1:315–317.

7 Cartlidge PHT, Rutter N: Percutaneous respiration in the new-born infant. Effect of ambient oxygen concentration on pulmonary oxygen uptake. Biol Neonate 1988;54:68–72.

Mark W. Davies, FRACP
Grantley Stable Neonatal Unit, Royal Brisbane and Women's Hospital, The University of Queensland
Brisbane, QLD 4029 (Australia)
Tel. +61 736 368 918, Fax +61 736 365 259
E-Mail Mark_Davies@health.qld.gov.au

Esquinas AM (ed): Applied Technologies in Pulmonary Medicine. Basel, Karger, 2011, pp 19–27

Extracorporeal Membrane Oxygenation for Respiratory and Heart Failure in Adults

J. Pat Herlihy[a] · Pranav Loyalka[b] · Timothy Connolly[a] · Biswajit Kar[b] · Igor Gregoric[c]

[a]Department of Pulmonary and Critical Care, and [b]Department of Cardiology, and [c]Department of Cardiovascular Surgery, The Texas Heart Institute at St. Luke's Episcopal Hospital, Baylor College of Medicine, University of Texas Health Science Center, Houston, Tex., USA

Abbreviations

ARDS	Acute respiratory distress syndrome
CESAR	Conventional Ventilatory Support vs. Extracorporeal Membrane Oxygenation for Severe Adult Respiratory Failure
CHF	Congestive heart failure
ECMO	Extracorporeal membrane oxygenation
ELSO	Extracorporeal Life Support Organization
ILA	Interventional Lung Assist
LA	Left atrium
LV	Left ventricle
LVADs	Left ventricular assist devices
MV	Mechanical ventilation
SIRS	Systemic inflammatory response syndrome
VA	Veno-arterial
VILI	Ventilator induced lung injury
VV	Veno-venous

By the late 19th century, French and German scientists had developed devices that effectively oxygenated blood outside of the body [1]. In 1931, John Gibbon, then a Harvard fellow in surgery at The Massachusetts General Hospital, began a lifetime of work to bring 'extracorporeal oxygenation' into the service of cardiac surgery after witnessing a failed embolectomy of massive pulmonary embolism in a young woman. In 1953, his 'heart and lung apparatus' successfully supported an 18-year-old through surgical closure of a large atrial septal defect by pumping the patient's blood from the vena cava through an oxygenator and back into the aorta by way of intravascular cannulae and tubing [2]. Gibbon's innovations, together with the work of other investigators from many different institutions, resulted in practical, effective 'cardiopulmonary bypass' and allowed all manners of 'open heart' surgery to be performed by the 1960s [3, 4].

Efforts to bring the newly successfully extracorporeal oxygenation technology to the rescue of patients suffering from primary respiratory failure, who were beyond the help of mechanical ventilation (MV), began in 1965 [5]. The first successful report of such was by Hill et al. [6], in 1972, using a novel 'membrane oxygenator'. A series of trials beginning in the 1970s and continued through the 1990s demonstrated the effectiveness of ECMO in the neonatal population (77% survival rate), as well as for pediatric patients (55% survival rate) suffering from a variety of pathologies causing primary respiratory failure [7, 8]. However, a large trial of ECMO for adult respiratory distress syndrome in the 1970s resulted in a 90% mortality [9]. Reasons for the stark outcome differences were not clear at the time. Nevertheless, as such, ECMO use for adults, the primary subject of this review, was relegated to rare and desperate circumstances over the next 30 years. However, the successful use of ECMO to treat ARDS in the recently completed CESAR trial [10, 11], as well as recent reports of effective use of ECMO to support acute heart failure, and refractory cardiac arrest [12, 13], promises to bring ECMO into more common and widespread use for adult patients. Before reviewing these studies and their implications for practice, it would seem helpful to first look at several of the technical advances in key tools for ECMO delivery, i.e. oxygenators, vascular access catheters and blood pumps, that to a large degree have allowed the current successes of ECMO. We will also briefly touch on some advances in understanding the pathophysiology of lung injury and CHF, as well as innovations in MV and cardiac support that have additionally contributed to ECMO success.

The original extracorporeal oxygenators used were 'direct contact' oxygenators wherein oxygen gas was bubbled through blood, or applied to blood drawn into a thin layer. These were the so-called 'bubble', 'screen', and 'film' oxygenators. These devices functioned adequately to oxygenate blood for heart surgery, but their use was complicated by the creation of gas bubbles and blood trauma, and could therefore only be used for a few hours. With the help of advancing material science, the 1970s ushered in 'membrane oxygenators' which employed ultrathin, gas-permeable sheets, initially of silicon rubber, to create tiny channels through which extracorporeal blood flowed, juxtaposed to an oxygen gas source. This technology allowed oxygen to diffuse into blood without direct contact and its associated problems, thus promoting better clinical tolerance and facilitating the longer use of oxygenators necessary to support respiratory failure [1, 3]. The 1980s saw the widespread introduction of microporous hollow polypropylene fibers into the design of membrane oxygenators. Oxygen gas flows through the center of these fiber membranes and blood around the oxygen, allowing much more efficient gas transfer [3]. Plasma leakage through these membranes, however, complicated their use and necessitated their frequent change, a situation not ideal for long-term ECMO [14]. Within the last several years however, microfiber, microporous, polymethylpentene membrane oxygenators have been commercially deployed which provide high-performance gas exchange with low resistance to flow and relatively little blood trauma, but without the plasma leakage. These devices have been found to perform very well for ECMO for more than a week at a time [15–17]. Very recently, these oxygenators have been produced with protein and heparin molecules lining the membrane in order to decrease the systemic inflammation and blood clotting associated with passage of blood through extrinsic surfaces. Certainly, this has led to decreased level of systemic anticoagulation required to prevent thrombus formation in the oxygenator. Whether these innovations will promote better outcomes for ECMO is, of yet, unclear [14, 18].

Originally, vascular access for the creation of the ECMO circuit in open heart surgery involved 'central cannulation' of either the vena cava or right atrium and the ascending aorta with large bore cannulae placed under direct visualization in an open chest. Initial protocols for ECMO in the support of respiratory failure used peripherally placed cannulae [19, 20]. These catheters used a femoral or internal jugular vein insertion site to allow catheter access to blood from the vena cava as inflow to the oxygenator and a carotid or femoral arterial cannula to provide outflow of the oxygenated blood to the proximal aorta. However, by the 1990s, VA ECMO was largely abandoned for use in respiratory failure in deference to a VV approach whereby venous blood from the distal inferior vena cava was pumped to the oxygenator and returned to the proximal vena cava or right atrium, using two different femoral venous catheters or both a femoral and an internal jugular venous catheter. This was because thromboembolic events from arterial catheters were found to be common and potentially devastating, as in the circumstance of a stroke. Furthermore, VV ECMO, aided by catheter systems with ever better flow characteristics, proved just as effective, in work largely done with the neonatal and pediatric populations [21, 22].

ECMO, when deployed to support of heart failure, utilizes a VA circuit [20]. The circuit can utilize a central vascular approach with catheters already in place for the circumstance of post-cardiotomy, or heart transplant failure, or a peripheral cannulae approach for rapid deployment for cardiac arrest or medically refractory CHF. Central catheters provide inflow to the oxygenator from the right atrium and outflow to the proximal ascending aorta with the advantage of providing oxygenated blood in a position where it carries well to the coronary and cranial arteries. Of course, bleeding and infectious complications are of high concern when VA ECMO is so configured for any significant length of time. Peripheral VA ECMO circuits consist of jugular or femoral venous access to the vena cava as inflow to the oxygenator and carotid or femoral artery catheter access to the aorta for outflow delivery. Carotid catheters have the advantage of delivering oxygenated blood to the ascending aorta, but their use can be complicated by thromboembolic stroke. Femoral artery catheters terminate in the proximal descending aorta, and provide antegrade flow of oxygenated blood into the aortic arch. With this approach, well-oxygenated blood may not carry well to the coronary arteries, brain or upper extremities. For this reason, when such a circuit is used, it is recommended to place a right radial arterial line as a monitor for upper extremity, and hence heart and brain, blood oxygenation. New catheter devices that permit access to the left atrium promise another route of inflow to the oxygenator and in the circumstance of CHF may offer some advantages that we will touch on later [23].

Pumps to move blood through the ECMO circuit were originally of the roller pump design. Two problems with this technique were direct blood trauma caused by squeezing the blood between the tubing walls, and spalling, hence embolization, of plastic microfragments from the tubing wall [24]. The blood trauma led to hemolysis, intravascular coagulation and activation of systemic inflammation. Design innovations to minimize these complications have included impeller blades which, though an improvement, still create significant blood turbulence and can promote air retention in the blood returning to the patient. Most current ECMO protocols incorporate centrifugal pumps which promote laminar flow with lessened blood trauma and air retention [13].

Catheters and pumps produced currently for ECMO have biologic and antithrombotic coatings to further reduce thromboembolic events and, as in the case of oxygenators, to lessen systemic inflammation that results from blood contact with an extracorporeal surface. Less systemic anticoagulation needs to be used with these systems, mitigating bleeding, a major complication of ECMO [20].

Several major advances in the understanding of acute lung injury, ARDS, and MV in support of these pathologies have been made since the 1970s, which, no doubt, have contributed in a major way to the current success with ECMO. In the 1980s it was discovered that positive pressure MV settings that were heretofore considered safe and effective were in fact often injurious to lungs, especially those already injured [25]. In fact, ventilators can promote ARDS and even SIRS. Current generation ventilators are built with the principles of preventing VILI, and clinical protocols for avoiding 'volutrauma' and other forms of VILI are in widespread use. Interestingly, MV of neonates and pediatric patients has, since almost the beginning of positive pressure ventilation, incorporated pressure limitation strategies [26]. One wonders if the difference between adult volume-cycled ventilation and pressure-cycled ventilation for pediatrics accounted in some significant degree for the outcome differences between pediatric and adult series of ECMO in the 1970s. During the late 1980s and early 1990s there also came a realization that ARDS progressed through two pathophysiologic phases, the early 'exudative' phase and subsequently the 'fibroproliferative' phase [27]. If the lung did not go down the path of normal architecture restoration, but instead to fibrosis and scar formation, outcomes were much worse. This understanding has figured in selection of patients more likely to benefit from ECMO.

ECMO for ARDS and Primary Respiratory Failure

In February 2008, results of the CESAR trial were released at the international Society of Critical Care Medicine meeting [10]. The full report was published in *The Lancet* in late 2009 [11]. This study, however, may already be promoting a paradigm shift in the management of severe lung injury. Essentially this randomized prospective study showed significantly improved outcomes using ECMO to manage severe and early ARDS compared to the standard current approach of MV, at what is currently thought to be noninjurious levels. Specifically, the entry criteria to the study was potentially reversible lung injury of high severity as determined by a Murray score >3.0 (severe hypoxia, extensive pulmonary infiltrates by chest x-ray, need for high levels of MV, and poor pulmonary compliance) or uncompensated hypercarbia resulting in a pH <7.2. Exclusion criteria included late ARDS as determined by a requirement of high FiO_2 (>80%), or high ventilator measured airway pressure (plateau pressure >30 cm H_2O) for >7 days. Moribund patients and those with contraindications to heparin were also excluded. For patients randomized to ECMO, survival without severe disability, the primary endpoint of the study was 63% as opposed to those receiving conventional MV for whom it was 47%. These data are consistent with that reported in the ELSO registry maintained by the University of Michigan [www.elso.med.umich.edu] which shows current survival rates of ECMO for adult ARDS of >50% [28].

These data suggest that ECMO has arrived as therapy for early and severe ARDS, and other potentially acute, reversible severe lung injuries such as cryptogenic organizing pneumonia [23], among other pathologies [29]. The CESAR trial concept was not only to support patients through respiratory failure but to intervene early to prevent toxic use of MV and allow the lung its best chance of recovery. Late ARDS, presumably in the fibroproliferative phase, with its poorer prognosis, was notably excluded. It is also salient that 22 of 90 patients, essentially a quarter of those eligible for the ECMO protocol, never received it because they improved. Separating those patients with early severe ARDS who will benefit from ECMO and those who will spontaneously improve will likely prove very difficult, if not impossible, at the bedside with our current diagnostic and prognostic tools.

ECMO for Primary Cardiac Failure

Management of the failing heart has come a long way from the 1960s when the first successful heart transplant was performed, and the first attempt at artificial heart support was made. Percutaneous coronary intervention has, of course, revolutionized the management of acute cardiogenic shock from coronary occlusion. LVADs have come into frequent use in heart transplant centers as a bridge to transplant, and the current generation of devices is now even approved as destination therapy [30]. Other mechanical support devices in early clinical application or development, such as the total artificial heart, are encouraging [31]. Understanding of ventricular remodeling and heart recovery from injury has also come a long way since the early days when damaged heart tissue was thought to be adynamic and fixed in dysfunction [31, 32]. Current clinical standards of CHF management incorporate many of these concepts, such as the critical importance of afterload reduction for optimal cardiac function and recovery from injury. Potentially revolutionary new therapies, such as stem cell implantation and myocardial cell apoptosis suppression, are being investigated by us at the Texas Heart Institute and many others throughout the world [32].

These advances have spurred the burgeoning interest in ECMO as a temporary support device for medically refractory CHF, cardiogenic shock, and failed resuscitation of cardiac arrest, until either heart recovery or implementation of a longer term solution such as cardiac transplant or LVAD insertion. It seems a bit ironic that ECMO is coming back to serve its original purpose of cardiac support, but outside of the operating room, and for a much more extended period of time.

Following initial successes in supporting neonatal and pediatric respiratory failure, cardiologists have been using ECMO in this age group over the past 20 years for severe CHF, pulmonary hypertension, and intracardiac shunts. Survival to discharge for these patients, who of course benefit from further interventions in addition to ECMO, is 40% [12]. Data for ECMO use in adult CHF and cardiogenic shock that has come out within the last decade have consistently shown remarkable survival rates of 50–60% [13, 33–36]. Disease states that ECMO alone may be sufficient for, given the oftentimes temporary nature of the pathology, include: the low cardiac output syndrome post-cardiotomy, post-partum cardiomyopathy, viral myocarditis, arrhythmia-induced cardiomyopathy, and severe pulmonary hypertension with right ventricular failure resulting from pulmonary embolism or post-pulmonary artery surgical thrombectomy [37]. In patients who do not recover sufficient intrinsic heart function, ECMO has served well as bridge therapy until it is clear that the patient is beyond recovery for reasons of neurologic injury or multiple system organ failure, or cardiac transplantation/mechanical heart assist device placement can be performed [38]. We have even reported using ECMO as bridge to heart lung transplant in a patient with severe refractory primary pulmonary hypertension [39]. The last several years have seen ECMO applied to cases of refractory cardiac arrest, and data from ELSO show the survival rate in this circumstance to be an amazing 27% [40].

Practical Aspects

At this point, some practical aspects of providing ECMO for lung or heart patients are worth reviewing. First of all, ECMO is an extraordinary resource and labor-intensive process. Institutions and individual providers need to be prepared for such. That being said, there are indications that, at least for ARDS, ECMO may prove economically viable relative to current standard therapy [11]. In addition to the equipment for ECMO a dedicated team of specialists experienced in ECMO is recommended. ELSO recommends that institutions perform 20 cases a year to achieve and maintain optimal skill levels. The team should include: perfusionists, for continual maintenance and monitoring of the ECMO system; interventionalists, for catheter placement; pulmonologists and respiratory therapists, to monitor lung injury and maintain appropriate ventilator settings; cardiologists, to monitor and manage central hemodynamics, hematologists, to help for anticoagulation, and to monitor for coagulopathy, thrombocytopenia and bleeding complications; nephrologists, to monitor and manage renal function and volume status; infectious disease specialists, to monitor the many potential sources or infections and to treat such early and aggressively; nutritionists, to prevent malnutrition; potentially neurologists, to asses neurologic change; and of course, the bedside

ICU nurse, whose array of assessment, intervention and communication skills make it all work. Patients who survive ECMO need a variety of support services, as do their families. Social service support is key over the long haul of illness and recovery. High level rehabilitation services are typically involved at the earliest opportunity in our patients' post-ECMO as they often demonstrate severe deconditioning or myopathy, neuropathy of critical illness.

Vascular access for ECMO has been discussed above. Essentially, VV ECMO is the current standard for support of primary respiratory failure. VA ECMO is used for primary cardiac failure. However, it is worth noting here that this configuration causes significant afterload for the left ventricle [13]. This is at least counterproductive for a ventricle with potential for recovery and may be catastrophic resulting in pulmonary hemorrhage. Often, in this circumstance, an IABP is placed to off-load the ventricle. Unfortunately, this counterpulsation device may interfere with the ECMO arterial catheter delivering oxygenated blood. Several solutions have been proposed for this problem. Creation of an atrial shunt to by percutaneous transeptal perforation, and direct cannulation of the LA or LV as a vent to unload the LV have been reported [13]. Additionally, a percutaneous LVAD, specifically the Impella Recovery (Abiomed Inc., Danvers, Mass., USA), has been placed to effectively unload the LV in conjunction with ECMO to good effect [41]. We have reported the use of the TandemHeart System (CardiacAssist Inc., Pittsburg, Pa., USA) catheters to access the LA as the delivery point for ECMO-treated blood in a patient with severe pulmonary hypertension and right ventricular failure [23]. It may be possible to use the LA access of the TH system as inflow to ECMO and thereby reduce LV load and wall stress.

Once vascular access for ECMO has been established, the three key components of ECMO requiring fairly continuous adjustment are the blood flow through the oxygenator, regulated by the pump, the countercurrent gas flow through the oxygenator, known as the 'sweep', and the FiO_2 of the gas. Initial blood flow is approximately 70 ml/kg/min (or 5 l/min for an average-sized man). For large individuals a second ECMO system may be required. Initial sweep should match the blood flow. So if 5 l/min of blood is flowing through the system, then the sweep should be 5 l/min. Initially the sweep gas should be 100% FiO_2. Flow through the oxygenator can be increased to improve oxygenation of the blood or improve O_2 delivery. Increasing sweep can also improve oxygenation of the blood as well as offload CO_2. A primary goal of ECMO for respiratory failure is to allow lung injury recovery. A secondary goal of ECMO in the circumstance of cardiac failure is to allow ventilator settings that are noninjurious to the lung. Both goals are served by adjusting MV to a Vt of 4–8 ml/kg of ideal body weight (in the case of volume-cycled ventilation), disallowing a plateau pressure of >30 cm H_2O, and using an FiO_2 of 30% or less. This is usually accomplished gradually while adjusting ECMO to compensate for lost gas exchange.

A trial of wean from ECMO, in the circumstance of primary respiratory failure, is made when the chest x-ray has sufficiently cleared and pulmonary compliance is has sufficiently improved [11]. At that point, sweep is turned down, and eventually off, to see if gas exchange can be maintained by the ventilator alone, on nontoxic settings (as delineated above) that limit volutrauma and an FiO_2 of 60% or less. In the case of ECMO for cardiac support the key test of weanability is whether CO can be maintained at a sufficient level for tissue O_2 delivery, as determined by a combination of objective measurements of (>2.2 l/min/m^2) and clinical markers of sufficient oxygenation, such as lactic acid level and organ function, while the pump flow is decreased. Blood flow of <2 l/min through the ECMO circuit can prompt stasis in the system, so that is the usual lower limit of pump flow in a wean trial.

Continuous sedation of patients undergoing ECMO is necessary for tolerance. Fentanyl, with its relatively favorable hemodynamic profile, has worked well for us. Paralysis is also sometimes required. Potential complications of ECMO are many [8, 14, 20] but include, in order of practical importance: bleeding from administered anticoagulation as well as coagulopathy and thrombocytopenia induced by the ECMO system; intracranial bleeds are of particular concern; thromboembolic events, both venous and arterial; deep venous thrombosis can occur at venous catheter insertion sites and embolize; arterial access sites can thrombose and embolize causing, depending upon the location of the catheter, limb ischemia or vital organ infarcts including CVAs (10% incidence in adults on VA ECMO); hepatopathy and ischemic bowel from poor splanchnic perfusion, sepsis from lung, catheter, urinary and abdominal sources; SIRS, and multisystem organ failure. Device malfunctions which occur in up to 18% of cases include: oxygenator failure requiring change out (usually due to thrombus formation), and oxygenator or tubing rupture, resulting in air emboli.

Promising Developments

There are several exciting and very promising developments in the area of lung assist devices. The ILA (Novalung GmbH, Talheim, Germany) has recently been approved for clinical use in Europe. This polymethylpentene membrane oxygenator is significantly smaller than traditional oxygenators, has excellent gas exchange characteristics, and is constructed in such a way that it presents very little resistance to blood flow through it. As such, it is pumpless, and driven by arterial flow in patients with intact hemodynamics, when placed in a femoral artery to ILA to femoral vein circuit. Typically only 1–2 l/min of blood flows through the oxygenator or about 20% of cardiac output. However, with high flow of sweep gas the ILA can result in dramatic improvements in gas exchange. It has been used in primary hypoxemic and hypercarbic respiratory failure with survival rates of 41%, a significant improvement over expected mortality in these patients using conventional therapy [42]. Interestingly it has been applied to chest trauma and blast victims because of its rapid application and lack of need for a pump, to excellent effect [14, 43]. It has also been used successfully as a bridge to lung transplant [43].

The first clinical case reports using paracorporeal artificial lung have just come out [44, 45]. This device is essentially a membrane oxygenator placed in parallel to the pulmonary circulation with connection to the pulmonary artery and to the left atrium. It has been used in the specific circumstance of right ventricular failure secondary to pulmonary hypertension, when standard ECMO is failing. It performed well in these circumstances supporting 1 patient for 63 days. There are hopes that, at a now distant point, this approach may ultimately result in a device that can be used long term, even out of the hospital [46].

Intravascular oxygenator systems such as the intravascular oxygenator [47, 48] and the Hattler catheter [49] are in the early stages of development, or subclinical testing. These systems are designed for implantation in the vena cava with or without blood pumps and using an external gas source for oxygenation.

Conclusion

ECMO appears poised to take a place in best practice clinical algorithms for managing severe acute lung injury, and medically refractory heart failure as a bridge to recovery, implantable mechanical cardiac assist device, or heart, lung or heart lung transplantation.

References

1 Lim MW: The history of extracorporeal oxygenators. Anaesthesia 2006;61:984–995.

2 Zareba KM: John H. Gibbon, Jr, MD: a poet with an idea (1903–1973). Cardiol J 2009;16:98–100.

3 Haworth WS: Gibbon's heart-lung machine. The development of the modern oxygenator. Ann Thorac Surg 2003; 76:S2216–S2219.

4 Daly RC, Dearani JA, McGregor CG, Mullany CJ, Orszulak TA, Puga FJ, et al: Fifty years of open heart surgery at the Mayo Clinic. Mayo Clinic Proc 2005;80: 636–640.

5 Rashkind WJ, Freeman A, Klein D, et al: Evaluation of a disposable plastic, low volume, pumpless oxygenator as a lung substitute. J Pediatr 1965;66:94–102.

6 Hill JD, O'Brien TG, Murray JJ, Dontigny L, Bramsom ML, Osborn JJ, et al: Prolonged extracorporeal oxygenation for acute post-traumatic respiratory failure (shock-lung syndrome). Use of the Bramson membrane lung. N Engl J Med 1972;286:629–634.

7 Dalton HJ, Rycus PT, Conrad SA: Update on extracorporeal life support 2004. Semin Perinatol 2005;29:24–33.

8 Schuerer DJ, Kolovos NS, Boyd KV, Coopersmith CM: Extracorporeal membrane oxygenation: current clinical practice, coding, and reimbursement. Chest 2008;134:179–184.

9 Zapol WM, Snider MT, Hill JD, et al: Extracorporeal membrane oxygenation in severe acute respiratory failure: a randomized prospective study. JAMA 1979; 242:2193–2196.

10 Peek G: CESAR: adult ECMO vs. conventional ventilation trial. Society of Critical Care Medicine – 37th Critical Care Congress, Honolulu, February 2–6, 2008.

11 Peek GJ, Mugford M, Tiruvoipati R, et al: Efficacy and economic assessment of conventional ventilatory support versus extracorporeal membrane oxygenation for severe adult respiratory failure (CESAR): a multicentre randomised controlled trial. Lancet 2009;374:1351–1363.

12 Cooper DS, Jacobs JP, Moore L, Stock A, Gaynor JW, Chancy T, et al: Cardiac extracorporeal life support: state of the art in 2007. Cardiol Young 2007;17(suppl 2):104–115.

13 Matsumiya G, Saitoh S, Sawa Y: Extracorporeal assist circulation for heart failure. Circ J 2009;73(suppl A).

14 Pesenti A, Zanelli A, Patroniti N: Extracorporeal gas exchange. Curr Opin Crit Care 2009;15:52–58.

15 Toomasian JM, Schreiner RJ, Meyer DE, et al: A polymethylpentene fiber gas exchanger for long-term extracorporeal life support. ASAIO J 2005;51:390–397; erratum in ASAIO J 2008;54:137.

16 Formica F, Avalli L, Martino A, Maggioni E, Muratore M, Ferro O, et al: Extracorporeal membrane oxygenation with a poly-methylpentene oxygenator (Quadrox D). The experience of a single Italian centre in adult patients with refractory cardiogenic shock. ASAIO J 2008;54:89–94.

17 Agati S, Ciccarello G, Fachile N, et al: DIDECMO: a new polymethylpentene oxygenator for pediatric extracorporeal membrane oxygenation. ASAIO J 2006; 52:509–512.

18 Palatianos GM, Foroulos CN, Vassili MI, Astras G, Triantafillou K, Papadakis E, et al: A prospective, double-blind study on the efficacy of the bioline surface-heparinized extracorporeal perfusion circuit. Ann Thorac Surg 2003;76:129–135.

19 Hill JD: Acute pulmonary failure: treatment with extracorporeal oxygenation. Med Instrum 1977;11:198–201.

20 Marasco SF, Lukas G, McDonald M, McMillan J, Ihle B: Review of extracorporeal membrane oxygenation support in critically Ill adult patients. Heart Lung Circ 2008;17(suppl 4);S41–S47.

21 Knight GR, Dudell GG, Evans ML, Grimm PS: A comparison of venovenous and venoarterial extracorporeal membrane oxygenation in the treatment of neonatal respiratory failure. Crit Care Med 1996;24:1678–1683.

22 Pettignano R, Fortenberry JD, Heard ML, Labuz MD, Kesser KC, Tanner AJ, et al: Primary use of the venovenous approach for extracorporeal membrane oxygenation in pediatric acute respiratory failure. Pediatr Crit Care Med 2003;4:291–298.

23 Herlihy JP, Loyalka P, Jayaraman G, Kar B, Gregoric, ID: Extracorporeal membrane oxygenation using the TandemHeart System's catheters. Tex Heart Inst J 2009;36:337–341.

24 Kopp R, Steinseifer U, Rossant R: Extracorporeal lung assist for ARDS: past, present and future; in Vincent, J-L (ed): Intensive Care Medicine Annual Update 2008. New York, Springer Science + Business Media, 2008, pp 235–247.

25 Tremblay LN, Slutsky AS: Ventilator-induced lung injury: from the bench to the bedside. Intensive Care Med 2006; 32:24–33.

26 AARC Clinical Practice Guidelines: Neonatal time-triggered, pressure-limited, time-cycled mechanical ventilation. Respir Care 1994;39:808–816.

27 Luh S, Chiang C: Acute lung injury/acute respiratory distress syndrome: the mechanism, present strategies and future perspectives of therapies. J Zhejiang Univ Sci B 2007;8:60–69.

28 Conrad SA, Rycus PT, Dalton H: Extracorporeal Life Support Registry Report 2004. ASAIO J 2005;51:4–10.

29 Kahn J, Muller H, Marte W, Rehak P, Wasler A, Prenner G, et al: Establishing extracorporeal membrane oxygenation in a university clinic: case series. J Cardiothorac Vasc Anesth 2007;21:384–387.

30 Lahpor J: State of the art: implantable ventricular assist devices. Curr Opin Organ Transplant 2009;14:554–559.

31 Jugdutt BI, Current and novel cardiac support therapies. Curr Heart Fail Rep 2009;6:19–27.

32 Khovnezhad A, Jalali Z, Tortolani AJ A synopsis of research in cardiac apoptosis and its application to congestive heart failure. Tex Heart Inst J 2007;34:352–359.

33 Koerner MM, Jahanyar J: Assist devices for circulatory support in therapy-refractory acute heart failure. Curr Opin Cardiol 2008;23:399–406.

34 Luo XJ, Wang W, Hu SS, Gao HW, Long C, Song YH, et al: Extracorporeal membrane oxygenation for treatment of cardiac failure in adult patients. Interact Cardiovasc Thorac Surg 2009;9:296–300.

35 Hoefer D, Ruttman E, Poelzl G, Kilo J, Hoermann C, Margreiter R, et al: Outcome evaluation of the bridge-to-bridge concept in patients with cardiogenic shock. Ann Thorac Surg 2006;82:28–33.

36 Murashita T, Eya K, Miyatake T, et al: Outcome of the perioperative use of percutaneous cardiopulmonary support for adult cardiac surgery: factors affecting hospital mortality. Artif Organs 2004;28: 189–195.

37 Ogino H, Ando M, Matsuda K, Sasaki H, Nakanishi N, et al: Japanese single-center experience of surgery for chronic thromboembolic pulmonary hypertension. Ann Thorac Surg 2006;82:630–636.

38 Copeland J: Invited commentary. Ann Thorac Surg 2006;82:33–34.

39 Gregoric ID, Chandra D, Myers TJ, Sheinin SA, Loyalka P, Kar B: Extracorporeal membrane oxygenation as a bridge to emergency heart-lung transplantation in a patient with idiopathic pulmonary arterial hypertension. J Heart Lung Transplant 2008;27:466–468.

40 Thiagarajan RR, Brogan TV, Scheurer MA, Laussen PC, Rycus PT, Bratton SL: Extracorporeal membrane oxygenation to support cardiopulmonary resuscitation in adults. Ann Thorac Surg 2009;87: 778–785.

41 Vlasselaers D, Desmet M, Desmet L, Meyns B, Dues J: Ventricular unloading with a miniature axial flow pump in combination with extracorporeal membrane oxygenation. Intensive care Med 2006;32:329–333.

42 Bein T, Weber F, Philipp A, et al: A new pumpless extracorporeal interventional lung assist in critical hypoxemia/hypercapnia. Crit Care Med 2006;34:1372–1377.

43 Meyer A, Struber M, Fisher S: Advances in extracorporeal ventilation. Anesthesiol Clin 2008;26:381–391.

44 Schmid C, Philip A, Hiker M, Arit M, Trabald B, Pfeiffer M, et al: Bridge to lung transplantation through a pulmonary artery to left atrial oxygenator circuit. Ann Thorac Surg. 2008;85:1202–1205.

45 Camboni D, Philipp A, Arit M, Pfeiffer M, Hilker M, Schmid C: First clinical experience with a paracorporeal artificial lung in humans. ASAIO J 2009;55: 304–306.

46 Zwischenberger BA, Clemson LA, Zwischenberger JB: Artificial lung: progress and prototypes. Expert Rev Medical Devices 2006;3:485–497.

47 Zwischenberger JB, Tao W, Bidani A: Intravascular membrane oxygenator and carbon dioxide removal devices: a review of performance and improvements. ASAIO J 1999;45:41–46.

48 Cattaneo G, Strauss A, Reul H: Compact intra- and extracorporeal oxygenator developments. Perfusion 2004;19:251–255.

49 Hattler BG, Lund LW, Golob J, et al: A respiratory gas exchange catheter: in vitro and in vivo tests in large animals. J Thorac Cardiovasc Surg 2002;124:520–530.

J. Pat Herlihy, MD
Department of Pulmonary and Critical Care
The Texas Heart Institute at St. Luke's Episcopal Hospital
Baylor College of Medicine, University of Texas Health Science Center
6624 Fannin Street, Suite 1730
Houston, TX 77030 (USA)
Tel. +1 713 255 4000, Fax +1 713 255 4050, E-Mail jph@houstonlungdocs.com

Esquinas AM (ed): Applied Technologies in Pulmonary Medicine. Basel, Karger, 2011, pp 28–34

Automatic Control of Mechanical Ventilation Technologies

Fleur T. Tehrani

Department of Electrical Engineering, California State University, Fullerton, Calif., USA

Abbreviations

ASV	Adaptive support ventilation
ATC	Automatic tube compensation
Edi	Neural drive signal to the diaphragm
FiO_2	Fraction of inspired oxygen
HFJV	High-frequency jet ventilation
HFOV	High-frequency oscillatory ventilation
NAVA	Neurally adjusted ventilatory assist
PAV	Proportional assist ventilation
PEEP	Positive end-expiratory pressure
PPS	Proportional pressure support ventilation
VAPS	Volume-assured pressure support

Mechanical ventilation is a life-saving technology that has evolved remarkably in the past several decades. In particular, positive pressure mechanical ventilation in many different forms and by using various modalities is employed as an essential medical treatment in the ICU settings of hospitals all over the world. Without this technology, the treatment of many illnesses and most major surgical operations would not be possible. However, if this treatment is not provided properly or the duration of mechanical ventilation is unduly prolonged due to non-optimal treatment, many medical complications such as ventilator-associated pneumonia may result. Those complications can significantly increase the mortality and morbidity rates of patients on this medical treatment. Therefore, any useful innovation in mechanical ventilation technology that can improve and expedite the treatment can significantly impact the quality of healthcare for ICU patients.

The following provides a brief overview of different mechanical ventilation technologies and a discussion of several innovative techniques that have been employed in practice in mechanical ventilators in recent years. The potential impacts on healthcare by several newer techniques including closed-loop ventilation technologies will be analyzed by discussing the applications of those techniques along with their main strengths and weaknesses.

An Overview of Various Mechanical Ventilation Technologies

Mechanical ventilation is used in various forms and by using different technologies. In what is called negative pressure ventilation, the patient's thoracic area or his entire body up to his neck is enclosed in an airtight chamber and the volume of the chamber is expanded, thereby inflating the lungs using negative pressure. Examples of such devices are tank ventilators, jacket ventilators, and cuirasses. However, negative pressure ventilation devices are not used in many applications today. Instead, positive pressure ventilation in which the patient's lungs are inflated by application of positive pressure to his airways is considered as today's dominant technology. This kind of treatment can be applied non-invasively, by use of a facial mask or a mouthpiece, or it can be given invasively by using an endotracheal tube or by use of tracheostomy.

Positive pressure ventilation can be provided by using high-frequency ventilation techniques such as HFJV and HFOV. In high-frequency ventilation, the oxygenated air is delivered at high rates and small volumes to the patient's airways, vibrating the alveoli at high frequencies to avoid injuring the lung tissue. High-frequency ventilation is used predominantly in the neonatal and pediatric patient populations with less frequent applications in adult patient groups. The more commonly used type of positive pressure ventilation is referred to as conventional ventilation. This kind of ventilation can be given in both invasive and non-invasive forms. In conventional mechanical ventilation, the respiration frequency can be selected to be close to the natural breathing rate of the patient [1]. The methods used in conventional ventilation are many, and it is not the purpose of this article to describe those modalities. The focus of this article is on newer automated modalities of conventional ventilation that have impacted ventilatory treatment in recent years.

Importance of Automation in Conventional Positive Pressure Mechanical Ventilation

In the past few decades, mechanical ventilators have become more advanced with many options and modalities. The purpose of offering various options in these machines is to make them more responsive to patients' needs and thereby improve treatment. However, the majority of advanced ventilators are still open-loop controlled machines in which the main outputs of the ventilator are manually set by an operator. In using these ventilators, the clinician needs to know various options and limitations of the advanced ventilators, and based on the patient's illness and requirements chooses a suitable treatment option among many alternatives and sets the main ventilatory parameters. The clinician's decisions which in many cases can make the difference between life and death for the patient need to be made in the ICU setting within a short period of time.

It has been reported that in the USA alone there are between 44,000 and 98,000 injuries resulting from medical errors per year [2]. The human costs of serious injuries and mortalities associated with medical errors cannot be measured financially and the financial costs of such incidents are between USD 17 and 29 billion per year in the USA alone [2]. It is needless to say that by expecting so much from clinicians, such errors become inevitable. Medical technology has to be employed more aggressively to address this issue. As was discussed above, mechanical ventilation is an essential treatment technique that is mainly used in the ICU settings of hospitals. Provision of optimal ventilatory treatment can expedite weaning and prevent prolonged ventilation therapy. Such treatments not only will improve the quality of care and help reduce medical complications associated with prolonged mechanical ventilation such as incidents of ventilator-associated pneumonias, but they will significantly reduce the costs of ICU ventilatory treatments at the same time.

Automatic control of this technology can be used to reduce errors associated with the treatment. Several innovative automatic ventilation techniques have been employed in mechanical ventilators to this date [1]. Those technologies and their strengths and weaknesses are discussed below.

Advanced Mechanical Ventilation Technologies

There have been many advanced features included in mechanical ventilators in recent years. In a mode called VAPS, which is available in Bird 8400STi model, the ventilator's output is controlled automatically during each breath to assure the delivery of a target volume set by the clinician. In this mode, the first portion of the breath is pressure-limited. However, if the target tidal volume cannot be delivered, inspiration is continued based on a peak flow setting to deliver the target volume to the patient. In another technique called ATC that is incorporated in a number of different ventilators including the Drager Evita series, the Viasys Avea ventilators, and the Nellcor Puritan Bennett 840 model, the ventilator is designed to compensate for the imposed additional work of breathing due to the endotracheal tube. By using ATC, the pressure drop across the endotracheal tube is calculated based on the measured flow and the tube characteristics, and the ventilator compensates for that pressure drop. Use of ATC reduces the work of breathing and makes it easier for the patient to start breathing on his own. While VAPS is designed to assure delivery of adequate ventilation to the patient and to prevent the untoward effects of hypoxemia and hypercapnia, ATC is designed to facilitate weaning patients from mechanical ventilation. These techniques like other innovative modes of ventilation such as synchronized intermittent mandatory ventilation, pressure-regulated volume control and many others have been used in practice in ventilators for some time and are designed to improve mechanical ventilation treatment and expedite weaning.

Despite the application of automation in various forms in today's ventilators and their many advantages, still the main outputs of these machines such as tidal volume, respiratory rate, minute ventilation, FiO_2, and PEEP are manually set by clinicians in most advanced modes of ventilation. Therefore, using such techniques still requires the clinician to make the important choices about the treatment by trial and error. However, due to the advancements in sensor technology and the pressing need for more automation of ventilation, there have been many attempts by a number of researchers to more aggressively control the main outputs of ventilators automatically in different phases of treatment. Many researchers have developed systems for automatic control of patient's oxygenation by closed-loop control of FiO_2, PEEP, or both. Examples of such systems have been reviewed [3]. A number of other researchers have designed automatic systems for adjusting ventilation, respiration rate, or control of weaning, and in some more recent systems automatic control of ventilation or weaning has been combined with closed-loop adjustment of PEEP and/or FiO_2 [3].

Despite many attempts by a number of researchers to develop automatic ventilation systems for control of the main outputs of ventilators, only a few of such systems have been used in practice to this date. Those major automatic systems are: (i) ASV used in Hamilton Medical ventilators; (ii) PAV (or PPS) used in several different ventilators including Drager Evita series, Puritan Bennett 840 model, and Respironics BiPAP ventilators; (iii) SmartCare offered by Drager Evita ventilators, and (iv) NAVA designed to use the patient's own neural respiratory drive that is adapted in Maquet ventilators. An overview and discussion of these commercially available systems are provided below.

Major Automatic Ventilation Technologies

Adaptive Support Ventilation

ASV is a closed-loop technique for automatic adjustment of tidal volume and respiratory rate in mechanical ventilation. This technique was invented in 1980s and was described as one of the embodiments of a patent issued in 1991 [1, 4]. ASV is used by Hamilton Medical ventilators. Figure 1 shows a schematic block diagram of this system.

In the ASV mode, the required minute ventilation is calculated from an input called %MinVol and the patient's ideal body weight. The patient's respiratory mechanics are measured on a breath-by-breath basis and provided to the controller to

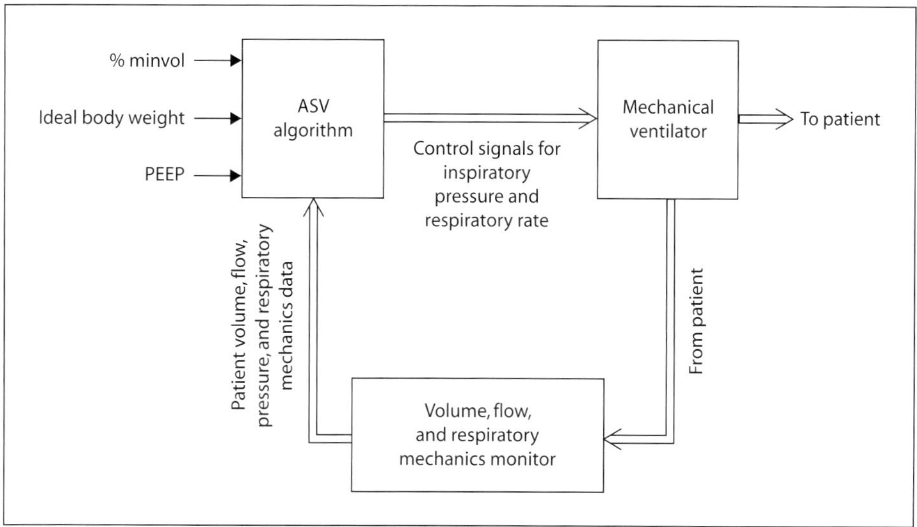

Fig. 1. Schematic diagram of the ASV system.

calculate the required tidal volume and respiratory rate of the patient. In this mode, if the patient triggers the breaths and can breathe spontaneously, the machine provides additional pressure support to meet the calculated tidal volume target. For passive patients, the ventilator delivers the required tidal volume by using pressure control ventilation at the calculated optimal rate of breathing. The optimal frequency of breathing in this method is calculated on a breath-by-breath basis by using the measured respiratory mechanics data to minimize the respiratory work rate. By providing a more natural breathing rate to the patient, ASV aims at reducing asynchrony between the machine and the patient and thereby to stimulate spontaneous breathing and expedite weaning. The expiration time in ASV is also adjusted when necessary to make sure that lungs are effectively emptied during expiration and the buildup of intrinsic PEEP is prevented. ASV can be used for passive as well as active patients and a minimum required ventilation can be guaranteed by using this mode. Despite the advantages of ASV, still several main outputs of the ventilator need to be manually adjusted in this mode. ASV does not provide continuous automatic adjustment of minute ventilation, and PEEP and FiO_2 are manually controlled.

Proportional Assist Ventilation

PAV is a patented technique in which the ventilator measures the patient's ongoing volume and rate of flow of inspiratory gas and applies additional pressure support in proportion to the patient's own inspiratory effort [5]. Some variations of this mode are offered in Puritan Bennett 840 ventilators as PAV+, in Drager Evita series as PPS, and as a non-invasive mode in Respironics BiPAP ventilators. Figure 2 shows a schematic block diagram of PAV. Proper use of this technique requires constant and accurate measurement of respiratory elastance and airway resistance in order to prevent a runaway situation. In that case, the PAV controller of figure 2 also receives the respiratory mechanics data and processes that along with volume and flow rate data to adjust the level of pressure support to the patient.

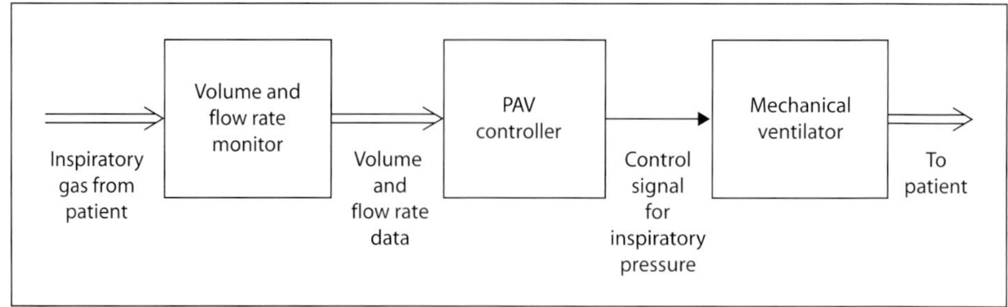

Fig. 2. Schematic diagram of the PAV system.

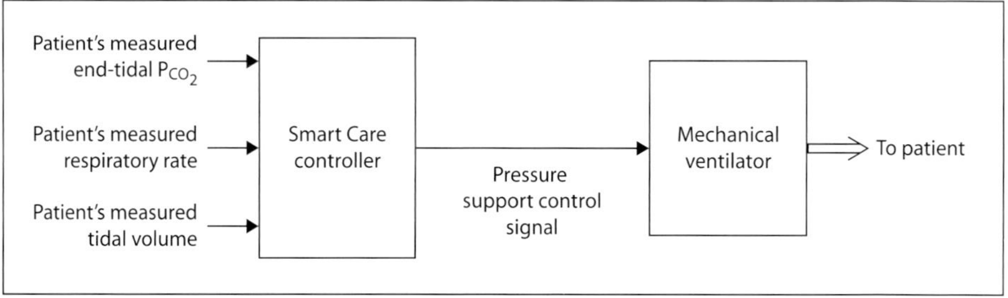

Fig. 3. Schematic diagram of the SmartCare system.

The main advantage of PAV is the synchrony between the patient and the machine. This synchrony is quite significant since it tends to reduce the fighting that occurs between the ventilator and a spontaneously breathing patient. Therefore, by providing this synchrony, PAV can give more comfort to the patient and expedite weaning.

PAV is fundamentally a weaning method and cannot be used for passive patients. Its proper operation requires accurate measurement of respiratory mechanics during spontaneous breathing. It is suited to patients with relatively strong spontaneous activity and should be watched carefully for ventilatory leaks. PEEP and FiO_2 need to be manually adjusted in this mode.

SmartCare

SmartCare is a weaning technique available in Drager Medical Evita ventilators. Figure 3 shows a schematic block diagram of this system. In this technique which was first introduced in 1992 [6], three patient parameters are monitored by the ventilator, namely tidal volume, respiratory rate, and the end-tidal pressure of carbon dioxide. The system's function is to keep these variables within a predefined 'comfort zone'. Using SmartCare, the ventilator that operates in the pressure support mode, increases the level of support incrementally if respiratory rate increases beyond a prescribed range, or tidal volume decreases below a certain level, or end-tidal pressure of CO_2 increases above an acceptable value. If the measured values of these three parameters remain within their predefined ranges, then the level of support is reduced incrementally until the patient is ready to be extubated. This system provides automated support during weaning and is designed to expedite the procedure by using established protocols. The system in

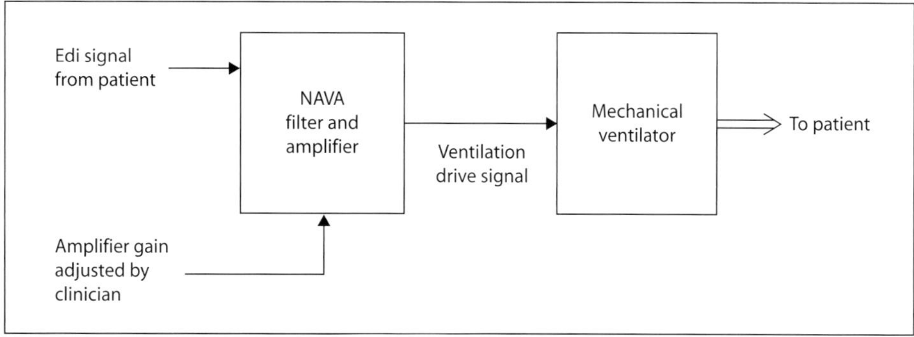

Fig. 4. Schematic diagram of the NAVA system.

SmartCare does not take into account the effects of variations in patient's respiratory mechanics on the acceptable ranges of breathing frequency and tidal volume and there is no guarantee in the system that the patient receives adequate minute ventilation during weaning. PEEP and FiO_2 are manually adjusted in this mode.

Neurally Adjusted Ventilatory Assist

NAVA is a fundamentally different ventilatory mode compared with the other methods described above, in the sense that it uses the patient's own respiratory neural drive signal to control the ventilator. The principles of this technology were first introduced in 1970 [7]. That early technique was enhanced and patented many years later in 1990s [8], and has been adapted in Maquet ventilators in recent years. Figure 4 shows a schematic block diagram of NAVA. In this technique, the patient's respiratory neural drive signal to the diaphragm (Edi) is detected by electrodes mounted on a nasogastric tube which needs to be properly positioned at the lower esophagus. This signal is filtered to eliminate noise due to moving artifacts, electrocardiogram, and other disturbances and is amplified by a gain set manually by the clinician before being applied to drive the ventilator. The main advantage of NAVA is the synchrony between the machine and the patient which improves patient comfort, reduces the fighting that develops between the ventilator and a spontaneously breathing patient due to asynchrony, and can expedite weaning. NAVA cannot be used in all patients and its effectiveness may be affected if strong sedatives are administered. The insertion of a nasogastric tube is an additional required invasive procedure in this mode that needs to be done with care and precision [9]. The amplification factor applied to the Edi signal which determines the level of support provided by the ventilator is adjusted manually by the clinician. PEEP and FiO_2 values are also controlled manually in NAVA.

Conclusion

Significant progress has been made in the design and development of automatic ventilation techniques in the past few decades. Several modalities in which some of the main outputs of ventilators are automatically controlled are currently in use in the ICU settings. When applied properly, these technologies tend to improve treatment and help facilitate the complex tasks handled by ICU clinicians. Despite these significant improvements, there are still some drawbacks associated with the available automatic techniques of ventilation that can be addressed by newer technologies and there are a number of remaining ventilatory tasks that can be automated.

Recommendations

The following are some recommendations for improvement of automation of mechanical ventilation:

- Inclusion of more innovative technologies in mechanical ventilation to address the shortcomings of the present automatic techniques.
- Emphasizing on technologies that increase synchrony between the patient and the ventilator without increasing the invasiveness of the treatment.
- Incorporation of more innovative sensor technologies to prevent measurement errors during automatic control of ventilation.
- More emphasis on non-invasive ventilation when such treatment is applicable.
- Inclusion of more effective automatic weaning technologies in mechanical ventilation.

In summary, there is little doubt that the trend of automation in mechanical ventilation will continue in the future. However, no matter how well designed an automatic ventilation system may be, it is still an aide to the clinician and not a substitute for expert medical care. The automatic technologies that have been and will likely continue to be developed in mechanical ventilation, serve the purpose of helping to provide more optimal treatments to patients that can be more responsive to their needs. These technologies also serve to help clinicians further by constantly monitoring patients in a hectic environment and providing the ICU nurses, therapists, and physicians with more time to give higher attention to the kinds of care that machines cannot provide. Innovations in mechanical ventilation technology can improve ICU care by helping to prevent medical errors and unnecessary prolongation of mechanical ventilation. The innovations in this life-saving technology will likely have a significant impact on the quality of healthcare as they pertain to ICU treatments in the years to come.

References

1 Tehrani FT: Automatic control of mechanical ventilation. Part 2: The existing techniques and future trends. J Clin Monit Comput 2008;22:417–424.

2 Kohn LT, Corrigan JM, Donaldson MS (eds): To Err Is Human: Building a Safer Health System. Washington, Institute of Medicine, The National Academies Press, 2000.

3 Tehrani FT: Automatic control of mechanical ventilation. Part 1: Theory and history of the technology. J Clin Monit Comput 2008;22:409–415.

4 Tehrani FT: Method and apparatus for controlling an artificial respirator, US Patent No 4,986,268, issued January 22, 1991.

5 Younes M: Proportional assist ventilation, a new approach to ventilatory support. Am Rev Respir Dis 1992;145:114–120.

6 Dojat M, Brochard L, Lemaire F, et al: A knowledge-based system for assisted ventilation of patients in intensive care units. Int J Clin Monit Comput 1992;9:239–250.

7 Huszczuk A: A respiratory pump controlled by phrenic nerve activity. J Physiol 1970;210:183P.

8 Sinderby C, Grassino A, Friberg S, et al: Inspiratory proportional pressure assist ventilation controlled by a diaphragm electromyographic signal, US Patent No 5,820,560, issued October 13, 1998.

9 Barwing J, Ambold M, Linden, N, et al: Evaluation of the catheter positioning for neutrally adjusted ventilatory assist. Intensive Care Med 2009;35:1809–1814.

Prof. Fleur T. Tehrani, PhD, PE
Department of Electrical Engineering, California State University, Fullerton
800 N. State College Blvd, Fullerton, CA 92831 (USA)
Tel. +1 657 278 2658, Fax +1 714 281 1360
E-Mail ftehrani@fullerton.edu

Esquinas AM (ed): Applied Technologies in Pulmonary Medicine. Basel, Karger, 2011, pp 35–38

Corticosteroids to Prevent Post-Extubation Upper Airway Obstruction

Scott K. Epstein

Division of Pulmonary, Critical Care, and Sleep Medicine, Tufts Medical Center, Tufts University School of Medicine, Boston, Mass., USA

Abbreviations

CLV Cuff leak volume
UAO Upper airway obstruction

Extubation failure (reintubation) is associated with increased ICU mortality, increased length of hospital stay, greater need for tracheostomy and for long-term acute care, and increased costs [1]. Clinical deterioration between the time of extubation and the re-establishment of ventilatory support may provide the best explanation for increased morbidity and mortality. Therefore, strategies designed to prevent or treat extubation failure have the potential to improve outcome.

Prevalence of Post-Extubation UAO

Intubation, with placement of an endotracheal tube, often results in laryngotracheal injury manifested as inflammation, mucosal ulceration, edema, or granuloma formation. If severe, this results in glottic or subglottic narrowing leading to stridor, respiratory distress, or respiratory failure after removal of the endotracheal tube. Children are particularly susceptible to post-extubation UAO because: the larynx is smaller; fluid easily accumulates in the loose subglottic submucosal connective tissue, and the cricoid cartilage ring is less expandable. From 5 to 35% of patients will experience post-extubation UAO. This wide range results from the different patient populations studied, the variability in the definition of the entity, and the treatments employed after extubation (e.g. racemic epinephrine, noninvasive ventilation). Most studies use the presence of stridor as a surrogate for UAO or laryngeal edema. Others will only categorize a patient as having UAO if treatment was required (e.g. corticosteroids, racemic epinephrine, reintubation). Relatively few studies have used direct laryngoscopic assessment of the airway to define the presence of UAO. Up to 50% of patients who manifest post-extubation UAO will require reintubation though in some studies as few as 2–10% require reinsertion of an airway. Post-extubation UAO usually manifests within 8 h of extubation and almost always within 24–48 h of extubation. Numerous factors have been associated with increased risk for post-extubation UAO in adults (table 1) [2].

Table 1. Factors associated with post-extubation UAO in adults

Female gender (e.g. small tracheal diameter)
Trauma to upper airway
Multiple intubation attempts
Recent unplanned extubation
Age >70–80 years
Excessively mobile or overly large endotracheal tube size
Decreased ratio of patient height to tube diameter (e.g. large tube diameter placed in a short patient)
Ratio of endotracheal tube size to laryngeal diameter >45%
Increased duration of intubation (e.g. >6 days)
Tracheal infection
Low Glasgow Coma Scale score
Excess endotracheal tube cuff pressure
Reduced CLV (<24% of inspired tidal volume or <110 ml)

Detection of Increased Risk for Post-Extubation UAO

Because it is difficult to visualize the trachea in the presence of an endotracheal tube, detection of UAO is best performed using the quantitative cuff leak test [3]. During this maneuver the patient is ventilated on assist control (e.g. set tidal volume) with the endotracheal cuff deflated. The difference (CLV) between inspired and expired tidal volume, averaged over approximately six consecutive breaths is then compared. An obstructed upper airway results in similar inspiratory and expiratory tidal volumes while a patent airway results in a substantial difference as a large volume of gas escapes around the tube. This quantitative cuff leak is then reported as either a percentage of inspired tidal volume or as an absolute CLV. The risk for post-extubation stridor and reintubation is higher when CLV is less than approximately 12–25% of inspired volume or an absolute value of <110–130 ml. Some patients who appear to have UAO based on the cuff leak test can nevertheless be successfully extubated. This falsely low CLV can occur when secretions adhere to or pool around the external surface of the endotracheal tube. Another explanation is that with the cuff deflated, additional tidal volume may be inspired around the tube thus adding to tidal volume delivered by the ventilator. This additional inspired tidal volume is not measured by the ventilator leading to a falsely low measurement of inspired tidal volume. The resulting difference between inspired and expired tidal volume will be falsely low. Alternatively, if lung compliance is decreased, some of the inspired tidal volume immediately moves cephalad around the endotracheal tube rather than entering the lung. Thus delivered inspiratory tidal volume is falsely low resulting in a falsely low CLV. In this case, the risk for UAO may be underappreciated. Either of these sources of error can be eliminated by delivering the machine breath with the cuff inflated and then deflating the cuff just prior to expiration [4].

In pediatric patients the air leak test identifies the pressure (e.g. >30 mm Hg), measured using a manometer, at which an audible leak around the endotracheal tube occurs. The test has met with variable success [5].

Corticosteroids to Prevent Post-Extubation UAO

Corticosteroids are a logical therapeutic strategy to preventing UAO as inflammation is frequently the underlying cause. Studies published from

1989 to 1997 in pediatric and neonatal patients demonstrate that corticosteroids reduce post-extubation UAO by nearly 40%, and may reduce the need for reintubation [6]. In contrast, three randomized controlled trials in adults, published prior to 2000, all found intravenous corticosteroids administered prior to extubation did not reduce the incidence of post-extubation UAO or need for reintubation. Corticosteroids may not have worked in these studies for several reasons. The cohorts studied were not at high risk as reintubation rates in the control arms ranged from 0 to 2.6%. Corticosteroids were given immediately (30–60 min) prior to extubation and therefore were not likely to have sufficient time to exert a clinically significant anti-inflammatory effect. Lastly, only a single dose of corticosteroids was administered and the doses were relatively low.

Since 2006 there have been three well-conducted published randomized controlled trials that demonstrate that corticosteroids can effectively prevent post-extubation UAO and reduce the need for reintubation in adults. These studies differ from the older studies in that a high-risk cohort was selected and corticosteroids were given at higher doses, multiple doses were delivered, and administration began at least 12–24 h prior to extubation. The first study by Cheng et al. [7] randomized 128 medical and surgical patients, ventilated for at least 24 h, who were identified as being at elevated risk for post-extubation UAO based on a CLV <24% of inspired tidal volume. Three groups were studied: one group received 40 mg of methylprednisolone 24 h prior to extubation (one injection); one group received 40 mg of methylprednisolone every 6 h beginning 24 h prior to extubation (4 injections), and one group received placebo injections. Corticosteroids significantly decreased the percentage of patients with stridor (30% placebo, 2% one injection, 7% four injections) and the need for reintubation (19, 5, 7%).

The second study by Lee et al. [8] randomized 86 medical patients who were ventilated for at least 48 h and had a CLV <110 ml. Patients either received placebo or four doses of dexamethasone (5 mg) every 6 h for four doses. Patients were extubated 24 h after the last dose. Corticosteroids resulted in reduced post-extubation stridor (10 vs. 28%). There was no difference in the need for reintubation (2.5 vs. 5%) but a much larger cohort would have been necessary to demonstrate benefit given the low baseline event rate. An important observation is that treatment with dexamethasone led to a significant increase in CLV that persisted 24 h after the last dose (e.g., at the time of extubation).

The third trial randomized 761 patients who had been intubated for ≥36 h. Although no formal process was used to identify a high-risk cohort, the 22% incidence of stridor in the control group suggests an appropriate study population [9]. These investigators compared 20 mg of methylprednisolone, given every 4 h for 12 h prior to extubation, to placebo. Corticosteroid pretreatment was associated with decreased risk for post-extubation UAO (3 vs. 22%), need for reintubation (4 vs. 8%), and need for reintubation secondary to UAO (0.3 vs. 4%).

Since the publication of these trials a number of systematic reviews and meta-analyses have been published. The analysis of Jaber et al. [10] included five published randomized controlled trials and two abstracts totaling 1,846 patients. Overall, corticosteroids significantly reduced the risk of stridor (relative risk 0.48) and reintubation (relative risk 0.58) but the benefit was most pronounced in those deemed to be at high risk based on reduced CLV (stridor 35 vs. 19%, reintubation 20 vs. 9%). No clear benefit could be demonstrated in patients not deemed to be at high risk (using the CLV) or in those who only received corticosteroids 1 h prior to extubation. A subsequent meta-analysis included 14 studies of adults, children and neonates (approx. 2,600 patients) [6]. Overall, corticosteroids reduced post-extubation UAO and need for reintubation, with results consistent across all three patient populations. The effect was most pronounced when administration occurred at least 12 h prior to extubation. These meta-analyses identified no major complications associated with the use of corticosteroids.

Recommendations

Corticosteroids should be given to patients at high risk for post-extubation respiratory failure. High risk is best assessed by the quantitative cuff leak test using a reduced CLV of <24% of the inspired tidal volume or <110 ml. It must be remembered that some patients with a reduced CLV can be extubated successfully without other intervention though identifying these patients is difficult. Whether selection for high risk can be made using the factors in table 1, in the absence of reduced CLV, is unknown. Nevertheless, based on the safety of the published corticosteroid regimens, the threshold for treatment should be low. For adults, 20–40 mg of intravenous methylprednisolone should be administered every 6 h beginning at least 12–24 h prior to planned extubation. For pediatric and neonatal patients, intravenous dexamethasone 0.25–0.5 mg/kg should be given every 6 h at least 12 h prior to planned extubation. Of note, most pediatric/neonatal studies have continued corticosteroids for approximately 12 h after extubation.

References

1 Epstein SK: Decision to extubate. Intensive Care Med 2002;28:535–546.
2 Roberts RJ, Welch SM, Devlin JW: Corticosteroids for prevention of postextubation laryngeal edema in adults. Ann Pharmacother 2008;42:686–691.
3 Miller RL, Cole RP: Association between reduced cuff leak volume and postextubation stridor. Chest 1996;110:1035–1040.
4 Prinianakis G, Alexopoulou C, Mamidakis E, et al: Determinants of the cuff-leak test: a physiological study. Crit Care 2005;9:R24–R31.
5 Mhanna MJ, Zamel YB, Tichy CM, et al: The 'air leak' test around the endotracheal tube, as a predictor of postextubation stridor, is age dependent in children. Crit Care Med 2002;30:2639–2643.
6 McCaffrey J, Farrell C, Whiting P, et al: Corticosteroids to prevent extubation failure: a systematic review and meta-analysis. Intensive Care Med 2009;35:977–986.
7 Cheng KC, Hou CC, Huang HC, et al: Intravenous injection of methylprednisolone reduces. the incidence of postextubation stridor in intensive care unit patients. Crit Care Med 2006;34:1345–1350.
8 Lee CH, Peng MJ, Wu CL: Dexamethasone to prevent postextubation airway obstruction in adults: a prospective, randomized, double-blind, placebo-controlled study. Crit Care 2007;11:R72–R79.
9 Francois B, Bellissant E, Gissot V, et al: 12-Hour pretreatment with methylprednisolone versus placebo for prevention of postextubation laryngeal oedema: a randomised double-blind trial. Lancet 2007;369:1083–1089.
10 Jaber S, Jung B, Chanques G, et al: Effects of steroids on reintubation and post-extubation stridor in adults: meta-analysis of randomised controlled trials. Crit Care 2009;13:R49–R59.

Scott K. Epstein, MD
Office of Educational Affairs, Sackler 317
136 Harrison Avenue, Boston, MA 02111 (USA)
Tel. +1 617 636 2191, Fax +1 617 636 0894
E-Mail Scott.Epstein@tufts.edu

Esquinas AM (ed): Applied Technologies in Pulmonary Medicine. Basel, Karger, 2011, pp 39–45

FLEX: A New Weaning and Decision Support System

Fleur T. Tehrani

Department of Electrical Engineering, California State University, Fullerton, Calif., USA

Abbreviations

CO_2 Carbon dioxide
FiO_2 Concentration of oxygen in the inspiratory gas
O_2 Oxygen
PEEP Positive end-expiratory pressure
PS Pressure support

Choosing the right ventilatory mode and parameters for ICU patients can be a challenging task for many medical personnel. ICU clinicians are required to carefully review the patients' underlying illnesses as well as many available modes of ventilation, and set the ventilatory parameters to deliver optimum treatment to their patients in a timely manner. These tasks can be significantly simplified by use of effective automatic ventilation modes, or with the aide of properly designed decision support systems. Use of advanced closed-loop techniques or effective open-loop advisory systems for ventilation can lead to better care for critically ill patients, which can in turn result in significant reduction in the mortality and morbidity rates associated with provision of inappropriate or unduly prolonged mechanical ventilation.

Many different techniques for automatic control of mechanical ventilation have been developed and there are several such technologies used in commercial ventilators today [1–3]. With regard to open-loop decision support systems, although many techniques have been developed to this date [4], most of them have not been implemented in commercial ventilators. This may be attributed to lack of training for the systems or that they may not have been accessible to clinicians and researchers other than the groups that developed them. Another drawback of such systems has been the concern over their noise immunity and error propagation. Nonetheless, effective decision support systems as well as closed-loop systems for mechanical ventilation can be quite useful tools in helping clinicians with ventilatory treatment of their patients in the ICU environment where correct and timely decision on treatment can often make the difference between life and death.

Analysis

Choice of Ventilatory Parameters and the Weaning Technique

Mechanical ventilation can be provided using various techniques such as negative pressure ventilation, high-frequency oscillatory ventilation, or conventional positive pressure ventilation [5]. Among these techniques, conventional positive pressure ventilation provided invasively (i.e. by use of an endotracheal tube or a tracheostomy tube), or non-invasively (e.g., by use of a facial or nasal mask) are the more common types of ventilation adapted today. Conventional positive pressure ventilation can be provided by using various modalities [2]. Advanced mechanical ventilators are designed to provide wide ranges of ventilatory parameters in various modes of ventilation. Open-loop decision support systems can be helpful to clinicians to set the required ventilatory parameters manually. Also, automatic ventilation and weaning technologies that have become available in recent years can provide valuable assistance to clinicians by constant monitoring of the patients' conditions and automatically adjusting ventilatory parameters in response to their changing requirements. Furthermore, weaning from mechanical ventilation can be a difficult task especially for hard-to-wean patients. Mechanical ventilation can cause serious complications if unnecessarily prolonged, while its premature discontinuation can lead to reintubation which may have detrimental consequences. Therefore, a computerized system that can wean patients safely and effectively can be quite helpful to patients and clinicians and lead to reduction in the ICU stay and healthcare costs at the same time.

In this article, the main features of a more recent computerized weaning and decision support system for mechanical ventilation known as FLEX are described and a brief discussion of future trends in this field is provided.

FLEX Features

FLEX is a computerized system for mechanical ventilation that can be used as an open-loop advisory system or as a closed-loop control technique. It can be used in positive pressure ventilation including invasive and non-invasive modes. It can be applied in volume control/assist as well as pressure control/assist modalities in the management or weaning phases of ventilation. FLEX can be used for adult and pediatric patient populations and a modified version of the system can be employed in neonatal ventilatory treatment.

When used as a closed-loop control technique, FLEX takes input data from the clinician as well as from a data monitoring unit that receives patient's data from the ventilator and provides it to the FLEX algorithm automatically. The algorithm computes the optimal ventilatory parameters for the patient that include the amount of required ventilation, the peak inspiratory pressure, the rate of respiration if applicable, the level of PEEP, the required FiO_2 and any needed adjustment in the inspiratory to expiratory time ratio. The system then provides control signals to the ventilator in accordance with the computed parameter values to adjust the machine's outputs automatically.

If FLEX is used as an open-loop advisory system, the patient and ventilatory data do not need to be provided automatically and can be input by the clinician intermittently. In the open-loop mode, the system makes treatment recommendations to the clinician and does not control the ventilator automatically. Figure 1 shows the record window of FLEX in the advisory mode for an adult patient.

Figure 2 shows a flowchart of the FLEX algorithm. In the beginning, the input and internal parameters along with their acceptable ranges are defined. At this stage, the input data is processed, artifact detection methods are used, and erroneous data is discarded. Also, abstraction techniques are used to prepare input data for processing. This data abstraction is needed to prevent provision of inappropriate outputs or abrupt changes in ventilation to the patient.

At the next step, the required optimum ventilation and respiratory rate are computed. This is done based on patient's ideal body weight, his/her temperature, patient's blood CO_2 and O_2 levels, and respiratory resistance and compliance data.

The patient's CO_2 data which can be obtained by end-tidal CO_2 monitoring is optional for adult and pediatric patients but needs to be provided for neonates. The patient's O_2 level is monitored by using pulse oximetry, the respiratory mechanics data is monitored and provided to the system

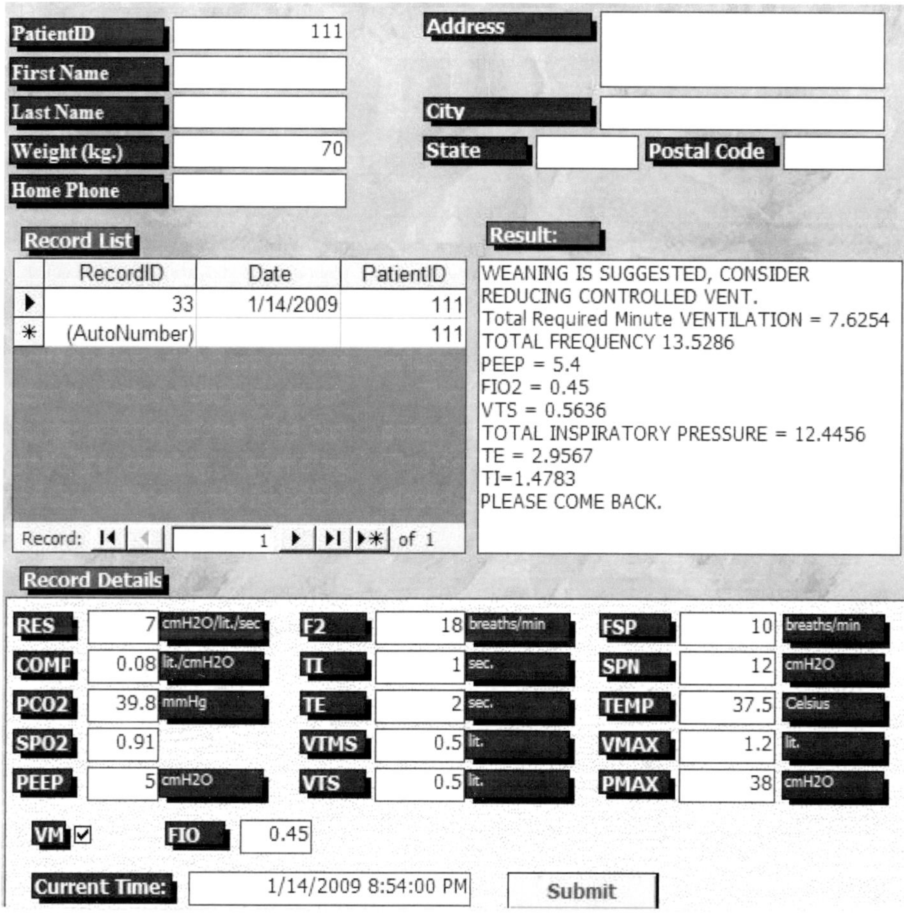

Fig. 1. A patient's record window of FLEX when used as an advisory system.

continuously or intermittently based on the mode of ventilation, and the patient's ideal body weight and temperature are input by the clinician. The patient's respiratory dead space is either measured or estimated by using empirical equations. The algorithm uses the above-mentioned data to compute the required alveolar ventilation and the optimum rate of respiration which is found to minimize the work rate of breathing. The technique of optimizing the respiratory rate and tidal volume to minimize the breathing work rate is a patented technology [6] that has been available in a mode of ventilation known as adaptive support ventilation. The system further adjusts the inspiratory to expiratory time ratio if necessary to prevent the build up of intrinsic PEEP based on the patient's respiratory mechanics data.

In the next step of the algorithm, the optimal values of FiO_2 and PEEP are computed. This is done to prevent hypoxemia, hyperoxemia, barotraumas, and reduction in the cardiac output. If the system is used in a closed-loop mode, a fine proportional- integral-derivative control scheme can be added to the algorithm to adjust

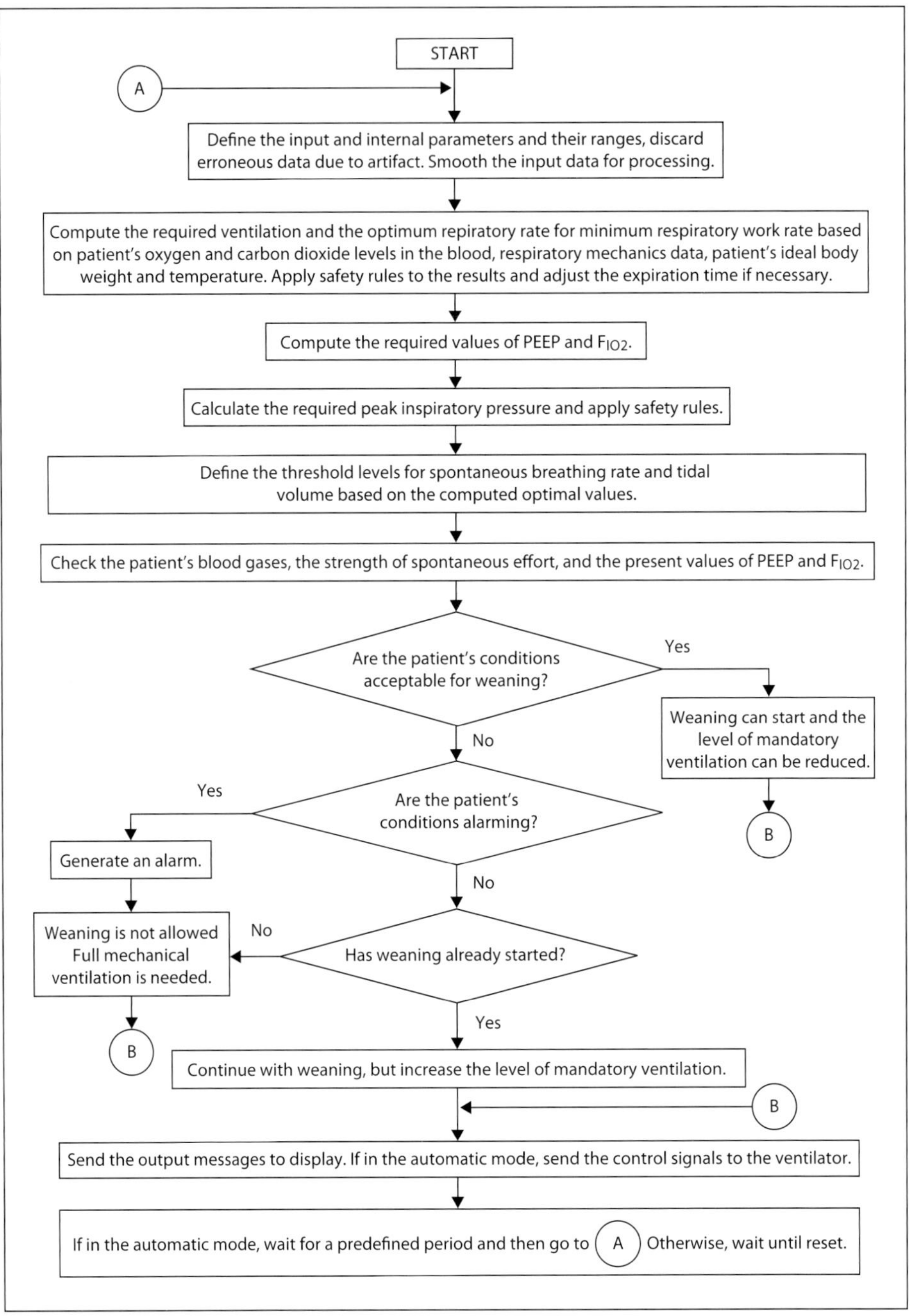

Fig. 2. A flowchart of the FLEX algorithm.

FiO_2 and PEEP [7]. Next, the required inspiratory pressure is computed and safety rules are applied. Then the threshold levels of tidal volume and respiratory rate are defined based on the computed required values. These threshold levels are needed in later steps to determine the strength of the patient's spontaneous breathing and to assess his/her readiness for weaning. Next, the program checks a series of conditions including the patient's blood gases, the strength of his/her spontaneous effort, and the levels of FiO_2 and PEEP to determine whether the patient is ready to be weaned. If the patient's conditions are acceptable, weaning is allowed and is started at the discretion of the clinician by reducing the level of ventilatory support. Otherwise, weaning is not started but the program checks to see whether the patient's conditions are alarming and also if weaning has already begun. If the patient's conditions are not alarming but the ventilatory treatment is already in the weaning phase, the level of support is increased. However, if the patient's conditions are found to be alarming, warnings are generated and full mechanical ventilation is provided.

This procedure is repeated automatically at prescribed intervals in the closed-loop mode and is performed intermittently at the discretion of the clinician in the open-loop advisory mode.

The details of the control scheme and the mathematical equations and procedures of the algorithm have been described in detail elsewhere [8], and therefore are not repeated here for brevity.

Discussion

Various open-loop techniques for adjustment of ventilatory parameters have been introduced in the past [4]. Also, a number of technologies for automatic control of mechanical ventilation have been developed that are designed to control patients' ventilation, oxygenation, or weaning [1–3]. Several automatic ventilatory techniques are already available in commercial ventilators [3]. In one of the more recent of these technologies known as neurally adjusted ventilatory assist ventilation [9], the patient's own respiratory neural drive signal is used to drive the ventilator. This signal which is detected by electrodes mounted on a nasogastric tube positioned at the lower esophagus of the patient, needs to be effectively cleared of artifact noise and amplified by a manually controlled gain factor to control the ventilator. Use of the patient's own respiratory drive signal provides good synchronization between the machine and the patient's respiratory system. However, this technique cannot be used in all patients, administration of neural depressants can interfere with the treatment, and the requirement of having a well-positioned nasogastric tube is not always convenient especially in non-invasive ventilation. In another technique known as proportional assist ventilation [10] the pressure applied by the ventilator is controlled by and follows the pressure developed by the patient's own respiratory system. This technique is suitable for use in the weaning phase of ventilatory treatment and cannot be used for passive patients or those whose spontaneous breathing effort is not reasonably strong. Proper application of this technique which can be employed in both invasive and non-invasive ventilation requires measurement of respiratory elastance and airway resistance in spontaneously breathing patients.

FLEX is a system which is designed to be flexible for use in a wide range of ventilatory modes. This system which is the subject of a new patent application can be used in the management phase of treatment for passive patients as well as weaning phase by application of PS. It incorporates the features of a patented mode known as adaptive support ventilation by automatically controlling tidal volume and respiratory rate and augments the features of that mode by closed-loop control of several additional ventilatory parameters including minute ventilation, PEEP and FiO_2. In the weaning phase of treatment, using modes such as PS, FLEX controls the pressure applied by the machine automatically while adjusting PEEP and FiO_2 at the same time. It can be used in non-invasive modes of ventilation such as continuous positive airway pressure, or bilevel positive airway pressure by controlling the PS level while improving oxygenation by automatically adjusting FiO_2. FLEX has shown good potential in closed-loop setups as well as open-loop clinical evaluations [8, 11]. However, more extensive clinical assessments are needed to evaluate the strengths and weaknesses of the system for different patient profiles and populations.

Recommendations

Application of automation in mechanical ventilation has gained increasing momentum in recent years and this trend will likely continue in the future. Despite the existence of several major automatic techniques in commercial ventilators, most ventilatory parameters are still manually adjusted. It is likely that more parameters for control of ventilation, weaning, or oxygenation will be automatically controlled using newly developed modes in the near future. The automatic techniques offer clear advantages over manual systems and are designed to prevent clinical errors, improve healthcare and reduce costs. However, the following points may be worth considering in choosing and using such systems:

- Every system has its advantages as well as drawbacks and needs to be chosen with the needs of the patient in mind. Although non-invasive ventilation is becoming increasingly popular, clinical indications should be clearly observed to choose between invasive and non-invasive ventilatory treatments. Likewise, in choosing a ventilatory mode or an automatic technology, it is essential to know what kind of patients the technique is intended for, for example (1) whether the mode is restricted to weaning or if it can be used for passive patients as well; (2) whether the ventilatory mode is targeted towards certain patient profiles such as those with acute respiratory distress syndrome or chronic obstructive pulmonary disease, or it can be used for various patient groups.
- Before using an automatic ventilatory technique, it is necessary to know what parameters it is designed to control automatically, which inputs are monitored and used by the system, and whether certain aspects of ventilation or parameters need to be carefully watched during the treatment.
- It is important to note that no automatic technique is designed to substitute for the expert clinical care. Rather, such systems are designed to assist the clinicians to choose better treatments for their patients. No matter how well an automatic system might have been developed, careful attention to the conditions of the patient and his/her response to treatment are essential for a successful outcome.

References

1 Branson RD, Johannigman JA, Campbell RS, et al: Closed-loop mechanical ventilation. Respir Care 2002;47:427–451.

2 Chatburn RL: Classification of ventilator modes: update and proposal for implementation. Respir Care 2007;52:301–323.

3 Tehrani FT: Automatic control of mechanical ventilation. Part 2: The existing techniques and future trends. J Clin Monit Comput 2008;22:417–424.

4 Tehrani FT, Roum JH: Intelligent decision support systems for mechanical ventilation. Artif Intell Med 2008;44:171–182.

5 Pilbeam SP, Cairo JM: Mechanical ventilation, physiological and clinical applications, ed 4. St Louis, Mosby Elsevier, 2006, pp 81–103.

6 Tehrani FT: Method and apparatus for controlling an artificial respirator. US Patent No 4,986,268, issued January 22, 1991.

7 Tehrani FT: Method and apparatus for controlling a ventilator. UK Patent Serial No 2423721, granted October 14, 2008 (patent pending in several other countries).
8 Tehrani FT, Roum JH: FLEX: a new computerized system for mechanical ventilation. J Clin Monit Comput 2008;22:121–130.
9 Sinderby C: Neurally adjusted ventilatory assist (NAVA). Minerva Anestesiol 2002;68:378–380.
10 Younes M: Proportional assist ventilation, a new approach to ventilatory support. Am Rev Respir Dis 1992;145;114–120.
11 Tehrani FT, Abbasi S: Evaluation of a computerized system for mechanical ventilation of infants. J Clin Monit Comput 2009;23:93–104.

Prof. Fleur T. Tehrani, PhD, PE
Department of Electrical Engineering, California State University, Fullerton
800 N. State College Blvd, Fullerton, CA 92831 (USA)
Tel. +1 657 278 2658, Fax +1 714 281 1360
E-Mail ftehrani@fullerton.edu

Esquinas AM (ed): Applied Technologies in Pulmonary Medicine. Basel, Karger, 2011, pp 46–50

Thermal Infrared Imaging during Polysomnography: Has the Time Come to Unwire the 'Wired' Subjects?

Jayasimha N. Murthy[a] · Ioannis Pavlidis[b]

[a]Divisions of Pulmonary, Critical Care and Sleep Medicine, University of Texas Health Science Center, and [b]Department of Computer Science, University of Houston, Houston, Tex., USA

Abbreviations

ATHEMOS	Automated thermal monitoring system
BCI	Bayesian credible interval
κ (kappa)	Chance-corrected agreement
Pn	Nasal pressure – airflow monitoring device routinely used in polysomnography
REM	Rapid eye movement
RERA	Respiratory effort-related arousals
SDB	Sleep disordered breathing – encompasses a wide variety of disorders characterized by breathing abnormalities during sleep such as obstructive sleep apnea, central sleep apnea, etc.
TIRI	Thermal infrared imaging

Untreated SDB is a very prevalent problem and can cause daytime sleepiness as well as have far-reaching socioeconomic and health-related consequences. A summary of statistics from three pooled studies estimated that 20% of adults with a body mass index between 25 and 28 kg/m^2 have SDB based on an apnea-hypopnea index of ≥5 per hour [1]. Sleepiness is believed to have played a major role in causing disasters such as the Chernobyl and the Three Mile Island tragedies [2] and has been reported to be the most common cause of fatalities associated with motor vehicle accidents [3]. Untreated SDB is also associated with cardiovascular diseases [4].

Diagnosis of sleep apnea typically involves an overnight sleep study with simultaneous monitoring of airflow channels (Pn, oro-nasal thermistor), electrocardiogram, sleep staging by electroencephalography, electrooculography, and chin and leg electromyography in accordance with the Level 1 recommendations of the American Academy of Sleep Medicine [5]. However, conventional polysomnography has the potential to interfere with the 'usual' sleep pattern. A sizeable proportion of patients and normal volunteers who have never had a prior sleep study, experience the 'first night effect' characterized mainly by a decrease in sleep efficiency, prolongation of sleep-onset time, increase in REM sleep latency and a reduction in the total amount of REM sleep [6]. Additionally, it has been demonstrated that instrumentation during polysomnography affects body position during sleep [7] and thus impacts the diagnosis of SDB, the severity of which can increase during supine sleep. Moreover, bedside manipulation of sensors, in an effort to obtain high-quality data, may further disturb sleep and hinder our ability to obtain a true representation of the patient's usual sleep pattern. Thus, decreasing subject contact with monitoring equipment and testing in the 'usual' sleep environment may help counteract polysomnography's interference with sleep and SDB.

American Academy of Sleep Medicine recommends the use of thermistor as the airflow sensor for the diagnosis of apnea and Pn for the diagnosis of hypopnea as well as RERA [5]. While Pn can overestimate pathological events, especially when subjects change from nasal to predominantly oral breathing, the thermistor on the other hand lacks the sensitivity as compared to Pn, to detect subtle flow abnormalities such as hypopnea and RERAs. Non-contact airflow monitoring technology such as TIRI has the capability to monitor airflow during sleep without subject contact. This concept can be extended to include both laboratory-based and home-based sleep studies.

Description of TIRI

The principle of operation of TIRI is close to that of the oro-nasal thermistor in that both these methods sense thermal radiation. However, it is important to note the following differences between the thermistor and TIRI:

(1) TIRI can sense thermal information at a distance (contact-free), while the thermistor needs to be physically placed and tethered to patient's oro-nasal area, in the proximity of the thermal signal.

(2) TIRI acquires thermal information through natural radiation from the source as opposed to the thermistor which acquires thermal information by conduction when placed in the path of airflow. Theoretically, conduction is bidirectional and has an associated measurement error based on where and when the measurements are made. The accuracy also depends on the intensity as well as the magnitude of change in the thermal signal that is being measured. This error can be detrimental to the detection of subtle airflow abnormalities. TIRI, on the other hand, is an array (imaging sensor) and not just a point sensor-like thermistor. Therefore, it can be used to obtain a thermistor-like signal across time by averaging the thermal signal from all the points in the cross-sectional area of the visible nares, as well as provide thermal information over an extended two-dimensional surface. Analysis of signal as an evolving two-dimensional surface across increases the sensitivity of TIRI and may increase its ability to detect subtle airflow-related phenomena.

Thus, on theoretical grounds alone, one would expect TIRI to be considered a 'virtual thermistor' to perform at least as good as the oro-nasal thermistor [8]. Despite these inherent advantages of TIRI as compared to the thermistor, the following significant challenges had to be overcome to realize the translation of this technology for airflow monitoring:

(1) *Virtual probing*: Since there is no physical probe involved in TIRI, a computational method is needed to segment the nostrils in the image, thus creating a 'virtual' probe, where the measurement can be performed. The difference in the temperature of inspired and expired air brings about a temporal variation in the thermal signature of the nostrils. This fluctuating thermal signal helps in the differentiation of the nostrils (or mouth, if the subject is mouth-breathing) from the rest of the facial tissue. The nostrils can thus be segmented from the face with the nasal cartilages forming 'colder' boundaries around the thermal signal (fig. 1).

(2) *Tracking*: Because there is no tethering and the subject is free to move, a computational method is needed to track changes in position, so that the virtual probe stays always in place and the accuracy of measurement is preserved. Functional imaging such as TIRI that maps randomly changing thermophysiological function in a non-restrained subject requires a collaborative network of particle filter trackers based on advanced statistics (coalitional tracking [9]) to compensate for subject movement.

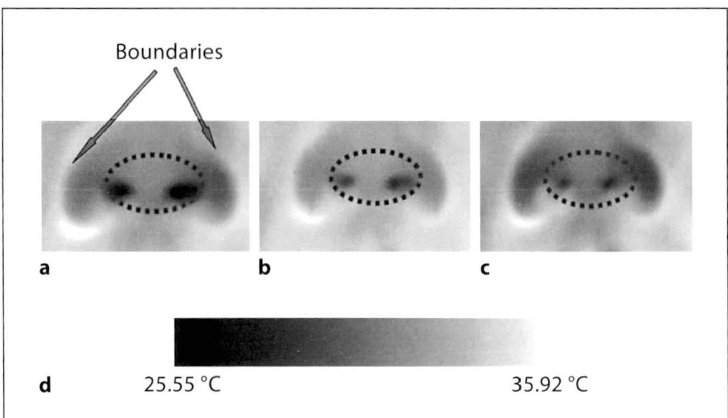

Fig. 1. Temporal variance of nostril region in thermal imagery during breathing: (**a**) inspiration phase, (**b**) transition phase, (**c**) expiration phase, and (**d**) thermal color map. Note the cold boundaries (labeled 'Boundaries') of the nasal cartilages that allow the segmentation of nostrils from the rest of the facial tissue.

(3) *Signal extraction:* Assuming that virtual probing and tracking work well, they create the opportunity for a good measurement, but not the measurement in itself. Since there is no physical transducer that can produce an electronic signal in response to thermal signal, the signal has to be computationally generated. This has been achieved by continuous wavelet transformation on the normalized thermal signal under the assumption that the breathing component is the strongest part of the varying thermal signal.

Integration of TIRI with Polysomnography

The integrated hardware and software system we used in our preliminary study [10] is called ATHEMOS. The thermal signal acquired by the infrared camera and processed by ATHEMOS as an airflow signal was recorded into an existing polysomnography system as an airflow channel, using a custom-made digital to analog converter. This allowed for easy display and comparison of all the airflow channels on a single screen. The camera was kept at about 2.45 m away from the patient during the recording.

Fourteen subjects (9 men and 5 women) without sleep apnea and 13 subjects (7 men and 6 women) with obstructive sleep apnea were studied for an average recording time of around 110 min. There was excellent κ (κ = 0.92, 95% BCI 0.86, 0.96; probability of κ being ≥0.70 [pκ] = 0.99) between TIRI and thermistor for the detection of apnea (defined as a ≥90% decrease in airflow for at least 10 s) and hypopnea (defined as a decrease in airflow signal by at least 50% from the baseline with a ≥4% oxygen desaturation from pre-event baseline). Likewise, there was a high degree of κ between TIRI and Pn (κ = 0.83, 95% BCI 0.70, 0.90; pκ = 0.98). When the performance of thermistor, Pn and TIRI was compared, the thermistor missed the most number of concordant events detected in the other two channels, while Pn missed the least. However, it is intriguing to note that TIRI missed only 3 concordant events detected by the thermistor and Pn while the thermistor missed 21 concordant events detected by TIRI and Pn. The better performance of TIRI as compared to the thermistor can be explained by the increased efficiency of detection of thermal signal by natural radiation, as opposed to conduction.

Discussion

There appears to be need to further advance the field of polysomnography with the use of non-contact-sensing methods in laboratory and home-based sleep studies. The need to obtain a true representation the usual sleep pattern motivates this shift in paradigm. Non-contact-sensing methods such as TIRI have the potential to advance the field in this direction. However, this technology should be thoroughly tested prior to its widespread clinical use. Even though the results of our initial evaluation of TIRI appear to be optimistic, significant concerns in the study design, including a small sample and a limited monitoring period, remain. TIRI, to our knowledge, has never been evaluated during an overnight polysomnography. A study of this nature is of vital importance to establish the resilience and accuracy of thermal imaging as airflow-sensing method during routine nocturnal sleep studies. Even if contact airflow-sensing devices are replaced by non-contact technology, we still have to contend with the remaining contact sensors that may continue to interfere with sleep during polysomnography. On the other hand, the role of TIRI in conducting home sleep studies should be explored and validated. Since TIRI is currently a prototype, the expense associated with this technology is relatively high. However, with further development and widespread use of this technology, here is potential for cost reduction.

Analysis of thermal imaging signal using algorithms that preserve the array structure of the sensor may help in the detection of subtle airflow abnormalities such as RERAs. In such a situation, direct comparison of TIRI with Pn in scoring RERAs would be necessary to further validate this technology.

TIRI is the only technology that can perform signal acquisition in a retrospective manner since signal transduction is done computationally. The operator can redefine a new region of interest and computationally transduce the thermal signal. This concept can be expanded to simultaneously monitor airflow from the oro-nasal region and artificial airways such as tracheostomies. The current tracking algorithms automatically compensate for mild to moderate subject movement. In the event of a drastic change in subject position, signal acquisition can still continue if the nostrils are within the camera frame. In such a scenario, the operator can remotely change the camera position on a tilt-pan stand, redefine the region of interest and resume data collection. Extreme changes in body position can also be handled by interfacing multiple cameras at different positions in the room. Only when a subject buries his or her face into a pillow or pulls a sheet over the face, will the signal be lost. This scenario will need a technician intervention to instruct the patient appropriately. On a similar note, masks also interfere with thermal signal acquisition and thus TIRI cannot be used simultaneously with a continuous positive airway pressure titration at the present time.

TIRI has the potential to make a significant impact in pediatric polysomnography, where contact oro-nasal sensors are difficult to place and maintain. Sterilization of equipment or consumables is not necessary for TIRI to operate.

Future studies should validate TIRI in laboratory-based nocturnal polysomnography in adults and children. Since the accuracy of TIRI in the detection RERAs and its resilience during overnight polysomnography are still uncertain, this technology at the present time should only be used for investigational purposes.

Recommendations

- There is a need to develop non-contact-sensing modalities such as TIRI during polysomnography to not only improve patient comfort and experience, but also to obtain a representative sample of the subject's usual sleep.
- Even though the preliminary study with TIRI is encouraging, further validation is required before this technology can be used in a clinically meaningful way.
- TIRI has the potential to be used for medical applications beyond polysomnography where airflow monitoring in a non-contact manner is necessary.

References

1 Young T, Peppard PE, Gottlieb DJ: Epidemiology of obstructive sleep apnea: a population health perspective. Am J Respir Crit Care Med 2002;165:1217–1239.

2 Mitler MM, Carskadon MA, Czeisler CA, et al: Catastrophes, sleep, and public policy: consensus report. Sleep 1988;11:100–109.

3 Young T, Blustein J, Finn L, et al: Sleep-disordered breathing and motor vehicle accidents in a population-based sample of employed adults. Sleep 1997;20:608–613.

4 Takama N, Kurabayashi M: Influence of untreated sleep-disordered breathing on the long-term prognosis of patients with cardiovascular disease. Am J Cardiol 2009;103:730–734.

5 Iber C, Ancoli-Israel S, Chesson A, et al: The AASM Manual for the Scoring of Sleep and Associated Events: Rules, Terminology and Technical Specifications, ed 1. Westchester/IL, American Academy of Sleep Medicine, 2007.

6 Tamaki M, Nittono H, Hayashi M, et al: Examination of the first-night effect during the sleep-onset period. Sleep 2005;28:195–202.

7 Metersky ML, Castriotta RJ: The effect of polysomnography on sleep position: possible implications on the diagnosis of positional obstructive sleep apnea. Respiration 1996;63:283–287.

8 Fei J, Pavlidis I: Thermistor at a distance: unobtrusive measurement of breathing. IEEE Trans Biomed Eng 2010;57:988–998.

9 Dowdall J, Pavlidis I, Tsiamyrtzis P: Coalitional tracking. Comput Vis Image Underst 2007;106:205–219.

10 Murthy JN, van Jaarsveld J, Fei J, et al: Thermal infrared imaging: a novel method to monitor airflow during polysomnography. Sleep 2009;32:1521–1527.

Jayasimha N. Murthy, MD
Divisions of Pulmonary, Critical Care and Sleep Medicine
University of Texas Health Science Center
6432 Fannin MSB 1.274, Houston, TX 77030 (USA)
Tel. +1 713 500 6828, Fax +1 713 500 6829, E-Mail Jayasimha.Murthy@uth.tmc.edu

Esquinas AM (ed): Applied Technologies in Pulmonary Medicine. Basel, Karger, 2011, pp 51–52

Cardiopulmonary Resuscitation with the Boussignac System

Georges Boussignac

Antony, France

More than 600,000 people suffer a cardiac arrest every year in Europe and the USA. This pathology has a very severe prognosis. Only 3–5% of the people who suffer a cardiovascular accident survive.

Guidelines (ILCOR/AHA, 2005) for cardiopulmonary resuscitation (CPR) have advanced considerably in the last 30 years: (i) in the 1980s there were 5 compressions for 1 ventilation; (ii) in the 1990s there were 15 compressions for 2 ventilations, and (iii) nowadays the ratio is 30 compressions for 2 ventilations, and once the patient is intubated a constant external cardiac massage follows at 10–12 V/min.

Recommendations have advanced more and more towards the predominance of the massage considered the best way of maintaining correct hemodynamics. However, two problems arise: (1) making the blood flow without oxygen is not an interesting option if we want to guarantee survival of the vital organs that are great consumers of oxygen, and (2) the type of present ventilation (oxygen cylinder facemask or ventilator) is not adapted to chest compression (desynchronization massage/ventilation can induce a barotrauma).

It will be interesting to find a new way to give oxygen to patients with CPR and maintain or improve hemodynamics.

Analysis

Ideal ventilation must be (i) automatic and (ii) help fill the lungs during decompression in order to avoid barotraumas. This is the concept of the CPR Boussignac system, which uses positive pressure to fill oxygen into the lungs during decompression. During each compression, the O_2 administered is expelled towards the outside because the CPR Boussignac system is an open system. In each compression the lung receives an insufflation without needing a ventilator or an oxygen cylinder facemask. Also, being an open system a risk of barotraumas is not possible. This concept is that of passive oxygenation. Passive oxygenation administered by the CPR Boussignac system can be performed by a specially designed intratracheal tube or by a supraglottic device that improves the interesting form of the gaseous interchanges [1] as well as hemodynamics [2, 3].

Discussion

For several years, application of a positive pressure during CPR has been rejected for being a factor of reduction of the venous return (reperfusion). The studies of Steen et al. [2] have demonstrated that the concept of passive oxygenation for the CPR Boussignac system did not reduce the venous return, but otherwise it was improved. These same studies in an animal model have demonstrated a 50% survival rate using classic ventilation and a 100% survival rate using passive oxygenation according to Boussignac. A study carried out in Belgium has demonstrated that the association of continuous chest compressions with a cardiac compressor with the concept of passive oxygenation by the CPR Boussignac system has made it possible to obtain a survival rate of 26.3% as opposed to 10% obtained with continuous chest compressions combined with classic ventilation.

To conclude: (i) a patient with cardiac arrest must be considered as an inert body; (ii) in the thoracic cavity there is a very important ΔP during CPR; (iii) there is 15–20 cm of water in the lung during compression and –5 to –8 cm during decompression, and (iv) in the mouth, pressure variability is very low with between 2 and 3 cm of water.

Recommendations

- Simplification of the attention to the patient: only massage.
- Defibrillate as soon as possible.
- Use passive oxygenation to supply the patient oxygen.
- Execute all these steps as quickly as possible (<10 min).

References

1 Brochard L, Boussignac G, Dubois Randé JL, Harf A, Bertrand C, Geschwind H: Cardiopulmonary resuscitation without a ventilator using a novel endotracheal tube in a human. Anesthesiology 1990;72:389.

2 Steen S, Liao Q, Pierre L, Paskevicius A, Sjöberg T: Continuous intratracheal insufflation of oxygen improves the efficacy of mechanical chest compression-active decompression cardiopulmonary resuscitation. Resuscitation 2004;62:219–227.

3 Gillis M, Keirens A, Steinkamm C, Verbelen J, Muysoms W, Reynders N: The use of Lucas and the Boussignac tube in the prehospital setting. ERC Congress, Ghent 2008.

Georges Boussignac, MD
1, rue de Provence
FR–92160 Antony (France)
Tel. +33 6 60 99 12 83, E-Mail georgesboussignac@orange.fr

Esquinas AM (ed): Applied Technologies in Pulmonary Medicine. Basel, Karger, 2011, pp 53–59

Respiratory Function Monitoring during Simulation-Based Mannequin Teaching

Georg M. Schmölzer[a–d] · Colin J. Morley[a,c,e]

[a]Neonatal Services, Royal Women's Hospital, [b]The Ritchie Centre, Monash Institute for Medical Research, Monash University, [c]Murdoch Children Research Institute, Melbourne, Vic., Australia, [d]Division of Neonatology, Department of Paediatrics, Medical University, Graz, Austria, and [e]Department of Obstetrics and Gynaecology, The University of Melbourne, Melbourne, Vic., Australia

Abbreviations

PEEP	Positive end-expiratory pressure
PIP	Peak inflation pressure
PPV	Positive pressure ventilation
RFM	Respiratory function monitor
t_E	Expiratory time
t_I	Inflation time
V_T	Tidal volume
V_{Te}	Expiratory tidal volume
V_{Ti}	Inspiratory tidal volume

Adequate ventilation remains the cornerstone of respiratory support during neonatal transition [1]. Internationally agreed consensus statements on neonatal resuscitation recommend that breathing should be assisted by giving PPV with a manual inflation device [2]. However, PPV can be difficult because the assessment of facemask seal, tidal volume (V_T) and effective ventilation is subjective relying on clinical impression of adequate chest rise and an increase in heart rate [2].

Neonatal life support courses are a mandatory part of neonatal training in many countries. Although they emphasise the importance of 'bag-and-mask' ventilation, the evaluation of how well the trainee applies the mask and ventilates the mannequin is subjective.

Facemask leak is both a common and unrecognised problem during PPV which can lead to failure of ventilation. Recently, a RFM was used to evaluate 'bag-and-mask' ventilation during simulation-based mannequin teaching [3–6]. Participants had large and unrecognised leaks between the face and the mask [6]. When the participants used a RFM they were able to adjust the mask position and facemask leak was halved [4].

During resuscitation the spontaneous V_T or the V_T being delivered during PPV is unknown. Various studies suggest a V_T within a range of 4–8 ml/kg. Insufficient V_T can lead to inadequate gas exchange, whereas excessive V_T can lead to volutrauma [7–11]. PPV is always pressure-limited, however the purpose of applying a peak pressure is to inflate the lung with an appropriate V_T. However, the V_T delivered is not fixed but dependent on the size, compliance, and resistance of the lungs, and the applied pressure. During resuscitation as the lung aerates the V_T delivered will change as the infant starts breathing. Recent studies have been shown that

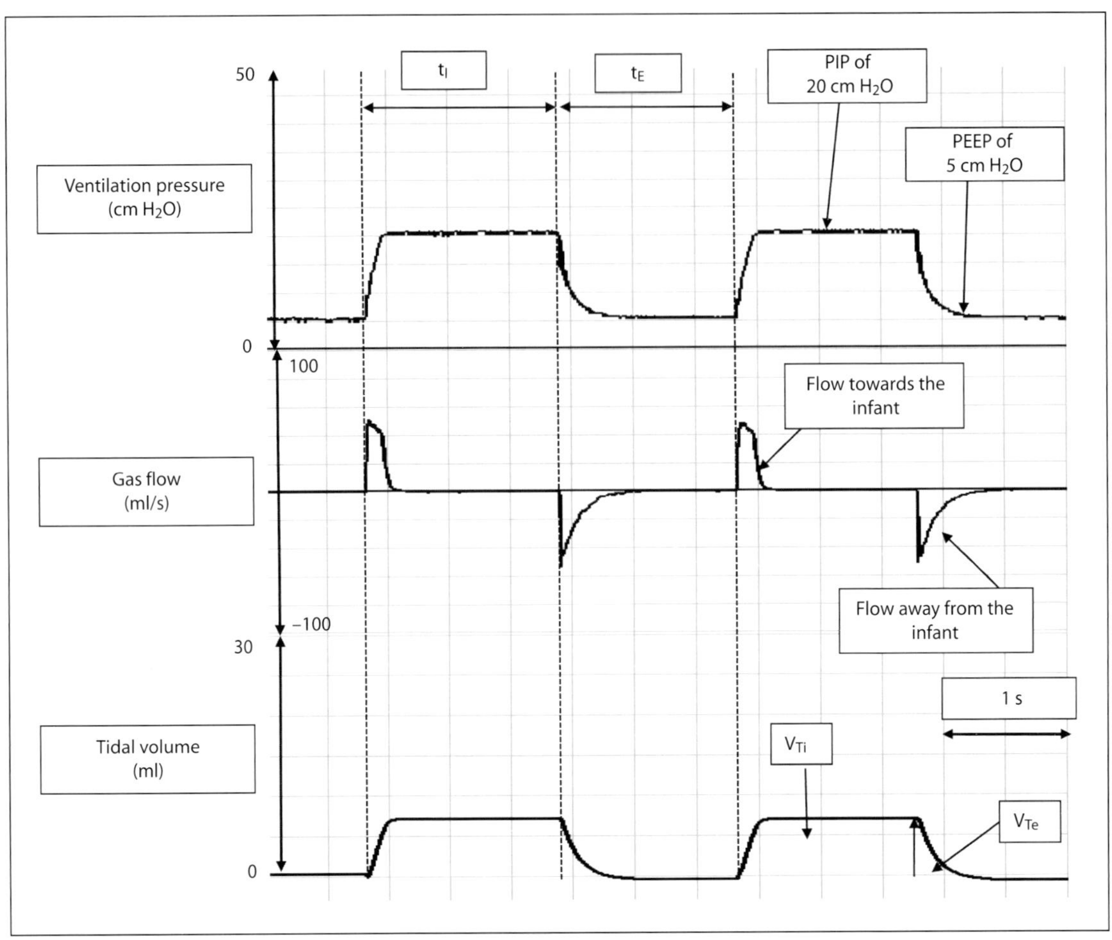

Fig. 1. PPV with a facemask and no leak. PPV with a set PEEP and PIP of 5 and 20 cm H_2O. Gas flow curves of inflation and expiration are returning to the baseline. This indicates sufficient inspiration and expiration time. The areas underneath both inflation and expiration gas flow curves are similar reflecting an equal amount of gas entering and leaving the lung. The V_T curve displays V_{Ti} and V_{Te}, showing an equal volume of gas entering and leaving the lung. In addition, no leak is present. V_{Ti} has reached a plateau indicating no further gas continues to enter the lung as inflation is continued.

operators are unable to deliver accurate and appropriate V_Ts during simulation-based PPV or during neonatal resuscitation [12, 13]. When the participants could see a display of the V_T they were able to achieve the desired volume more accurately [12].

In this chapter we discuss the potential use of a RFM during simulation-based mannequin teaching. A RFM can assist during mask ventilation: (i) it can help to identify correct mask hold and positioning techniques to reduce leak of gas between the mask and face; (ii) continuously measure and display the PIP and PEEP, (iii) enable the operator to adjust the pressure to deliver an appropriate V_T, and (iv) provide an objective assessment of the trainee's performance.

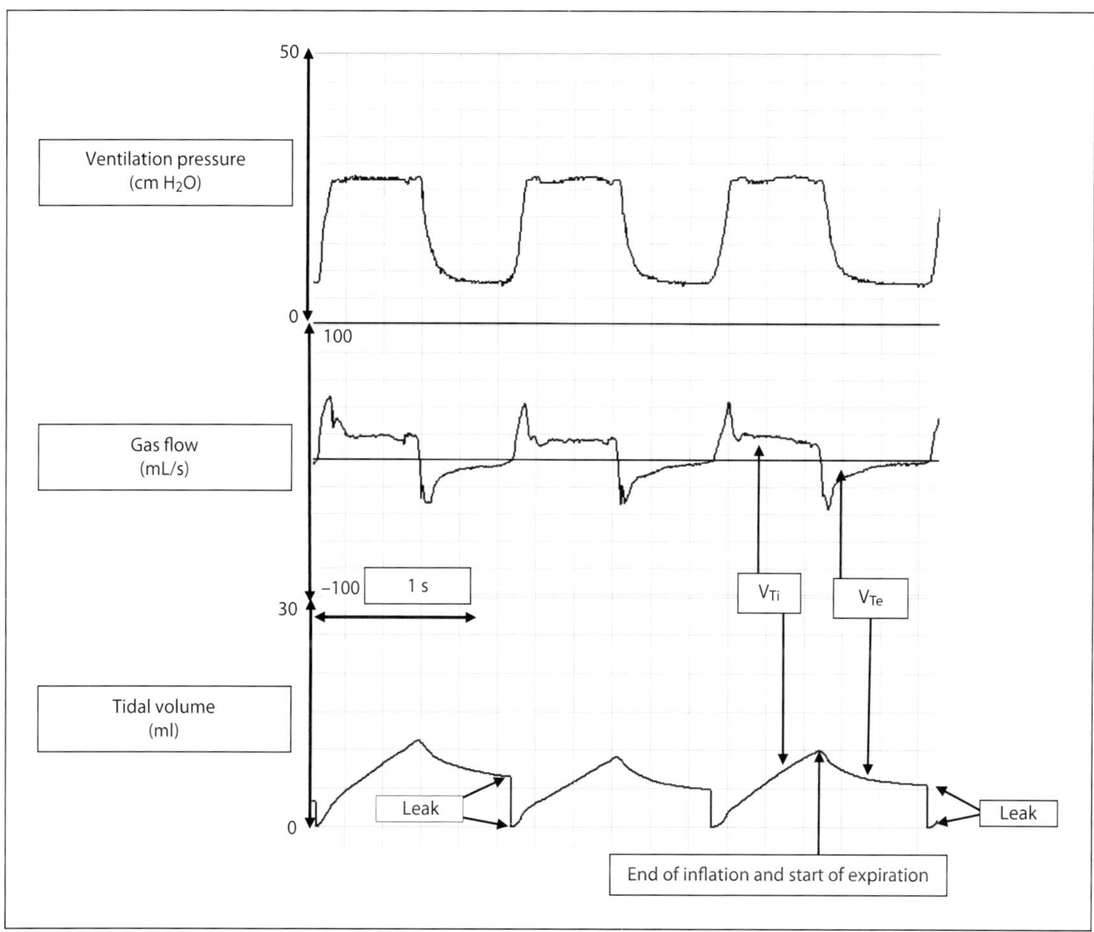

Fig. 2. Airway leak during PPV. The area underneath the inflation gas flow curve is larger than that under the expiratory gas flow curves. The V_T curve displays a larger V_{Ti} compared to V_{Te} and leak is shown as a straight line in the V_T curve.

Respiratory Function Monitor

Any RFM which measures and displays airway pressure, gas flow and V_T can be used during simulation-based mannequin training. The flow sensor is placed between the facemask and the ventilation device [3–6]. By integrating the flow signal, the V_{Ti} and V_{Te} passing through the sensor are automatically calculated. An airway pressure line is connected to measure and display the PIP and PEEP.

A RFM continuously displays airway pressure, gas flow and V_T waves. In addition, it measures and displays numerical values for PIP, PEEP, V_{Ti}, V_{Te}, respiratory rate, expiratory minute ventilation, t_I, and t_E (fig. 1). The percentage of leak between mask and face is calculated and displayed with the following equation: $[(V_{Ti} - V_{Te}) \div V_{Ti}] \times 100$ (fig. 2) [3].

All figures were obtained during PPV of a Laerdal neonatal mannequin (Laerdal Medical AS, Stavanger, Norway), which was made internally leak-free. PPV was performed using a round silicone facemask (Laerdal Medical AS) and a Neopuff Infant T-Piece Resuscitator (Fisher &

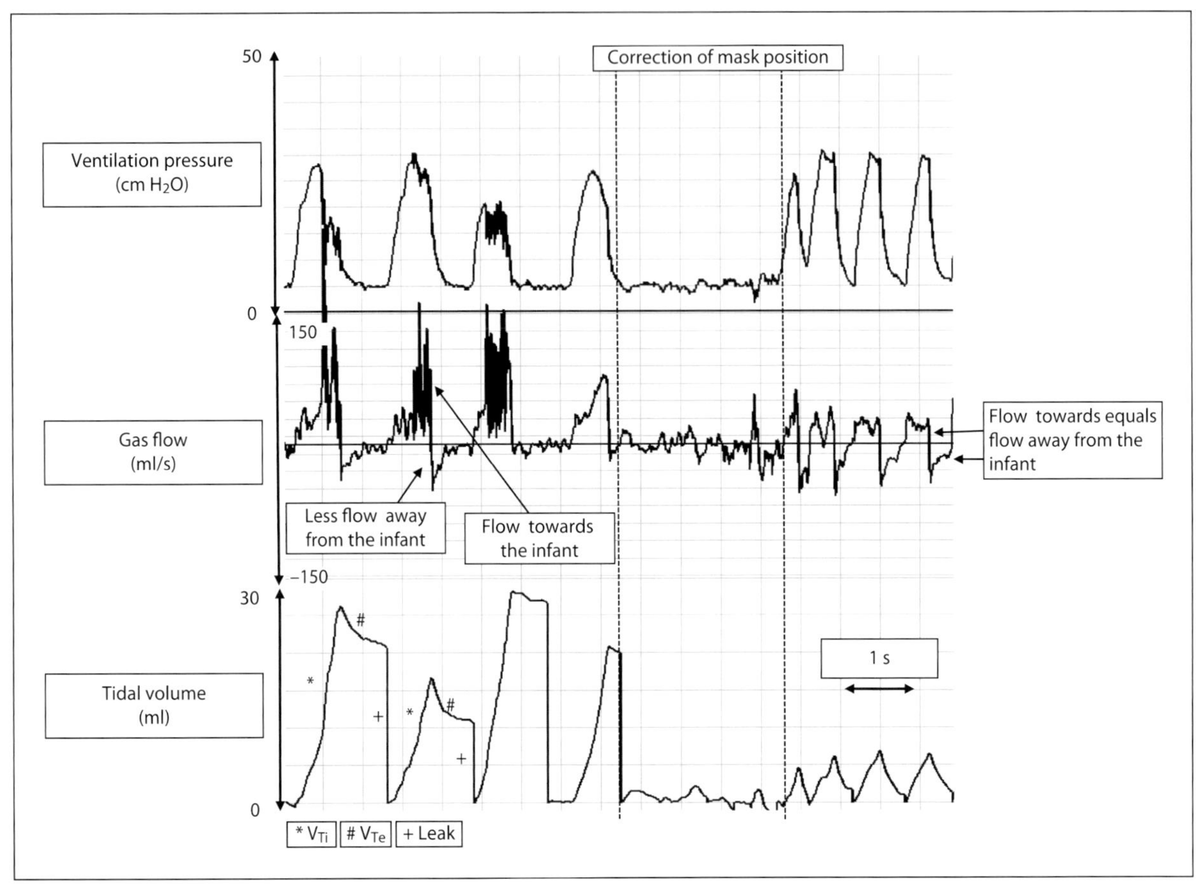

Fig. 3. Correction of facemask position. During PPV the airway pressure curve fails to achieve the set PIP of 30 cm H_2O. A returning inspiratory gas flow curve to baseline indicates gas flow towards the facemask. In contrast, there is much less expiratory gas flow indicating a leak around the facemask. The V_T curve reflects the gas flow curve and displays a leak of around 80%. There is almost no gas entering or leaving the lung. A significant reduction in the facemask leak is achieved after correction of facemask position. Adequate gas flow is entering and leaving the lung and the set PIP is delivered.

Paykel Healthcare, Auckland, New Zealand), a continuous-flow, pressure-limited, T-piece device with a built-in manometer and a PEEP valve.

Mask Hold and Positioning Techniques

During simulation-based mannequin training a RFM can be used to teach the best technique of positioning, holding and ventilating with a facemask (fig. 1). This can be easily demonstrated using a resuscitation mannequin that is internally leak-free and a flow sensor placed between the facemask and the ventilation device [3–5]. Any leak will be displayed as the difference between V_{Ti} and V_{Te} or the difference in area of the flow curve above and below zero (fig. 2) [3].

During PPV the trainee receives constant visual feedback because the RFM displays the amount of leak and the trainee can adjust the position of the facemask to minimise leak (fig. 3) [4].

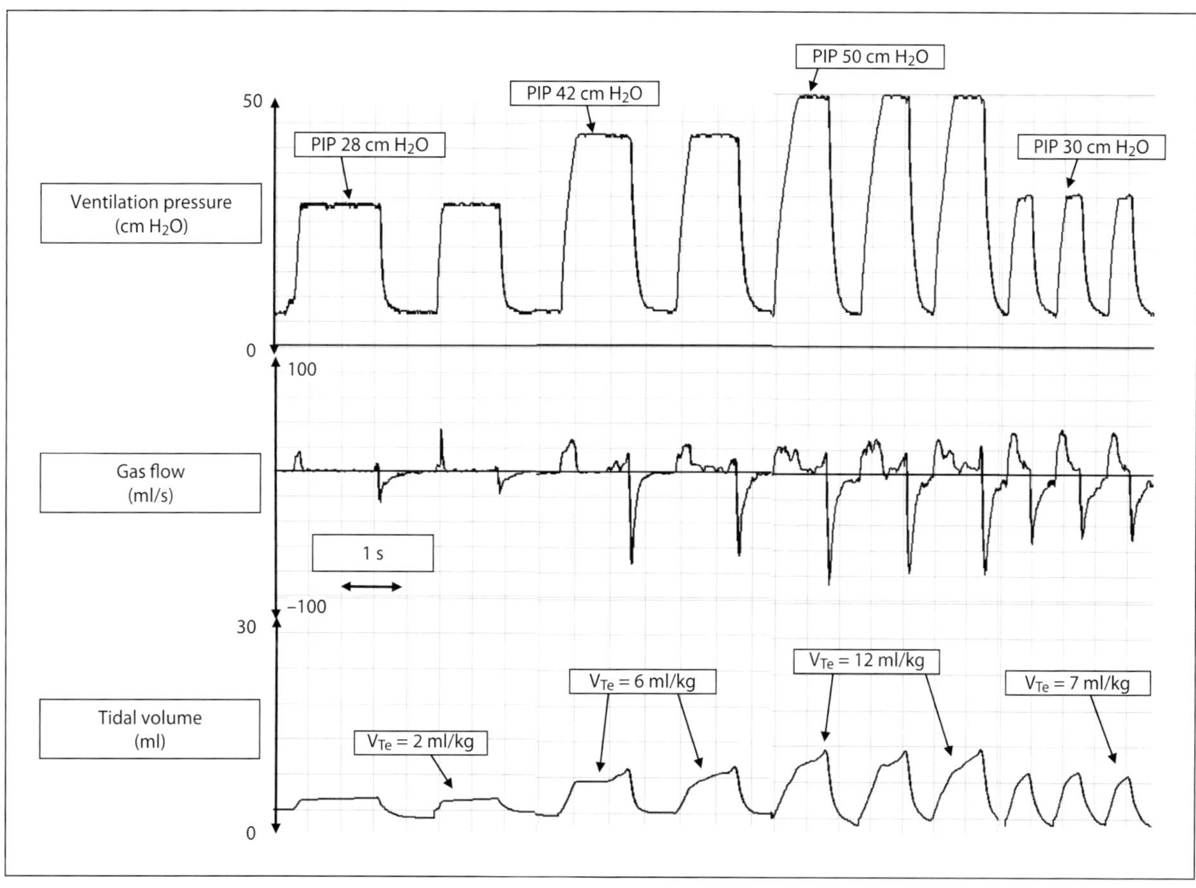

Fig. 4. Adjusting PIP to achieve appropriate V_Ts. Initially, the inflation and expiratory gas flow curves are small; the measured V_{Te} is approximately 2 ml/kg. An increase in V_{Te} to 6 ml/kg is achieved with an increase in PIP to 42 cm H_2O. The consequence of a further PIP increase to 50 cm H_2O is an increase in V_{Te} to 12 ml/kg, which is excessive. Decreasing the PIP to 30 cm H_2O resulting in a delivered V_{Te} of 7 ml/kg.

Assessment of PIP and PEEP

The purpose of applying any inflating pressure during PPV is to inflate the lungs with an appropriate V_T to create a functional residual capacity and thereby facilitate gas exchange. With a self- or flow-inflating bag the pressure delivered is unknown unless it is measured and displayed using a manometer [14–17]. The applied pressure is usually shown on a dial during PPV with a T-piece device. Although this is useful, as pressure rises and falls rapidly, it can be difficult to see the PIP and PEEP [17]. During simulation-based mannequin training with a RFM the trainee can easily assess the whole pressure wave and the numerical values of PIP and PEEP (fig. 1).

Adjusting PIP to Achieve Appropriate V_Ts

Once a trainee is able to obtain leak-free facemask ventilation, he then can concentrate on assessing the delivered V_T by adjusting the inflating pressure. With a self- or flow-inflating bag they will learn how hard they need to squeeze and with a T-piece device adjust the PIP they should set to deliver an appropriate V_T (fig. 4). Although mannequins are different from infants, the principles can be learned and then applied during real resuscitation [18].

Assessment of the Trainee's Performance

Assessment of a trainee's performance remains a substantial part of any neonatal resuscitation training courses. However, the assessment of adequate 'bag-and-mask' ventilation remains subjective. The 'instructor' judges mask position, ventilation rate, and chest rise to assess the adequacy of the trainees' performance of PPV. Recently, Schmölzer et al. [13] have shown that during neonatal resuscitation, operators were unable to judge their delivered V_{Te} or facemask leak by looking at chest rise. They showed that the majority of operators underestimated their delivered V_{Te} and facemask leak. A RFM can assist the 'instructor' to objectively assess the provider's performance during 'bag-and-mask' ventilation.

Conclusion

A RFM can aid during simulation-based mannequin training providing a quantitative assessment of the trainee's technique. A RFM can assist during 'bag-and-mask' ventilation: identifying correct mask hold and positioning techniques, assessment of PIP and PEEP, and adjusting the PIP to deliver an appropriate V_T provide objective assessment of a trainee's performance.

References

1 Singhal N, McMillan DD, Yee WH, et al: Evaluation of the effectiveness of the standardized neonatal resuscitation program. J Perinatol 2001;21:388–392.

2 2005 International Consensus on Cardiopulmonary Resuscitation and Emergency Cardiovascular Care Science with Treatment Recommendations. Part 7: Neonatal resuscitation. Resuscitation 2005;67:293–303.

3 O'Donnell CP, Kamlin CO, Davis PG, et al: Neonatal resuscitation 1: a model to measure inspired and expired tidal volumes and assess leakage at the face mask. Arch Dis Child Fetal Neonatal Ed 2005;90:F388–F391.

4 Wood FE, Morley CJ, Dawson JA, et al: A respiratory function monitor improves mask ventilation. Arch Dis Child Fetal Neonatal Ed 2008;93:F380–F381.

5 Wood FE, Morley CJ, Dawson JA, et al: Improved techniques reduce face mask leak during simulated neonatal resuscitation: study 2. Arch Dis Child Fetal Neonatal Ed 2008;93:F230–F234.

6 Wood FE, Morley CJ, Dawson JA, et al: Assessing the effectiveness of two round neonatal resuscitation masks: study 1. Arch Dis Child Fetal Neonatal Ed 2008;93:F235–F237.

7 Bjorklund LJ, Ingimarsson J, Curstedt T, et al: Manual ventilation with a few large breaths at birth compromises the therapeutic effect of subsequent surfactant replacement in immature lambs. Pediatr Res 1997;42:348–355.

8 Hillman NH, Moss TJ, Kallapur SG, et al: Brief, large tidal volume ventilation initiates lung injury and a systemic response in fetal sheep. Am J Respir Crit Care Med 2007;176:575–581.

9 Wada K, Jobe AH, Ikegami M. Tidal volume effects on surfactant treatment responses with the initiation of ventilation in preterm lambs. J Appl Physiol 1997;83:1054–1061.

10 Polglase GR, Hillman NH, Pillow JJ, et al: Positive end-expiratory pressure and tidal volume during initial ventilation of preterm lambs. Pediatr Res 2008;64:517–522.

11 Vilstrup CT, Bjorklund LJ, Werner O, et al: Lung volumes and pressure-volume relations of the respiratory system in small ventilated neonates with severe respiratory distress syndrome. Pediatr Res 1996;39:127–133.

12 Kattwinkel J, Stewart C, Walsh B, et al: Responding to compliance changes in a lung model during manual ventilation: perhaps volume, rather than pressure, should be displayed. Pediatrics 2009 vol, 123:e465–e470.

13 Schmölzer GM, Kamlin OC, O'Donnell CP, Dawson JA, Morley CJ, Davis PG: Assessment of tidal volume and gas leak during mask ventilation of preterm infants in the delivery room. Arch Dis Child Fetal Neonatal Ed 2010 (in press).

14 Oddie S, Wyllie J, Scally A: Use of self-inflating bags for neonatal resuscitation. Resuscitation 2005;67:109–112.

15 Bennett S, Finer NN, Rich W, et al: A comparison of three neonatal resuscitation devices. Resuscitation 2005;67:113–118.

16 Hussey SG, Ryan CA, Murphy BP: Comparison of three manual ventilation devices using an intubated mannequin. Arch Dis Child Fetal Neonatal Ed 2004;89:F490–F493.

17 O'Donnell CP, Davis PG, Lau R, et al: Neonatal resuscitation. 3. Manometer use in a model of face mask ventilation. Arch Dis Child Fetal Neonatal Ed 2005;90:F397–F400.

18 Schmölzer GM, Kamlin COF, Dawson JA, et al: Respiratory function monitoring of neonatal resuscitation. Arch Dis Child Fetal Neonatal Ed 2010;95:F295–F303.

Georg M. Schmölzer, MD
Department of Newborn Research, The Royal Women's Hospital
20 Flemington Road, Parkville, VIC 3052 (Australia)
Tel. +61 3 8345 3775, Fax +61 3 8345 3789
E-Mail georg.schmoelzer@me.com

Esquinas AM (ed): Applied Technologies in Pulmonary Medicine. Basel, Karger, 2011, pp 60–66

Technological Requirements for Inhalation of Biomolecule Aerosols

R. Siekmeier[a] · G. Scheuch[b]

[a]Federal Institute for Drugs and Medical Devices (BfArM), and [b]Activaero GmbH, Gemünden, Germany

Abbreviations

DPI Dry powder inhaler
MDI Metered dose inhaler

In the last decades, methods for recombinant synthesis of peptides and proteins were developed allowing the production of large amounts of these compounds for treatment of systemic diseases. Due to their biochemical properties (high molecular weight, hydrophilic properties, sensitivity against chemicals and proteolytic enzymes) they require parenteral administration resulting in negative effects on convenience and compliance of the patients in cases of chronic diseases (e.g. diabetes mellitus). Therefore, inhalant administration via the nose or mouth seems to be an alternate method. The best conditions for drug absorption are found in the lung periphery (i.e. the alveolar region) making it an important target for inhalant administration of drugs with a systemic mode of action: size of the alveolar surface about the half of a tennis court (132 m^2) depending on lung distension (much larger than that of the nose of about 180 cm^2), thin alveolar epithelium (thickness in most regions between 0.1 and 0.2 µm resulting in a total distance between epithelial surface and blood between 0.5 and 1.0 µm which is much less than in the bronchial tract where the deposited substances have to pass a distance of 30–40 µm and more between mucus surface and blood), low expression of proteases and peptidases when compared to the intestine, perfusion volume at rest of about 5 l/min and missing hepatic first pass effect (fig. 1, 2) [1–5].

General Problems of Inhalation Therapy

Problems in inhalation therapy can be caused by the pharmaceutical compound, the nebulizer used or the patient to be treated. Therefore, depending on the underlying cause, various approaches exist for optimization of the therapy. If the pharmaceutical compound is subject of rapid inactivation within the nebulization process (e.g. by aggregation and oxidation) or after pulmonary deposition (e.g. by proteolytic cleavage) or it is too large to penetrate the alveolar membrane, these problems can be solved for example by addition of stabilizers, proteinase inhibitors as well as absorption enhancers [5–7]. Nebulizer-related problems, e.g. low aerosol output, inadequate aerosol distribution width or high variability of the aerosol particle spectrum,

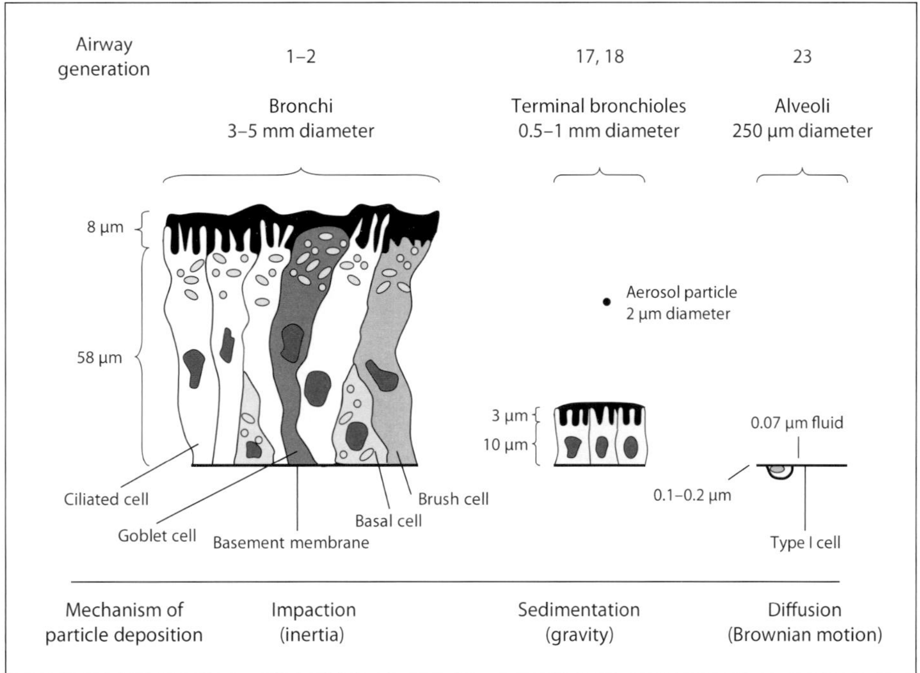

Fig. 1. Lung epithelium and mechanisms of particle deposition at different sites within the lungs [3]. Lung epithelial cells of the different lung regions are drawn at their relative sizes. The higher the number of the airway generation the deeper the particle is inspired into the lung (0: trachea, 1–2: bronchi, 3–5: bronchioles, 17–18: terminal bronchioles, 19–20: respiratory bronchioles, 21–22: alveolar ducts, 23: alveolar sacs). Mechanisms of particle depositions depending on the aerodynamic particle diameters (d_{ae}) are impaction (inertia), sedimentation (gravity) and diffusion (Brownian motion) in bronchi, terminal bronchioles and alveoli, respectively. A typical aerosol particle (d_{ae}: 2 µm) contains tens to hundreds of millions of insulin molecules or hundreds of millions/billions small molecules depending on its physical character (liquid or solid). Solid aerosol particles are too large to be absorbed in total and must dissolve to release their drugs for absorption. The deeper an aerosol particle penetrates into the lung the thinner becomes the airway epithelium and the larger becomes the lung surface. In consequence, the function of the epithelial absorption barrier decreases and the absorption increases as a function of the particle penetration depth into the lung. Typical cells in the bronchi are basal cells which serve as the stem or progenitor cells for the other epithelial cells in case of injury or apoptosis, ciliated cells which provide the mechanism for moving the mucus blanket, goblet cells which secrete the mucus and brush cells which are involved in drug metabolism. The same cells and the mucus layer are also found in the smaller airways but not as tall. The thinnest absorption barrier is found in lung alveoli. The basement membrane is not a membrane but an extracellular matrix of different biopolymers to which epithelial cells attach.

can be solved by use of another type of nebulizer, e.g. ultrasonic nebulizer or DPI. Finally, patient-related problems (e.g. lung function, pulmonary morphometry, breathing technique and compliance) can be improved by use of another nebulizer and optimization of the breathing maneuver [2, 8–10]. However, different problems may occur together and in consequence the optimal solution has to consider all underlying aspects (table 1).

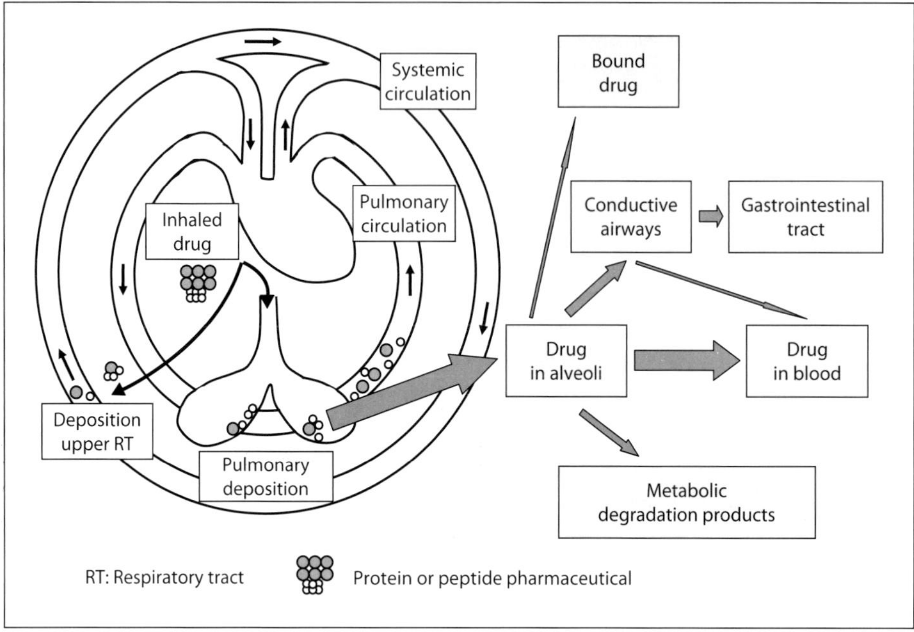

Fig. 2. Uptake of inhaled drugs after peripheral/alveolar deposition [1]. Most of the drug deposited in the alveoli is absorbed into the blood. Minor proportions are the subject of local degradation and transport into the conductive airways. From the latter the most is swallowed and degraded in the gastrointestinal tract and only a minor proportion is absorbed into the blood.

Physical Methods for Aerosol Administration

Inhalant drug administration requires high efficiency of drug delivery, reproducible dosing, targeted delivery of the inhaled drug to the site of action, ease of device operation, short duration of treatment, minimized risk to the patient and the medical personnel, environmental protection and cost-effectiveness [11]. A number of products have been developed for this purpose. However, there are strong differences regarding their suitability for nebulization and administration of the various compounds. In the past, often low rates of pulmonary drug absorption were achieved because the nebulizers used were not qualified for production of an adequate aerosol particle spectrum and the breathing patterns of the patients were not taken into account [4, 7, 10].

Dry Powder Inhalers

In DPIs, aerosols are produced by disaggregation of preformed (e.g. milled or spray-dried) micronized particles. The energy required for disaggregation is supplied by the inhalation maneuver or alternatively by means of an external energy source [2, 12]. The advantages of DPIs are the environmental sustainability (due to a propellant-free design) and the ease to use (not much patient coordination is needed). However, the disadvantages are the dependency of the deposition efficiency on the patient's inspiratory airflow, the potential for dose uniformity problems and the relative high complexity and costs for development and manufacture. DPIs are established for treatment of asthma and chronic obstructive pulmonary disease by means of β-mimetics, anticholinergics or steroids, but up to now there is only little experience on

Table 1. Problems in aerosol therapy and their solution [2, 4, 5, 8–10]

Source of the problem	Type of the problem	Solution of the problem
Compound	Formulation: Chemical/physical stability Aerodynamic diameter Adhesion force Electrical charge Biology: Permeability Metabolism Safety Immunogenicity	Optimization of manufacturing: Refinement of production processes Addition of stabilizing excipients Improvement of galenics: Addition of absorption enhancers and proteinase inhibitors and packing into particles
Device	Low aerosol output Aerosol distribution width Variability of aerosol particle spectrum Long treatment times for drug solutions	Vibrating mesh nebulizers Dry powder inhalers (DPIs) Metered dose inhalers (MDIs) Vibrating mesh nebulizers
Patient	Lung function Lung morphology Pulmonary diseases Breathing maneuver Compliance	Optimization of nebulizers (including their handling) Standardization of the breathing maneuver

inhalant administration of biomolecules except insulin (Exubera®) for systemic treatment [1, 12, 13]. This is caused by specific problems for the use of proteins or peptides occurring in the processes of lyophilization or spray drying, micronization, completeness of dispersion and disaggregation as well as the surveillance of the latter.

In passive systems the inspiratory air flow of the patient is an essential parameter. If it is not sufficient for complete disaggregation, large aggregates are inhaled which cannot reach the alveolar region. On the other hand, a high air flow rate increases oropharyngeal deposition which is also followed by a reduction of pulmonary aerosol deposition. Furthermore, humidity can be a large problem because it impairs protein stability and also affects disaggregation and dispersion [2, 12]. However, if the underlying problems especially in particle engineering are solved by novel techniques, fast dissolving dry powders might be considered as carriers for nanoparticles [14].

Metered Dose Inhalers

In MDIs, compounds are dissolved or suspended in a pressurized propellant (nowadays typically hydrofluoroalkanes) which has to be nontoxic, noninflammable, compatible with drugs formulated as suspensions or solutions and has appropriate boiling points and densities. Consistent dosing requires a constant vapor pressure throughout the product's life. After its release with high velocity the mixture rapidly expands forming an aerosol. Therefore, MDIs often require spacers for optimization of aerosol deposition [2, 15]. Aerosols from MDIs are well established in clinical treatment of patients with asthma or chronic obstructive pulmonary disease (e.g. by β-mimetics, parasympatholytics and steroids) for about 50 years [2, 15]. Unfortunately, MDIs cannot be used for treatment with macromolecules (e.g. peptides and proteins) because a number of prerequisites (stability of the drug within storage in the inhaler, no denaturation of the drug within the nebulization process, production of an aerosol with appropriate particle distribution pattern) are not sufficiently fulfilled.

Nebulizers

The appropriateness of nebulizers for administration of macromolecular compounds depends on their performance (e.g. aerosol output, distribution width and variability of the aerosol particle spectrum) as well as the stability of the compounds used for nebulization. In air-jet nebulizer's protein structure and function can be compromised independently from the molecular weight of the protein by surface denaturation, shear-stress-induced denaturation as well as desiccation of the aerosol droplets within the nebulization process [2]. However, additives like lipids, surfactant, amino acids, albumin, polyols as well as packing into liposomes may enhance protein stability [2, 16].

Ultrasonic nebulizers act by a disruption of liquid surfaces by means of ultrasound and allow a production of high concentration aerosols [16]. Usually, aerosol particles are produced with such nebulizers which are not appropriate for deep lung delivery.

In vibrating mesh nebulizers, a liquid aerosol with a high fine-particle fraction is produced by means of a vibrating mesh or plate with multiple apertures. Aerosols are generated as a fine mist without requirement of an internal baffling system [11, 16]. In comparison to conventional jet nebulizers and ultrasonic nebulizers, they have a number of advantages which are a higher efficiency for drug delivery to the respiratory tract, an effective aerosolization of solutions, a minimal residual volume of medication left in the device (cost economic effect) and a breath-actuated aerosol delivery which limits the release of aerosolized drug into the environment [11]. However, it is difficult to aerosolize suspensions (exception: nano-suspensions) and they sometimes fail when liposomal formulations should be aerosolized.

Novel Devices for Enhanced Pulmonary Drug Delivery

Numerous devices are based on the bolus inhalation technique [9, 10]. For example, MDIs and DPIs are supposed to deliver the aerosol cloud at the beginning of a breath which leads to a more efficient lung deposition than an aerosol inhalation over the entire inspiration because the clean air that follows the aerosol cloud transports the particles deeply into the lungs and extends their pulmonary residence time [9, 10]. The AERx® Pulmonary Drug Delivery System of Aradigm (USA) uses a bolus of aerosol particles produced by a piston that empties a small liquid reservoir into the inhalation air. The release of the bolus can be activated during a certain time point during an inspiration. Other devices, like the AKITA® Inhalation System (Activaero, Germany) and the I-neb® AAD® System (Philips Respironics, The Netherlands) use liquid nebulizer systems operating only at a certain time during an inhalation cycle and therefore also use the bolus inhalation technique to increase pulmonary particle deposition [10]. Currently, the AKITA® technology is the most advanced technology as it is the only one that actively controls the entire inhalation maneuver of the patient. This is done by means of a positive air pressure delivered by a computer-controlled compressor which is programmed on the basis of the patient's individual lung function data. By Activaero's SmartCard technology the lung function data can be submitted quickly after a prior lung function test to the AKITA® device. However, the design has been further improved in

Table 2. Advantages of individualized controlled inhalation for research and routine therapy

Advantages of individualized controlled inhalation	Benefit for clinical trials	Benefit for outpatient treatment
Reduction of side effects	Lower number of dropouts	Higher quality of life and compliance
Lower lung drug dose variability	Reduction in the number of patients to be included	Increase of efficiency
Better drug targeting	Increase of efficiency	
Electronic compliance control	Reduction in the number of patients to be included	Extended feedback for physicians
Higher drug exploitation	Lower drug costs	

the AKITA-2®, the next generation of this technology. The AKITA-2® operates with ultrasonic and ultrasonic mesh nebulizers. This new nebulizer is able to nebulize up to 99% of the filled dose into particles with mass median aerodynamic diameter <4 μm – measured for 0.9% NaCl solution.

Advantages of Individualized Controlled Inhalation

The optimization of the breathing maneuver by individualized controlled inhalation has a number of advantages. These include clinical trials with pulmonary drug administration as well as clinical routine of hospital and outpatient treatment. In brief, in clinical studies, improved pulmonary dosage, better drug targeting and reduced side effects may result in lower required drug doses, lower number of dropouts and a lower number of patients to be included which is followed by a relevant reduction of costs. Corresponding benefits for outpatient treatment also include an improved efficiency, lower costs and, important for many patients, a better quality of life (due to lower rate of side effects and shorter inhalation times) (table 2). A number of studies have demonstrated the improved pulmonary drug deposition as well as the good convenience and compliance of the treated patients using the Akita® inhalation device [17].

Conclusions

The improved understanding of aerosol physics and mechanisms of pulmonary aerosol deposition have been followed by development of modern devices for inhalant drug delivery. Both modern devices and optimized breathing patterns are prerequisites for optimal pulmonary drug delivery. The most recent step for optimization of pulmonary drug deposition is the consideration of the individual lung function which is a critical factor in inhalation therapy. Likely, future aerosol therapy in contrast to the past will not be based on a standard therapy with fixed application volumes and times in a large number of patients but on patient's individual anthropometric data and lung function. This will be followed by a further extension of clinical indications for aerosol therapy, e.g. inhalation of pharmaceuticals and biomolecules for treatment of local (e.g. tobramycin in cystic fibrosis patients) and systemic (e.g. insulin in diabetes mellitus and heparin for anticoagulation) diseases.

References

1 Agu RU, Ugwoke MI, Armand M, Kinget R, Verbeke N: The lung as a route for systemic delivery of therapeutic proteins and peptides. Respir Res 2001;2:198–209.
2 Niven RW: Delivery of biotherapeutics by inhalation aerosol. Crit Rev Ther Drug Carrier Syst 1995;12:151–231.
3 Patton JS, Byron PR: Inhaling medicines: delivering drugs to the body through the lungs. Nat Rev Drug Discov 2007;6:67–74.
4 Wolff RK: Safety of inhaled proteins for therapeutic use. J Aerosol Med 1998;11: 197–219.
5 Siekmeier R, Scheuch G: Systemic treatment by inhalation of macromolecules – principles, problems and examples. J Physiol Pharmacol 2008;59(suppl 6):53–79.
6 Hussain A, Arnold JJ, Khan MA, Ahsan F: Absorption enhancers in pulmonary protein delivery. J Control Release 2004; 94:15–24.
7 Yu J, Chien YW: Pulmonary drug delivery: physiologic and mechanistic aspects. Crit Rev Ther Drug Carrier Syst 1997;14:395–453.
8 Byron PR, Patton JS: Drug delivery via the respiratory tract. J Aerosol Med 1994;7:49–75.
9 Scheuch G, Kohlhaeufl MJ, Brand P, Siekmeier R: Clinical perspectives on pulmonary systemic and macromolecular delivery. Adv Drug Deliv Rev 2006; 58:996–1008.
10 Scheuch G, Siekmeier R: Novel approaches to enhance pulmonary delivery of proteins and peptides. J Physiol Pharmacol 2007;58(suppl 5):615–625.
11 Dhand R: New frontiers in aerosol delivery during mechanical ventilation. Respir Care 2004;49:666–677.
12 Telko MJ, Hickey AJ: Dry powder inhaler formulation. Respir Care 2005;50:1209–1227.
13 Siekmeier R, Scheuch G: Inhaled insulin – Does it become reality? J Physiol Pharmacol 2008;59(suppl 6):81–113.
14 Shoyele SA, Cawthorne S: Particle engineering techniques for inhaled biopharmaceuticals. Adv Drug Deliv Rev 2006; 58:1009–1029.
15 Newman SP: Principles of metered-dose inhaler design. Respir Care 2005;50: 1177–1190.
16 Köhler D, Fleischer W (eds): Theorie und Praxis der Inhalationstherapie. München, Arcis Verlag, 2000.
17 Fischer A, Stegemann J, Scheuch G, Siekmeier R: Novel devices for individualized controlled inhalation can optimize aerosol therapy in efficacy, patient care and power of clinical trials. Eur J Med Res 2009;14(suppl IV):71–77.

PD Dr. med. habil. Rüdiger Siekmeier
Federal Institute for Drugs and Medical Devices (BfArM)
Kurt-Georg-Kiesinger-Allee 3, DE–53175 Bonn (Germany)
Tel. +49 228 207 5360, Fax +49 228 207 5300
E-Mail r.siekmeier@bfarm.de

Esquinas AM (ed): Applied Technologies in Pulmonary Medicine. Basel, Karger, 2011, pp 67–76

Problems and Examples of Biomolecule Inhalation for Systemic Treatment

R. Siekmeier[a] · G. Scheuch[b]

[a]Federal Institute for Drugs and Medical Devices (BfArM), and [b]Activaero GmbH, Gemünden, Germany

Abbreviations

BAL	Bronchoalveolar lavage
G-CSF	Granulocyte colony-stimulating factor
GM-CSF	Granulocyte-monocyte colony-stimulating factor
IL-2	Interleukin-2
LMWH	Low molecular weight heparin
MW	Molecular weight

In recent decades a number of biomolecules, mostly peptides and proteins, have come into the focus of interest for inhalant administration as an alternative of parenteral delivery. Novel inhalation devices and optimization of the breathing technique enabled researchers to develop methods for the non-invasive administration of these compounds, especially for treatment of chronic systemic disorders (e.g. diabetes mellitus, anticoagulation). However, beside aspects of aerosol delivery and inhalation, a number of special biochemical and biological aspects must be considered. These include the physical and biochemical stability of the biomolecules within the nebulization process as well as after pulmonary deposition, and the alveolar absorption of the compound.

Stability of Biomolecules

Independent from the type and the MW of the biomolecule, aerosolization may result in denaturation and loss of functionality, for instance by oxidation. For example, aerosolization by means of an air-jet nebulizer may cause an inactivation of recombinant human G-CSF (MW: 18.8 kDa), interferon-α (MW: 19 kDa) and growth hormone (MW: 22 kDa), whereas α_1-antitrypsin (MW: 51 kDa), desoxyribonuclease (MW: 30 kDa) and heparin (MW: 3–20 kDa) are more stable [1, 2]. For enhancement of stability within the nebulization process, various additives may be added or a dry powder aerosol may be used instead of a liquid aerosol [1, 2].

Physiological Inhibitors of Absorption

The lung has been exposed to microorganisms and foreign substances from the environment for millions of years within the evolution process. In consequence, a complex defense system has been developed protecting the respiratory tract from the nostrils down until the alveoli. In upper airways and bronchi, defense mechanisms consist of anatomic barriers, cough, mucociliary apparatus, airway epithelium, secretory immunoglobulin A, dendritic cell network and lymphoid structure [3]. About 90% of inhaled particles with diameters >2–3 μm are deposited in the central airways on the mucus overlying the cilial epithelium from where they are rapidly transported to the trachea by means of the mucociliary escalator and then swallowed into the gastrointestinal tract [3–5]. The absorption of biomolecules deposited there is further reduced by the thickness of mucus layer and respiratory epithelium as well as local peroxidases.

Much better conditions for absorption are found in the lung periphery, i.e. the alveoli [1, 2, 6–8]. However, even there a number of defense mechanisms exist (fig. 1). The first barriers after contact are the mucus layer (a complex mixture of lipids and glycoproteins, but also surfactant from the lower respiratory tract) and the alveolar lining fluid (includes a large amount of surfactant with phospholipids and surfactant apolipoproteins acting as a surface-active substance). Amount, composition and thickness of the mucus layer depend on its localization in the respiratory tract, inflammatory and neuronal factors whereas synthesis and release of surfactant from type II pneumocytes are modulated by hyperventilation, endogenous and exogenous factors (pharmaceuticals) [1, 2]. Cells located in the respiratory tract (mostly macrophages representing about 85% of cells retrieved by BAL in healthy individuals) also counteract the absorption of deposited substances. They serve as an unspecific defense mechanism (e.g. against bacteria and inhaled particles) and act via phagocytosis, secretion of reactive oxygen species by means of respiratory burst and release of mediators of inflammation. However, even granulocytes (about 1–2% in normal BAL) may invade rapidly and serve as potent inhibitors of absorption, e.g. by phagocytosis, respiratory burst and secretion of proteases. Last but not least, lymphocytes (10–20% in normal BAL, mostly CD4+ lymphocytes) play a crucial role in the immunological response after antigen presentation by macrophages and dendritic cells. However, lymphocytes can also phagocytose and include granules containing proteases and proteolytic enzymes [1–3]. Type I pneumocytes which cover about 97% of the alveolar surface (the remaining area consists of type II pneumocytes) express carboxypeptidase which degrades a number of peptides and proteins. However, the total distance between the respiratory tract and circulation is only 0.5 μm facilitating the diffusion of gasses as well as penetration and transport of fluids and (inhaled) macromolecules. The latter can pass alveolar epithelium via different transport mechanisms, which are intracellular tight junctions, membrane pores and vesicular transport by type I and type II pneumocytes (fig. 1) [1, 2].

Another transport mechanism serving for the exchange of fluids and macromolecules are membrane pores. It is assumed that pores of different sizes exist, which can increase their diameter in case of an existing hydrostatic pressure gradient [1, 2].

In pneumocytes types I and II another mechanism of vesicular transport has been described, which is comparable to that in epithelial and endothelial cells. In detail, the vesicular transport mechanism of type I pneumocytes is pressure-independent and allows the transcellular transport of fluids and macromolecules. However, an estimation of the functional capacity of this transport mechanism is difficult, because (1) the number of vesicles increases in liquid-filled lung indicating their role in the transport of fluids, (2) the glycocalix affects the uptake of proteins via specific or unspecific binding mechanisms and a number of receptors and binding proteins were identified on capillary endothelia, (3) the definite processing of the vesicles inside the cells and the mechanisms for their movement (e.g. Brownian movement) are not conclusively identified, (4) the energetic mechanisms of membrane displacement and fusion of the vesicles are not yet conclusively

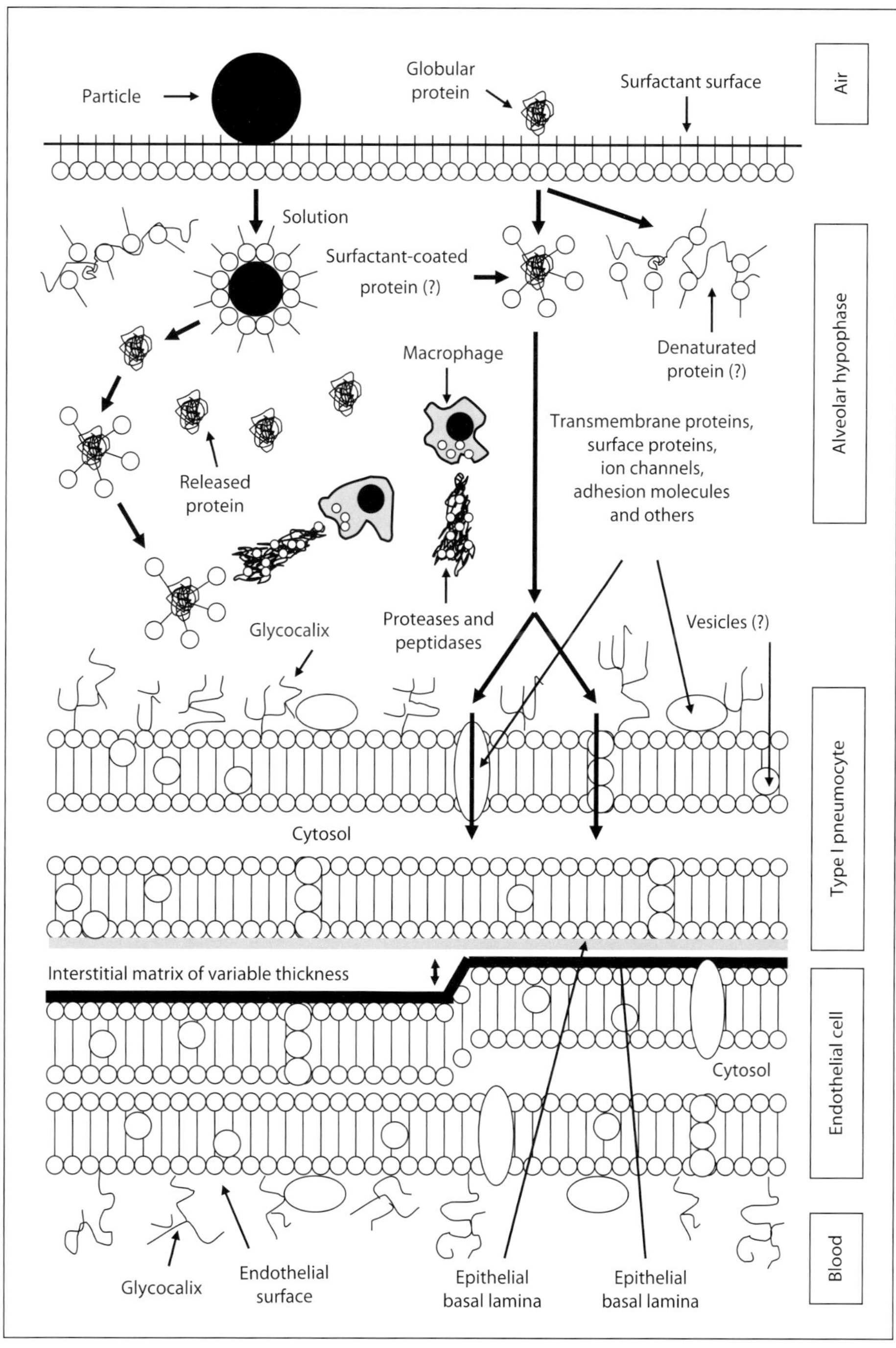

Fig. 1. Barriers for absorption of peptides and proteins after peripheral/alveolar deposition [1, 2].

elucidated, and (5) different types of vesicles (e.g. clathrin-coated and clathrin-uncoated) exist, which both play a role in transcytosis, but differ in respect to their characteristics of protein uptake [1, 2].

Surfactant produced from pneumocytes type II together with proteins plays an important role for the clearance of macromolecules by means of the alveolar lining fluid. Further cellular processing can take place with or without binding of the macromolecules on the cellular surface and depends strongly on the charge of the molecules. A large proportion of the material absorbed by endocytosis from type II pneumocytes is deposited in lamellar bodies. In addition, transcellular transport represents another mechanism for absorption of macromolecules [1, 2].

The basal lamina (thickness of about 20–25 nm) placed below the epithelium predominantly consists of glycoproteins (e.g. laminin and fibronectin) and has an anionic charge on its outer surface. Presumably, the latter regulates the permeation dependent on size and charge of the molecules. After their passage through the alveolar wall and alveolar basal lamina, inhaled substances reach the interstitium, where proteins can be bound by macromolecules or inactivated or phagocytosed by macrophages or transported to the lymphatic system. In the latter case, proteins can be detected after some hours in the circulation. Endothelial basal lamina and endothelium are also barriers for the absorption of macromolecules. However, compared to the other barriers described before they are less effective in inhibiting the absorption of biomolecules (fig. 1) [1, 2].

Factors Affecting the Absorption of Macromolecules

After alveolar deposition, proteins with a low MW are absorbed more rapidly than those with a high MW. The bioavailability of proteins with a MW up to 30 kDa (which includes the vast majority of proteins used in clinical therapy) is between 20 and 50%. However, because of proteolytic degradation the bioavailability of some proteins is much smaller [1, 2, 7–10]. Other variables affecting the absorption are pH value, electrical charge, surface activity, solubility and stability in the alveolar environment [1, 2, 7, 9]. In hydrophilic compounds (e.g. carbohydrates, peptides and proteins) the half-life time of alveolar absorption ($t_{0.5}$) as well as the time to reach the maximum serum concentration (t_{max}) increase as a function of their MW [2, 9, 10].

Improvement of Macromolecule Absorption

Biomolecules deposited in the alveoli can be absorbed by four distinct mechanisms: phagocytosis by alveolar macrophages, paracellular diffusion via tight junctions, vesicular endocytosis or pinocytosis, and receptor-dependent transcytosis [1, 2, 8]. Accordingly, the functional role of barriers and transport mechanisms and their control by physiological and pharmacological factors is very different and in consequence a large number of very different compounds and techniques for absorption enhancement were investigated [1, 2, 8, 11], some of which are described below in more detail.

Even though the activity of proteases and peptidases in the alveolar region is much lower than in the gastrointestinal tract, proteolytic degradation of susceptible proteins can cause a relevant reduction of the bioavailability [9]. Therefore, bioavailability can be increased by addition of protease inhibitors (e.g. nafamostat mesilate, aprotinin and *p*-amidinophenylmethanesulfonyl fluoride•HCl). However, the effects of the various protease inhibitors are very specific to the type of the protease or peptidase [2, 6, 10, 11].

The heterogenous group of surface-active compounds (e.g. bile acids, fatty acids, non-ionic detergents) is assumed to increase the alveolocapillary transport by an interaction with the cell membrane resulting in a liquefaction followed by an increased permeability and/or a modulation of cellular tight junctions followed by an increased paracellular permeability. Presumably, bile acids increase the absorption by alteration of the mucus layer, protection of proteins against enzymatic degradation, disaggregation of protein multimers, opening of epithelial tight junctions as well as solubilization of phospholipids and proteins out of the cell membrane followed by formation of micelles. However, a strong absorption-enhancing effect can result in damage to the epithelial surfaces, especially after treatment with higher doses and longer treatment times [2, 10, 11].

Cyclodextrins are cyclic polymers of glucose, which can form complexes with molecules fitting into their lipophilic inner structure. The underlying modes for absorption enhancement are solubilization and complexation of membrane lipids and proteins of epithelial cells, inhibition of proteolytic enzymes and modification of the physicochemical properties (e.g. solubility and partition coefficient) of the administered substances. However, the toxicity increases with the intensity of absorption enhancement, both depending on the structure of the compound [2, 6, 11].

Based on the observation that smaller particles are more rapidly phagocytosed than larger ones, methods were developed to bind macromolecules to microparticles [6, 9]. For this purpose, proteins are packed into the inner of biologically degradable polymers or lipids. This results in a reduction of physiological clearance in the alveolar region and proteolytic degradation of proteins after phagocytosis by alveolar macrophages. In addition, a sustained release of the compounds from the microparticles is achieved [9, 10]. Microparticles for drug administration can be classified into porous particles and liposomes [2, 6, 9–11]. Pharmacological properties of porous particles depend on the used material, particle size, porosity and surface structure, whereas those of liposomes depend on particle size and chemical properties (charge, MW) of the consisting phospholipids [2, 6, 11].

Liposomes are particles (size range from some nanometers up to a few micrometers) consisting of hydrophobic lipids and phospholipids forming a closed, concentric, bilayer-membrane vesicle with a hydrophilic aqueous center [2, 11, 12]. According to this structure, both hydrophobic and hydrophilic compounds can be packed into liposomes prior to transportation into the lung. Hydrophilic compounds (e.g. pharmaceuticals and larger biomolecules) are entrapped into the vesicle in the inner of the liposome, whereas lipophilic (hydrophobic) compounds are encapsulated into the membrane bilayer. Because of their strong chemical and structural similarity, liposomes merge with cell membranes and facilitate drug delivery into the interior of the cell (fig. 2). However, especially small liposomes are also absorbed via cellular phagocytosis [12]. Depending on their structure, liposomes have a high transport capacity and allow the transport of a large number of very different compounds. One more characteristic is the sustained release of the compounds transported by liposomes [2, 10–12]. Even though the majority of studies revealed no toxic effect of liposomes, it must be considered that both effects, absorption enhancement and lung toxicity, depend on their physicochemical properties (concentration, charge, chain length and MW of phospholipids) [2, 6, 11, 12].

Another approach is the modification of proteins by fusion to the Fc domain of an IgG_1 (IgG subtype 1) [2, 13, 14]. In contrast to rodents where the expression of the Fc receptor in the gut rapidly decreases after weaning and remains low in tissues of adult animals, the Fc receptor in humans keeps expressed in several absorptive tissues (e.g. lung, kidney, intestine) even in adulthood. IgG Fc fusion proteins are taken up into epithelial cells by pinocytosis. In detail, a coated vesicle is formed by invagination of the plasma membrane entrapping IgG and other solutes in its lumen. Obviously, only a small proportion of IgG binds

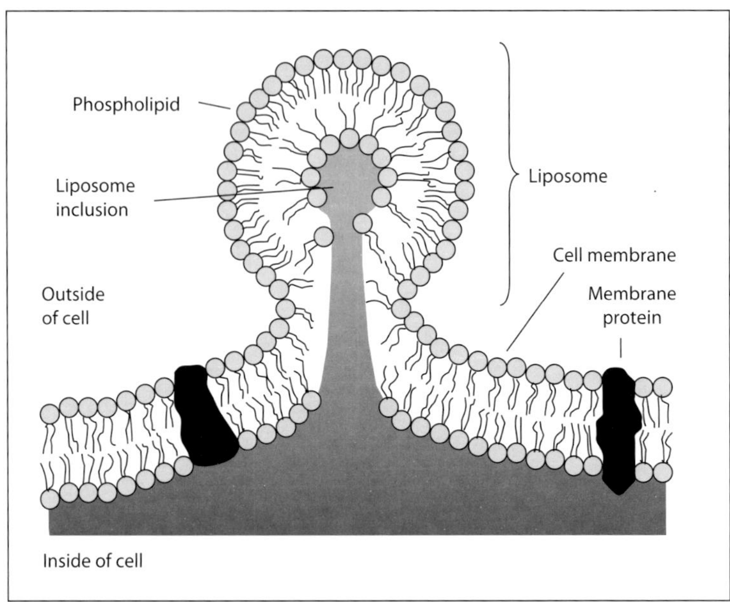

Fig. 2. Acceptance of a liposome into a cell. Liposomes consist of lipids and phospholipids [2, 12]. Each phospholipid has a polar hydrophilic 'head group' and two hydrophilic 'tails'. When phospholipid molecules are hydrated under low-shear conditions they spontaneously arrange themselves in sheets with their heads up and tails down. These sheets then join tails-to-tails and form a bilayer membrane that encloses water and – if added – water-soluble compounds (e.g. pharmaceuticals and larger biomolecules) in the center of the sphere. If liposomes come into contact with cell membranes consisting of phospholipids, lipids and proteins, the liposome membrane fuses with the cell membrane facilitating the entry of the encapsulated drug into the interior of the cell.

to FcRn at the plasma membrane, whereas most of the binding takes place intracellularly, because the majority of FcRn is localized in acidic endosomal vesicles inside the cell. The transport vesicles containing IgG bound to FcRn do not fuse with degradative lysosomes but rather pass unidirectionally through the epithelial cell, driven by the pH gradient between luminal and serosal exposures of the epithelial cells. As the binding of IgG to FcRn is pH-dependent (tight binding at slightly acidic pH), there is a release of IgG from FcRn after fusion of the transport vesicles with the plasma membrane at the basolateral site of the epithelial cells because of the neutral to slightly alkaline pH value of the interstitial space. Passage of IgG into the circulation is most likely primarily paracellular because of the absence of tight junctions between endothelial cells. The FcRn receptor is also responsible for the long half-life time of IgG in the bloodstream, because it protects IgG from degradation. As in epithelial cells, IgG is taken up from vascular endothelial cells by pinocytosis. However, in contrast to epithelial cells, IgG there is not subject of transcytosis, because the endocytic vesicles containing IgG bound to FcRn return to the plasma membrane of the endothelial cells, so that IgG is released back into the bloodstream resulting in a recycling process for IgG protecting IgG from lysosomal degradation. Fc fusion proteins can be efficiently administered as liquid aerosols and several studies have demonstrated a good tolerability, a high bioavailability even of larger proteins (e.g. erythropoietin) and an increased half-life time in the circulation in animals or humans [2, 13, 14].

Systemic Treatment with Inhaled Macromolecules

A number of studies investigated the feasibility of macromolecule inhalation for systemic treatment. A focus was set on hormones (insulin, calcitonin, growth hormones, somatostatin, thyroid-stimulating hormone, and follicle-stimulating hormone), growth factors (G-CSF and GM-CSF), different interleukins (e.g. IL-2) and heparin (unfractionated and LMWH) [6, 15–18]. However, in humans, most data are available for insulin, heparin and IL-2. In the following, some examples, except insulin which is described elsewhere in this book, are compiled.

Heparin, an acidic sulfated mucopolysaccharide, is characterized by a MW of unfractionated heparin between 2.8 and 58 kDa (mean value: 15 kDa) and between 2 and 6 kDa in case of fractionated LMWH. Both require parenteral administration and serve as an anticoagulant due to their binding to antithrombin III resulting in a conformation change of this protein. Beside this, a lot of other properties of heparin (e.g. interaction with growth factors, regulation of cell proliferation and angiogenesis, modulation of proteases and antiproteases) are of interest in medical research. Since 1965, a number of studies had investigated safety and feasibility of the inhalation of heparin and LMWH for anticoagulation. It was found that inhalant administration was effective, well tolerated and not followed by relevant pulmonary or systemic side effects [16, 19]. However, some studies showed a strong variability of the anticoagulative effect, e.g. due to an inadequate diameter of the produced aerosol particles in older nebulizers and a not sufficiently standardized inhalation maneuver. A more recent study investigated the anticoagulative effect (determined by measurement of the anti-FXa activity) of different doses of inhaled certoparin in healthy humans in comparison to subcutaneous administration. The study revealed a rapid onset of the anticoagulative effect after certoparin inhalation, a decrease of the interindividual variabilities after administration of higher doses (up to 9,000 IU) when compared to lower doses, a satisfactory anticoagulative effect after inhalation of 9,000 IU and a longer duration after inhalation of 9,000 IU when compared to subcutaneous administration of 3,000 IU which was achieved without side effects [16].

Erythropoietin, an erythrogenic growth factor (epoetin α: MW: 14.7 kDa; epoetin β, γ, δ, ε, ω: MW: 18.2 kDa) is used for stimulation of erythropoiesis in the bone marrow, e.g. in patients with end-stage renal failure and cancer. Due to its large MW the pulmonary absorption without methods for absorption enhancement is low [2, 14]. An interesting method based on Fc fusion proteins has been developed to improve pulmonary uptake and pharmacokinetics of erythropoietin (and also other proteins) [2, 13, 14]. In brief, in cynomolgus monkeys a better absorption of Epo-Fc dimers was observed after a shallow breathing pattern than after a deep inhalation due to the higher expression of Fc receptors in the central airways. After inhalation of the Epo-Fc dimer, the Epo-Fc monomer and unconjugated erythropoietin bioavailabilities of 5%, 35% (which is similar to that after subcutaneous administration) and 15% were observed, respectively. The low bioavailability of the Epo-Fc dimer was assumed to be caused by its higher MW or steric hindrance of IgG and erythropoietin. Independent from the mode of administration (inhalation, intravenous administration) the observed plasma half-life times ($t_{0.5}$) were higher for the Epo-Fc dimer and the Epo-Fc monomer than for unconjugated erythropoietin, demonstrating an increase of $t_{0.5}$ due to the fusion to the Fc residual of the immunoglobin. Functional analysis by measurement of reticulocytes in blood revealed that all types of inhaled erythropoietin and both fusion proteins were biologically active, although there were differences with respect to the strength of the reticulocyte-increasing effect [13, 18]. Some further experiments including measurement of pharmacokinetics after administration of different doses were also performed in healthy human volunteers and confirmed the absorption and a dose-dependent biological effect after inhalation of the Epo-Fc fusion protein [14, 18].

IL-2 is produced from T lymphocytes after antigen stimulation and serves as an immune modulator, e.g. activating cytotoxic T cells and natural killer cells making it to an interesting target in tumor research [20]. It was observed that IL-2 caused a suppression of metastases of malignant tumors, especially metastases from melanoma and kidney cancer. In the latter, persisting remissions were achieved in a number of patients. In consequence, IL-2 treatment received approval from the Food and Drug Administration (FDA) for treatment of metastasizing kidney cancer and melanoma in 1992 and 1998, respectively [20]. Most frequently, IL-2 was subject of systemic administration, however in a number of studies there was also an inhalant administration of IL-2 liposomes alone or in combination with other cytokines (e.g. interferon-α). Most data were published for patients with advanced kidney cancer, especially those with pulmonary or mediastinal metastases [20–23]. The inhalation (first-line and second-line therapy) was well tolerated showing fewer side effects than systemic treatment with cytokines and was followed by a relevant increase of survival time. Inhalation of high IL-2 doses (second-line therapy) was also followed by temporary regression of pulmonary metastases but not extrapulmonary metastases in patients with melanoma [21, 22].

Treatment with recombinant GM-CSF (MW: 14.6 kDa) has been approved for therapy of patients to recover neutrophils (e.g. after induction chemotherapy for treatment of acute myelogenous leukemia, mobilization of hematopoietic progenitor cells prior to cytapheresis and following transplantation of hematopoietic progenitor cells) [23]. However, several other potential clinical indications, e.g. use in antitumor therapy and treatment of alveolar proteinosis, have been investigated [23]. The glycoprotein is usually administered parenterally but in studies for treatment of cancer or alveolar proteinosis it has been administered by means of inhalation [18, 23]. The feasibility of aerosol administration of GM-CSF was proven in cynomolgus monkeys more than 15 years ago [18]. A number of studies investigated the effect of GM-CSF on pulmonary alveolar proteinosis which is an orphan disease (less than 500 reported cases until 2006 and first described in 1958). Since a first case report from 1996, several investigators demonstrated that inhalant administration of GM-CSF aerosol alone or if necessary in combination with whole lung lavage is a safe and efficient therapy for treatment of pulmonary alveolar proteinosis even for a longer treatment period resulting in a therapy-dependent improvement of clinical behavior and lung function parameters [18, 24, 25]. Other studies investigated the effect of various study regimens and doses of inhaled recombinant GM-CSF on different types of cancer, e.g. metastases of kidney carcinoma, osteosarcoma and melanoma [18]. Usually, inhalation of lower doses was not followed by relevant changes of lung function and side effects. In addition, there were also only minor increases of white blood cells and neutrophils under therapy. However, treatment with aerosolized GM-CSF resulted in a relevant disease regression or reduction of disease progression in some patients [18]. In a more recent study, escalating doses of up to 2,000 μg b.i.d. were administered in patients with lung metastases of melanoma. The investigators observed an acceptable toxicity of inhaled GM-CSF, the greatest changes of antitumor immunity in patients receiving the highest drug doses and longer times of progression-free survival in patients developing an immune response [26].

Cyclosporin A, a cyclic peptide (MW: 1,200 Da) serves as an immunosuppressant for prevention of graft rejection in patients after organ transplantation as well as in patients with autoimmune diseases [27]. In a number of studies predominantly performed in lung transplant recipients, the effect of cyclosporin liposome inhalation was investigated [27]. After inhalation the lipophilic compound is rapidly absorbed. However, the pharmacokinetics indicate a temporary uptake of the compound by alveolar macrophages as well as its interaction with pulmonary surfactant or membranes of alveolar epithelium [28]. Depending on the deposited lung dose of inhaled cyclosporin A, an improved transplant function (determined by measurement of the forced expiratory volume in 1 s) was observed in lung transplanted patients with graft rejection. At the same time, patients treated with aerosolized cyclosporin A required lower doses of other immunosupressants when compared to the control group. However, inhalant immunosuppressive therapy was well tolerated and there were no higher rates of pulmonary infections as well as no hepatotoxic or nephrotoxic effects [29]. More recent data of the same study group demonstrated that deposition of sufficient pulmonary doses of cyclosporin A can prevent the decrease of graft function and the occurrence of bronchiolitis obliterans (which is largely affecting the long-time prognosis after lung transplantation) and in consequence improve the long-time outcome in lung transplanted patients [30].

Safety of Macromolecule Inhalation

Safety and tolerability of pulmonary administered compounds can be largely different from those after subcutaneous administration. Inhaled pharmaceuticals as well as additives for absorption enhancement may induce an incompatibility (e.g. immunization in case of proteins and induction of specific effects on the target organ lung in case of hormones) as well as damage of lung epithelium directly (e.g. bile acids, cyclodextrins and other absorption enhancers) or via production of reactive oxygen species (e.g. in case of cationic liposomes). Last but not least, pulmonary diseases may complicate or prevent inhalant drug therapy under some circumstances [2, 6, 11, 17].

Conclusions

In recent decades, inhalation of biomolecules has come into the focus of interest. However, prior to studies investigating the inhalation of these compounds, the physical and physiological background for reproducible administration of sufficient drug doses into the lung had to be elucidated. After solving these basic questions, the feasibility of inhalative administration was investigated for a large number of biomolecules (mainly peptides and proteins). However, up to now, data regarding the long-time effects of inhaled macromolecules except insulin and heparin are sparse. In addition, there are also few data regarding the feasibility and safety of carriers (e.g. microparticles and liposomes) as well as stabilizers and absorption enhancers for pulmonary drug administration. Therefore, future studies are required for further investigation of long-time effects and optimization of inhalative drug administration. Then it is likely that inhalation-based methods for drug administration will serve as a safe and convenient alternative of subcutaneous injection in patients with systemic diseases.

References

1 Niven RW: Delivery of biotherapeutics by inhalation aerosol. Crit Rev Ther Drug Carrier Syst 1995;12:151–231.

2 Siekmeier R, Scheuch G: Systemic treatment by inhalation of macromolecules – principles, problems and examples. J Physiol Pharmacol 2008;59(suppl 6): 53–79.

3 Nicod LP: Pulmonary defence mechanisms. Respiration 1999;66:2–11.

4 Scheuch G, Kohlhaeufl MJ, Brand P, Siekmeier R: Clinical perspectives on pulmonary systemic and macromolecular delivery. Adv Drug Deliv Rev 2006; 58:996–1008.

5 Scheuch G, Siekmeier R: Novel approaches to enhance pulmonary delivery of proteins and peptides. J Physiol Pharmacol 2007;58(suppl 5):615–625.

6 Agu RU, Ugwoke MI, Armand M, Kinget R, Verbeke N: The lung as a route for systemic delivery of therapeutic proteins and peptides. Respir Res 2001;2:198–209.

7 Patton JS, Byron PR: Inhaling medicines: delivering drugs to the body through the lungs. Nat Rev Drug Discov 2007;6: 67–74.

8 Wolff RK: Safety of inhaled proteins for therapeutic use. J Aerosol Med 1998;11: 197–219.

9 Byron PR, Patton JS: Drug delivery via the respiratory tract. J Aerosol Med 1994;7:49–75.

10 Yu J, Chien YW: Pulmonary drug delivery: physiologic and mechanistic aspects. Crit Rev Ther Drug Carrier Syst 1997;14: 395–453.

11 Hussain A, Arnold JJ, Khan MA, Ahsan F: Absorption enhancers in pulmonary protein delivery. J Control Release 2004; 94:15–24.

12 Dhand R: New frontiers in aerosol delivery during mechanical ventilation. Respir Care 2004;49:666–677.

13 Bitonti AJ, Dumont JA, Low SC, Peters RT, Kropp KE, Palombella VJ, Stattel JM, Lu Y, Tan CA, Song JJ, Garcia AM, Simister NE, Spiekermann GM, Lencer WI, Blumberg RS: Pulmonary delivery of an erythropoietin Fc fusion protein in non-human primates through an immunoglobulin transport pathway. Proc Natl Acad Sci USA 2004;101:9763–9768.

14 Bitonti AJ, Dumont JA: Pulmonary administration of therapeutic proteins using an immunoglobulin transport pathway. Adv Drug Deliv Rev 2006; 58:1106–1118.

15 Laube BL: The expanding role of aerosols in systemic drug delivery, gene therapy, and vaccination. Respir Care 2005; 50:1161–1176.

16 Scheuch G, Brand P, Meyer T, Herpich C, Müllinger B, Brom J, Weidinger G, Kohlhäufl M, Häussinger K, Spannagl M, Schramm W, Siekmeier R: Anticoagulative effects of the inhaled low molecular weight heparin certoparin in healthy subjects. J Physiol Pharmacol 2007;58 (suppl 5):603–614.

17 Siekmeier R, Scheuch G: Inhaled insulin – does it become reality? J Physiol Pharmacol 2008;59(suppl 6):81–113.

18 Siekmeier R, Scheuch G: Treatment of systemic diseases by inhalation of biomolecule aerosols. J Physiol Pharmacol 2009;60(suppl 5):15–26.

19 Köhler D: Aerosolized heparin. J Aerosol Med 1994;7:307–314.

20 Eklund JW, Kuzel TM: A review of recent findings involving interleukin-2-based cancer therapy. Curr Opin Oncol 2004; 16:542–546.

21 Enk AH, Nashan D, Rübben A, Knop J: High-dose inhalation interleukin therapy for lung metastases in patients with malignant melanoma. Cancer 2000;88: 2042–2046.

22 Huland E, Heinzer H: Renal cell carcinoma – innovative medical treatments. Curr Opin Urol 2004;14:239–244.

23 Thipphawong J: Inhaled cytokines and cytokine antagonists. Adv Drug Delivery Rev 2006;58:1089–1105.

24 Seymour JF, Presneill JJ: Pulmonary alveolar proteinosis. Progress in the first 44 years. Am J Respir Crit Care Med 2002;166:215–235.

25 Wylam ME, Ten R, Prakash UBS, Nadrous HF, Clawson ML, Anderson PM: Aerosol granulocyte-macrophage colony-stimulating factor for pulmonary alveolar proteinosis. Eur Respir J 2006; 27:585–593.

26 Markovic SN, Suman VJ, Nevala WK, Geeraerts L, Creagan ET, Erickson LA, Rowland KM, Morton RF, Horvath WL, Pittelkow MR: A dose-escalation study of aerosolized sargramostim in the treatment of metastatic melanoma: an NCCTG Study. Am J Clin Oncol 2008;31: 573–579.

27 Corcoran TE: Inhaled delivery of aerosolized cyclosporine. Adv Drug Deliv Rev 2006;58:1119–1127.

28 Burckart GJ, Smaldone GC, Eldon MA, Venkataramanan R, Dauber J, Zeevi A, McCurry K, McKaveney TP, Corcoran TE, Griffith BP, Iacono AT: Lung deposition and pharmacokinetics of cyclosporine after aerosolization in lung transplant patients. Pharm Res 2003;20: 252–256.

29 Iacono AT, Smaldone GC, Keenan RJ, Diot P, Dauber JH, Zeevi A, Burckart GJ, Griffith BP: Dose-related reversal of acute lung rejection by aerosolized cyclosporine. Am J Respir Crit Care Med 1997;155:1690–1698.

30 Iacono AT, Johnson BA, Grgurich WF, Youssef JG, Corcoran TE, Seiler DA, Dauber JH, Smaldone GC, Zeevi A, Yousem SA, Fung JJ, Burckart GJ, McCurry KR, Griffith BP: A randomized trial of inhaled cyclosporine in lung-transplant recipients. N Engl J Med 2006;354:141–150.

PD Dr. med. habil. Rüdiger Siekmeier
Federal Institute for Drugs and Medical Devices (BfArM)
Kurt-Georg-Kiesinger-Allee 3, DE–53175 Bonn (Germany)
Tel. +49 228 207 5360, Fax +49 228 207 5300
E-Mail r.siekmeier@bfarm.de

Esquinas AM (ed): Applied Technologies in Pulmonary Medicine. Basel, Karger, 2011, pp 77–83

Diabetes Treatment by Inhalation of Insulin – Shine and Decline of a Novel Type of Therapy

R. Siekmeier[a] · G. Scheuch[b]

[a]Federal Institute for Drugs and Medical Devices (BfArM), and [b]Activaero GmbH, Gemünden, Germany

In recent decades, techniques for protein production by means of recombinant DNA technology have been developed and largely improved enabling us to produce sufficient quantities of peptides and proteins for novel medical treatment and administration options. Many decades were required to solve the problems of a reproducible and efficient drug dosing by inhalation, even in the case of insulin. However, shortly after approval and market launch, distribution was stopped due to low market penetration. This article briefly describes the history, problems and experience on insulin inhalation until market withdrawal.

History of Insulin Inhalation

Insulin was isolated in 1921 by Banting and Best, and 1 year later on January 11, 1922, it was introduced into medical treatment [1–3]. Initially it was the subject of intramuscular injection. However, other techniques for drug application (transdermal, ocular, oral, buccal, nasal, pulmonal, rectal, vaginal and transuterine) were investigated [4–6]. In 1924 and 1925 – only 2 years after the start of the therapeutic insulin era – the first studies on insulin inhalation were published. The first paper described the effect of intratracheally in comparison to subcutaneously (sc) administered insulin in rabbits. The authors observed a glucose-lowering effect and a more rapid onset of action after intratracheal than after sc administration, but higher drug doses were required [7]. A first study on inhaled insulin in patients was performed by Heubner et al. [8], also in 1924. They reported a dose-dependent effect of insulin inhalation on blood glucose. Again, the required dose was 30 times higher after inhalation. Independently from this group, Gänsslen [9] also studied the effect of insulin inhalation in patients. He also observed that inhaled insulin effectively lowered the concentration of blood glucose. His required amounts of insulin were not as high as those described above by Heubner et al. [8]. It took 46 more years until Wigley et al. [10] published their pivotal study of insulin inhalation offering the proof of principle of this therapy. They were able to demonstrate that pork-beef insulin administered by a nebulizer caused a prompt increase in plasma-immunoreactive insulin and that hypoglycemia showed a temporal relationship. However, pulmonary delivered insulin was far away from approval and several studies performed in the next decades were necessary to develop this therapy option [6]. For example, devices were developed for optimized drug deposition in the alveoli (standard nebulizers mainly deposit the aerosol in the bronchial system) [1, 11, 12]. At about 1990 the technical prerequisites for the pulmonary delivery of insulin were established. Based on different technical and pharmacological solutions (e.g. different inhalation systems, powder aerosol or liquid aerosol), several companies developed inhalation devices (table 1) [1, 6]. Exubera® from Pfizer/Nektar was the first to receive approval from the US Food and Drug Administration and the European Drug Agency in early 2006 for patients with diabetes mellitus types 1 and 2. However, 1 year after marketing start, Pfizer announced it would withdraw Exubera® from the market in October 2007, citing that the drug had failed to gain market acceptance. A few months later most other developers stopped their programs on inhaled insulin. However, one company, Pharmaceutical Discovery Corp./Mannkind Pharmaceuticals, continued [6].

Carriers of Insulin for Inhalation

Most of the recent pulmonary delivery methods were based on insulin powder aerosols. One exception was (AERx® iDMS) where a liquid packaging was used (table 1). In some of the novel techniques, insulin is formulated into microspheres (liposomes, particles, large porous particles) in order to improve its pharmacological properties (e.g. inhalation, absorption). Most of the published clinical data regarding the inhalation of particles were based on Technosphere®. An advantage of microparticles is that they are phagocytosed less rapidly [1, 6, 13]. Insulin packed in the inner part of biologically degradable polymers and lipids (microparticles and liposomes, respectively) is subject of a slow alveolar clearance and peptide degradation by alveolar macrophages resulting in an increased bioavailability. There may also be an altered pharmacokinetics which is subject of a slow release from these particles. However, prerequisites for use of these excipients are rapid degradation after inhalation and immunological and toxicological inertness [6, 13].

Liposomes are only used experimentally for pulmonary insulin administration so far, but may be an alternative [6, 13–15].

Solid particles (microspheres or large porous particles) are chemically and physically more stable than liposomes and allow higher drug loading [13, 16]. Pharmacological properties of microparticles (size range: <500 nm) depend on the used material, preparation technique, particle size, porosity and surface structure as well as the delivery device [6, 14, 16, 17]. Microspheres can be produced by a number of distinct methods based on supercritical fluid technology, emulsion-solvent evaporation, spray-drying and phase separation. Examples for the clinical use of microspheres for insulin inhalation are (ProMaxx®, Epic Therapeutics; Technosphere®, Pharmaceutical Discovery Corp., and calcium phosphate-polyethylene glycol particles, BioSante Pharmaceuticals) [6, 14].

Large porous particles are characterized by geometric diameters >5 μm, low particle density (generally <0.1 g/ml) and aerodynamic diameters <5 μm. They have good flow and aerosolization properties due to their low aerodynamic diameter. There was one system for insulin inhalation based on large porous particles (AIR®, Alkermes) [6, 14].

Improvement of Insulin Bioavailability by Addition of Absorption Enhancers

The bioavailability of biomolecules after alveolar deposition can be improved by addition of compounds affecting the absorption (e.g. bile acids) and compounds inhibiting the proteolytic degradation (e.g. aprotinin). However, many of these substances were found to be toxic [2, 6, 13, 16, 18].

Only few studies have investigated the effect of absorption enhancers in humans or other

Table 1. Devices for inhalant administration of insulin [modified according to 1, 6]: the table reflects the situation in 2006, i.e. before market withdrawal of Exubera®

Trade name (developer/partner)	Status of development	Principle or pharmaceutical form
Exubera® (Nektar/Pfizer)	Market approval 2006	Dry powder insulin packed into blisters of 1 mg (≈3 U insulin) or 3 mg. Dosing via the number of blisters. Pneumatic release of the aerosol out of the blister in an inhalation chamber. Particle diameter of 2.5 μm.
AERx® iDMS (Aradigm/ NovoNordisk)	Phase III	Liquid insulin packed into single strips and dosed in single units. Regulation of breathing maneuver by means of microprocessors and electronic optimization of insulin release within inspiratory flow. Particle diameter of 1–3 μm.
HIIP® (Alkermes/Eli Lilly)	Phase III	Dry powder insulin packed into blisters. Mechanical system with breath activated release of particles. Porous particles of low density with a geometric diameter of 5–30 μm (aerodynamic diameter of <5 μm).
Technosphere® (Pharmaceutical Discovery Corp./ Mannkind Pharmaceuticals)	Phase III	Dry powder recombinant insulin combined with a derivative of diketopiperazine. Self-assembly into an ordered lattice array at low pH value. Mass median aerodynamic diameter 2–4 μm. Dissolution of particles and insulin release at neutral pH value on alveolar surface. Dry powder inhaler and passive disagglomeration (MedTone®).
Microdose DPI® (Microdose Technologies/ Elan Corp.)	Phase II	Dry powder insulin packed into blisters. Disaggregation of drug powder by means of a piezo vibrator. Mass median aerodynamic diameter approximately 1.5 μm, 84% of the particles <4.7 μm.
Unknown (Abbott (formerly Kos Pharma.)/–)	Phase II	Dry crystals of a recombinant insulin formulation. Administration by means of a handheld breath actuated inhaler (BAI) driven by a propellant.
Aerodose® (Aerogen/–)	Phase II (stopped in 2003)	Liquid insulin. Administration by means of a breath activated multiple dose inhaler. Mean particle diameter of 3.2 μm, 87% of the particles between 1 and 6 μm.
Bio-Air® (BioSante Pharmaceuticals/–)	Phase I	Coated dry particles based on calcium phosphate nanoparticle carriers. Administration by means of a calcium phosphate nanoparticulate delivery system.
Alveair® (CoreMed/Fosun and Xuzhou)	Phase I	Liquid insulin. Administration by means of a generic handheld device delivering inhaled insulin with the same units as injected insulin.
Unknown (Epic Therapeutics/–)	Phase I	Microspheres of recombinant human insulin (ProMaxx®). Administration by means of a dry powder inhalation device (Cyclohaler) >90% insulin. 95% of the microspheres with diameters 0.95–2.1 μm (mean: 1.5 μm), 95% of the particles <4.7 μm.
Spiros® (Elan Pharma (formerly Dura Pharma)/–)	Phase I (stopped in 2004)	Dry powder insulin blisters. Release by means of a hand-held, battery-driven, multiple-dose inhalator. Novel powder dispersion system (Spiros-S2) without electromechanical components of the Spiros for administration at low inspiratory flow rates (15–30 l/min).

mammals except rats. For example, sodium citrate, mannitol and glycine are excipients used in Exubera® [6, 19]. However, even these data are unequivocal. For example, Heinemann et al. [20] observed only a small increase in bioeffectivity if a powder aerosol of insulin was administered in combination with an endogenous bile acid in healthy humans, whereas Johansson et al. [21] found a strongly increased bioavailability of insulin in dogs if the substance was administered as a fluidic aerosol containing also taurocholate [16, 18].

Pharmacokinetics of Inhaled Insulin in Individuals without Lung Diseases

Many studies investigated pharmacokinetics and pharmacodynamics of inhaled insulin in healthy subjects and found significant differences caused by inhaler use, administered formulations and doses of insulin. After inhalation, regular insulin is usually absorbed faster than sc administered insulin (time to peak concentration (t_{max}): 7–90 min vs. 42–274 min [1, 6, 11, 18, 22]. A biphasic pharmacokinetics has been found with a first peak rapidly after inhalation followed by a slow release. Within the first hour after administration the area under the concentration vs. time curve (AUC) is larger for inhaled insulin than for sc insulin. On the other hand, a larger total AUC is observed for sc insulin if an observation period of 6 h is used, suggesting a therapeutic benefit of inhaled insulin in treating of prandial or postprandial hyperglycemia. Additionally, inhaled insulin bears a lower risk for postprandial hypoglycemia because of increased clearance [18].

Dose-response studies in patients with diabetes mellitus type 1 revealed a widely linear dose response. However, even when the maximum insulin concentration (C_{max}) increased with administered dose there was an increasing time delay to peak concentration in plasma (t_{max}), which indicates the existence of a dose-dependent uptake mechanism [6, 18, 22]. A number of studies were also performed with the insulin derivative lispro. Lower doses of lispro were required to achieve the same insulin concentration and onset of action was more rapid. Both effects may be caused by a breakup of the hexamer into monomers.

Many studies determined relative bioavailability by comparing of AUC after inhalation with sc administration. Other investigators calculated the bioeffectivity (hypoglycemic effect of inhaled insulin compared to a defined sc administered insulin dose). However, both methods result in an underestimation of the therapeutic effect of the inhaled insulin fraction itself (only a small insulin fraction is deposited in the lung periphery where it can be absorbed). In controlled studies, bioavailabilities and bioeffectivities for inhaled insulin were found between 9 and 22% as well as 8 and 16%, respectively. In consequence, the inhaled insulin doses required to achieve the same therapeutic effect are up to 11 times higher compared to that after injection [6, 18]. Only about 30–40% of the filled insulin doses reach the lungs and from these over 50% are deposited in the airways (bronchial system) and underlie mucociliary transport and/or degradation. And from the particles reaching the alveoli, about 40–50% are rapidly absorbed into the circulatory system [6, 18].

This shows that deep lung deposition is a major predictor of bioavailability. The best deposition will be achieved if the aerosol is inhaled at the beginning of a slow and deep breath, enabling the particles to reach the alveolar region. However, not only the total amount of alveolar insulin deposition, but also the intraindividual reproducibility of this therapy is affected by the individual breathing of the patients. A number of studies have shown a similar or even better reproducibility of insulin administration by inhalation than sc injection. This shows that sc administration also has a high variability [2, 6, 18, 22–25].

Effect of Smoking on the Pharmacokinetics of Inhaled Insulin

A number of studies have described a higher absorption (up to 3–5 times) of inhaled insulin in smokers compared to non-smokers (higher absorption (C_{max}), AUC and bioavailability as well as a higher peak concentration (C_{max}) and a shorter time to peak (t_{max})) [1, 5, 6, 18, 22, 25, 26]. Smoking cessation reduced absorption, an effect which was reversed by smoking resumption [6, 26]. These changes are caused by an increased permeability of the alveolo-capillary barrier due to chronic cigarette smoking. However, acute cigarette smoking significantly blunts the enhanced insulin absorption. The underlying mechanisms of these effects are not understood. It is assumed that inhaled nicotine and pulmonary neutrophils may play a relevant role. Because of these complex effects, inhalant insulin therapy was not approved in current smokers and ex-smokers [6, 19].

Effect of Pulmonary Diseases on the Pharmacokinetics of Inhalant Insulin

Because it was assumed that lung diseases may affect pulmonary drug absorption, such patients were excluded from routine treatment with inhaled insulin. However, acute respiratory infections had no relevant effect on pharmacokinetics and pharmacodynamics in otherwise healthy individuals [6, 18]. In contrast, asthma patients showed a mild decrease of C_{max} and a distinct decrease of AUC (bioavailability) and plasma glucose concentration (bioeffectivity). Furthermore, asthma patients showed a higher variability of C_{max} and AUC after insulin inhalation. In principle, these changes can be caused by increased drug deposition in the bronchi. In contrast, published data on the pharmacokinetics of inhaled insulin in patients with chronic obstructive pulmonary disease are limited and conflicting. It was found higher or lower absorption of insulin compared to healthy subjects without chronic obstructive pulmonary disease [6]. In consequence, due to the high frequency of chronic obstructive pulmonary disease in the population, its effect on insulin absorption should be investigated prior to a re-launch.

Safety of Inhalant Insulin

The safety of inhaled insulin was subject of many investigations. Most data regarding the long-term tolerability were published for the Exubera® system and the AERx iDMS® system for study periods of up to 2 years and more in patients with diabetes mellitus types 1 and 2 [2, 6, 18, 22, 25, 27]. Inhalation of insulin caused only a minimal change of spirometric parameters of lung function (e.g. forced expiratory volume in 1 s, forced vital capacity) as well as parameters of diffusion capacity for carbon monoxide and blood gas analysis [1, 2, 5, 6, 18, 25, 27]. However, the manufacturer recommended spirometric measurement of lung function before treatment, after 6 months and thereafter at least annually in the product information for Exubera® [28]. In principle, the observed low pulmonary toxicity may be explained by the distribution of the inhaled doses of 4–5 mg t.i.d. on a total alveolar surface of about 80–120 m^2 and the following rapid decrease of its concentration due to absorption and distribution in the body fluid as well as proteolytic degradation [1, 2, 5, 6, 18, 23, 24].

Beside its strong metabolic effect, insulin also acts as a weak growth factor (effectivity only 1/100 of insulin-like growth factor-1) after binding to the receptor for insulin-like growth factor-1 [18]. About 6 months after the end of marketing of Exubera® the Food and Drug Administration published a press release reporting a potentially increased risk for bronchial cancer in ex-smokers treated with inhaled insulin [29]. However, the number of reported cases is extremely small and even though investigations were continued, no relevant data seem to confirm the theory of an increased lung cancer risk in smokers due to insulin inhalation.

In a number of insulin inhalation studies, increased serum titers of non-neutralizing IgG antibodies were found which had no therapeutic relevance, i.e. there were no correlations to the metabolic control, lung function and adverse events [1, 2, 4, 6, 18, 25, 27, 30, 31]. Most likely the induction of these antibodies is caused by insulin formulation and dose (inhaled insulin is given in higher doses and more frequently for treatment of postprandial hyperglycemia than sc insulin) as well as the lung as the target of delivery (presence of macrophages, dendritic cells and lymphocytes in the lung) [5, 6, 25, 30, 31].

Mild to moderate cough occurred rapidly after inhalation of dry powder insulin (seconds to minutes) in up to 20–30% of patients. However, the symptoms were transient, settled with continuation of the therapy and seldom resulted in treatment withdrawal [6].

In summary, there was no relevant difference regarding the risk for occurrence of hypoglycemia between inhalant and sc insulin. However, the risk was expectedly higher in patients treated with inhalant insulin when compared to those treated with oral antidiabetics [6].

Acceptance and Costs of Inhaled Insulin

The development of pen injector systems has largely improved diabetes treatment in the last decades. However, all these medical products are invasive which is important in patients suffering from needle phobia (about 10% of patients). Therefore, pulmonary administration of insulin was assumed to be a revolution in the treatment of insulin-dependent diabetes. Indeed, patients favored the inhaler even though it is more complex to handle [19, 27]. However, these advantages are opposed by (1) the small bioavailability of inhaled insulin and higher required insulin doses, (2) repeated pulmonary function tests (both resulting in extra costs depending on the required doses [32]), (3) an ongoing requirement of blood sampled by finger punction for the measurement of glucose concentration, and (4) no relevant improvement of metabolic control [19, 27, 32]. Based on these arguments, the National Institute for Health and Clinical Excellence (NICE, UK) and the Institute for Quality and Efficiency in Health Care (IQWiG, Germany) declined funding for inhalant insulin in Great Britain and Germany, respectively. It is likely that these decisions were substantial reasons that this therapy option failed in the market.

Conclusions

More than 80 years after the first studies, inhaled insulin (Exubera®) was approved and introduced into the market. Marketing has been rapidly stopped because of the unexpectedly low sales. In the short time of its marketing, Exubera® was accepted by the patients (although not reimbursed by most health insurance companies) and well tolerated without adverse effects. Beside Exubera® a number of other devices for inhalation of insulin were under development. However, due to the rapid stop of the distribution of Exubera® and the consecutive stop of the development of similar products by all competitors except Mannkind Pharmaceuticals, some questions are not completely answered. These include the effect of long-time inhalation on lung function and the effect of pulmonary diseases on deposition, absorption and pharmacokinetics of inhaled insulin as well as the potentially increased risk for lung cancer in ex-smokers. However, if there will be a re-launch of this interesting non-invasive method of drug administration, the open questions should be further investigated before.

References

1 Cefalu WT: Concept, strategies, and feasibility of non-invasive insulin delivery. Diabetes Care 2004;27:239–246.
2 Owens DR: New horizons – alternative routes for insulin delivery. Nat Rev Drug Discov 2002;1:529–540.
3 Wilde MI, McTavish D: Insulin lispro: a review of its pharmacological properties and therapeutic use in the management of diabetes mellitus. Drugs 1997;54: 597–614.
4 Belmin J, Valensi P: Novel drug delivery systems for insulin. Clinical potential for use in the elderly. Drugs Aging 2003;20: 303–312.
5 Heinemann L, Pfützner A, Heise T: Alternative routes of administration as an approach to improve insulin therapy: update on dermal, oral, nasal and pulmonary insulin delivery. Curr Pharm Des 2001;7:1327–1351.
6 Siekmeier R, Scheuch G: Inhaled insulin – does it become reality? J Physiol Pharmacol 2008;59(suppl 6):81–113.
7 Laqueur E, Grevenstuk A: Über die Wirkung intratrachealer Zuführung von Insulin. Klin Wochenschr 1924;3:1273–1274.
8 Heubner W, de Jongh SE, Laqueur E: Über Inhalation von Insulin. Klin Wochenschr 1924;3:2342–2343.
9 Gänsslen M: Über Inhalation von Insulin. Klin Wochenschr 1925;4:71.
10 Wigley FW, Londono JH, Wood SH, Ship JC, Waldman RH: Insulin across respiratory mucosae by aerosol delivery. Diabetes 1971;20:552–556.
11 Niven RW: Delivery of biotherapeutics by inhalation aerosol. Crit Rev Ther Drug Carrier Syst 1995;12:151–231.
12 Gonda I: The ascent of pulmonary drug delivery. J Pharm Sci 2000;89:940–945.
13 Siekmeier R, Scheuch G: Systemic treatment by inhalation of macromolecules – principles, problems and examples. J Physiol Pharmacol 2008;59(suppl 6):53–79.
14 Cryan SA: Carrier-based strategies for targeting protein and peptide drugs to the lungs. AAPS J 2005;7:E20-E41.
15 Sakagami M, Byron PR: Respirable microspheres for inhalation. The potential of manipulating pulmonary disposition for improved therapeutic efficacy. Clin Pharmacokinet 2005;44:263–277.
16 Hussain A, Arnold JJ, Khan MA, Ahsan F: Absorption enhancers in pulmonary protein delivery. J Control Release 2004; 94:15–24.
17 Agu RU, Ugwoke MI, Armand M, Kinget R, Verbeke N: The lung as a route for systemic delivery of therapeutic proteins and peptides. Respir Res 2001;2:198–209.
18 Patton JS, Bukar JG, Eldon MA: Clinical pharmacokinetics and pharmacodynamics of inhaled insulin. Clin Pharmacokinet 2004;43:781–801.
19 Guntur VP, Dhand R: Inhaled insulin: extending the horizons of inhalation therapy. Respir Care 2007;52:911–922.
20 Heinemann L, Klappoth W, Rave H, Hompesch B, Linkeschowa R, Heise T: Intra-individual variability of the metabolic effect of inhaled insulin together with an absorption enhancer. Diabetes Care 2000;23:1343–1347.
21 Johansson F, Hjertberg E, Eirefelt S, Tronde A, Hultkvist Bengtsson U: Mechanisms for absorption enhancement of inhaled insulin by sodium taurocholate. Eur J Pharm Sci 2002;17:63–71.
22 Sakagami M: Insulin disposition in the lung following oral inhalation in humans. A meta-analysis of its pharmacokinetics. Clin Pharmacokinet 2004;43: 539–552.
23 Scheuch G, Kohlhaeufl MJ, Brand P, Siekmeier R: Clinical perspectives on pulmonary systemic and macromolecular delivery. Adv Drug Deliv Rev 2006; 58:996–1008.
24 Scheuch G, Siekmeier R: Novel approaches to enhance pulmonary delivery of proteins and peptides. J Physiol Pharmacol 2007;58(suppl 5):615–625.
25 Valente AXCN, Langer R, Stone HA, Edwards DA: Recent advances in the development of an inhaled insulin product. Biodrugs 2003;17:9–17.
26 Becker RHA, Sha S, Frick AD, Fountaine RJ: The effect of smoking cessation and subsequent resumption on absorption of inhaled insulin. Diabetes Care 2006;29: 277–282.
27 Ceglia L, Lau J, Pittas AG: Meta-analysis: Efficacy and safety of inhaled insulin therapy in adults with diabetes mellitus. Ann Intern Med 2006;145:665–675.
28 NDA 21-868/Exubera®: US package insert, 2006. New York, Pfizer Labs (available from http://www.pfizer.com/pfizer/download/uspi_exubera.pdf).
29 Food and Drug Administration MedWatch Alert, 2008. Exubera® Inhalation Powder (available from http://www.drugs.com/fda/exubera-insulin-human-rdna-origin-inhalation-powder-12372.html).
30 Fineberg SE, Kawabata T, Finco-Kent D, Liu C, Krasner A: Antibody response to inhaled insulin in patients with type 1 or type 2 diabetes. An analysis of initial phase II and III inhaled insulin (Exubera®) trials and a two-year extension trial. J Clin Endocrinol Metab 2005;90: 3287–3394.
31 Stoever JA, Palmer JP: Inhaled insulin and insulin antibodies: a new twist to an old debate. Diabetes Technol Ther 2002; 4:157–161.
32 Black C, Cummins E, Royle P, Philip S, Waugh N: The clinical effectiveness and cost-effectiveness of inhaled insulin in diabetes mellitus: a systematic review and economic evaluation. Health Technol Assess 2007;11:1–126.

PD Dr. med. habil. Rüdiger Siekmeier
Federal Institute for Drugs and Medical Devices (BfArM)
Kurt-Georg-Kiesinger-Allee 3, DE–53175 Bonn (Germany)
Tel. +49 228 207 5360, Fax +49 228 207 5300
E-Mail r.siekmeier@bfarm.de

Esquinas AM (ed): Applied Technologies in Pulmonary Medicine. Basel, Karger, 2011, pp 84–88

Endobronchial Ultrasound

Devanand Anantham · Mariko Koh Siyue

Department of Respiratory and Critical Care Medicine, Singapore General Hospital, Singapore

Abbreviations

EBUS Endobronchial ultrasound
EUS Endoscopic ultrasound
TBNA Transbronchial needle aspiration

EBUS has revolutionized bronchoscopy because it extends the endoscopist's vision beyond the airway walls. EBUS is made possible by miniaturized ultrasound transducers that can be inserted via the working channel of a flexible bronchoscope. This is termed radial EBUS and facilitates evaluation of airway walls, as well as location of peripheral lung lesions. Alternatively, a linear transducer has been built in a dedicated bronchoscope to permit real-time TBNA biopsies. This is termed EBUS-TBNA and has become an accepted modality for the invasive staging of the mediastinum in non-small cell lung cancer.

Radial EBUS

Radial EBUS has a 20-MHz (12–30 MHz available) rotating transducer. 'Central' probes with balloon sheaths are used in the proximal airways for either bronchial wall assessment or to guide TBNA of lymph nodes. 'Peripheral' probes without balloon sheaths are used to identify parenchymal lung lesions for biopsy. In radial EBUS, a 360° image that is perpendicular to the long axis of the airway is produced (fig. 1). The resolution of the image is <1 mm and a depth of 40–50 mm is scanned.

In thoracic tumors, EBUS has been shown to be superior to even computed tomography in distinguishing airway wall invasion from extrinsic compression with a sensitivity of 89% and specificity of 100% [1]. When airway walls are examined, up to 7 layers can be distinguished. The mucosa, endochondium, perichondium and adventitia are hyperechoic (white) while the intervening submucosa, cartilage and connective tissue layer are hypoechoic (gray) [1]. The relationship of lymph nodes relative to the airways can also be visualized using radial EBUS. Once a target lesion is identified, the probe is removed from the bronchoscope and regular TBNA can be performed to obtain biopsy specimens. Although radial EBUS facilitates such guided biopsies, it is limited by the absence of real-time sampling. The reported diagnostic yields with radial EBUS directed TBNA is 72–86% and this procedure has been shown to improve diagnostic rates over 'blind' conventional TBNA in obtaining a histological diagnosis from paratracheal lymph node stations [2, 3].

When radial EBUS is used to guide bronchoscopic biopsies of peripheral lung lesions, it increases the diagnostic yield of transbronchial lung biopsies of small (<30 mm) lesions [4]. Diagnostic

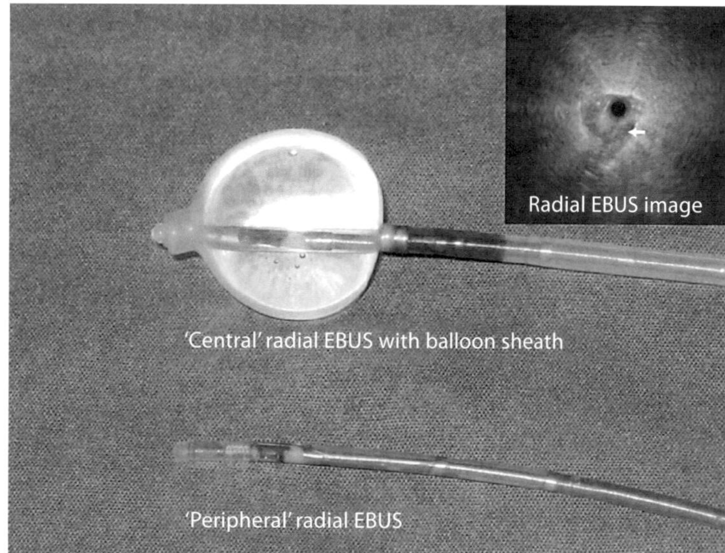

Fig. 1. 'Central' and 'peripheral' radial EBUS probes. Inset: ultrasound image of a peripheral lung lesion (arrow).

sensitivities of 61–80% that are independent of lesion size have been reported [3, 4]. EBUS also appears to remove variables that usually influence the ability to obtain a positive histological diagnosis. These variables include underlying disease, presence of the bronchus sign and lobar location [5]. The transducer probe is inserted through a guide sheath into the bronchi where the lesion is suspected based on pre-procedure computed tomography imaging. Normal air-filled alveoli produce a whitish snowstorm image with 'comet-tail' artifacts. Lung lesions are usually more hypoechoic or gray. When a tumor is located, the transducer is removed and regular biopsy forceps are used to take biopsies through the guide sheath that has been maintained in position within the lesion.

Linear EBUS-TBNA

The EBUS-TBNA bronchoscope has a 7.5-MHz transducer mounted on its distal tip. This transducer is convex and produces a 50° sector view parallel to the long axis of the bronchoscope extending 20–50 mm in depth (fig. 2). The EBUS-TBNA scope has an external diameter of 6.9 mm which is larger than a standard flexible bronchoscope. Therefore, oral rather than nasal intubation is necessary. Furthermore, the endoscopic viewing optics is at a 30° oblique angle and operator compensation is required during bronchoscopy. This bronchoscope has a 2.0-mm working channel that is designed to house a dedicated 21- to 22-gauge biopsy needle with a depth of penetration can be varied up to 40 mm by a safety lock. There is a balloon fitted over the transducer probe that can be filled with saline to facilitate coupling. However, this is not always needed if good contact can be maintained between the airway mucosa and the probe. Lymph nodes appear more echoic (gray) than blood vessels and Doppler can be used in making the distinction. Once the target lymph nodes are identified on EBUS, real-time TBNA is performed. The needle sheath that houses the TBNA needle is pushed forward first such that it is visualized on the endoscopic image before the 'jabbing' technique is used to perform TBNA under real-time guidance. Once the TBNA needle is

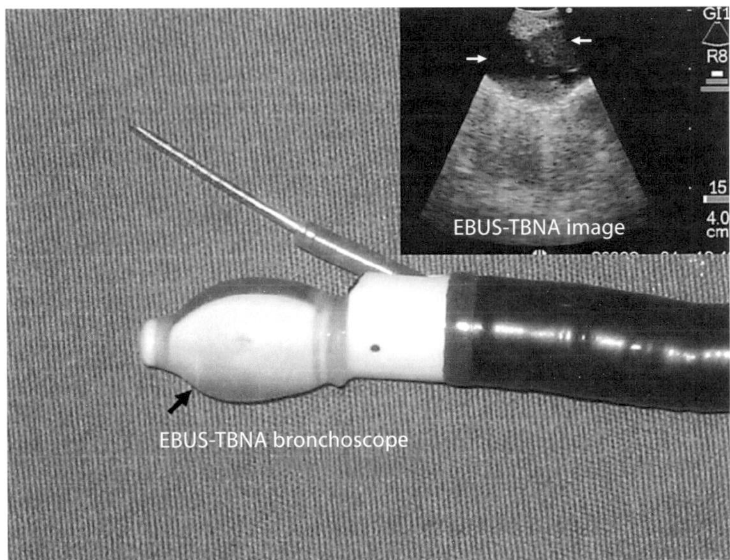

Fig. 2. EBUS-TBNA bronchoscope with balloon sheath (arrow) and 22-gauge needle. Inset: ultrasound image of tumor (right arrow) invading a blood vessel (left arrow).

within the target, the stylet of the needle is agitated to dislodge any airway debris. The stylet is then removed before biopsies can be aspirated. All mediastinal and hilar lymph nodes are accessible to EBUS-TBNA except the aortopulmonary (station 5), paraaortic (station 6), paraesophageal (station 8) and pulmonary ligament (station 9) nodes. For mediastinal staging of non-small cell lung cancer, 3 cytology aspirations per lymph node station is recommended. If adequate core specimens are obtained, then 2 passes will suffice [6].

EBUS-TBNA has been shown to have a higher diagnostic yield than conventional 'blind' TBNA and may be comparable in sensitivity to cervical mediastinoscopy [3, 7]. The pooled diagnostic sensitivity of EBUS-TBNA is 90% and specificity is 100%, but the false negative rate is about 20% [8]. This discordance between sensitivity and negative predictive value is attributed to the high prevalence of malignancy in the reported studies. The high false negative rates mandate that all negative results need to be either followed up clinically or subject to further testing using alternative modalities such as mediastinoscopy to confirm that the results are true negatives. Re-staging of the mediastinum with EBUS-TBNA after neoadjuvant chemotherapy has had less success with a much lower diagnostic sensitivity [3].

The histological staging of a radiologically normal mediastinum with either lymphadenopathy ≤10 mm or negative positron emission tomography has been shown to be feasible with sensitivities approaching 90% [9]. These data would suggest that systematic staging is possible as opposed to the targeted sampling that is widely practiced. However, such studies were performed by experts on patients under general anesthesia and the widespread applicability of the data is still not established because EBUS-TBNA is usually performed under moderate sedation. Nevertheless, EBUS clearly has the potential to identify lymphadenopathy that has been missed on computed tomography. In addition, the 22-gauge needle can obtain samples that are sufficient for genetic and molecular analysis such as epidermal growth factor receptor mutations.

By combining EBUS-TBNA with another endoscopic procedure, i.e. transesophageal EUS-guided fine-needle aspiration, complete staging of the mediastinum is possible with access to lymph node stations not accessible to either technique on its own. EBUS offers greater access to the paratracheal and hilar lymph nodes while EUS can target inferior mediastinal lymph nodes and adrenal metastases. Diagnostic sensitivities of 93–94% have been reported for the combined EBUS and EUS procedure [3].

EBUS-TBNA has also been used to successfully obtain biopsy specimens from primary tumors located in the paratracheal and peribronchial region with a diagnostic sensitivity of 82–94% [3, 10]. As long as there is no intervening aerated lung, these tumors can be identified as soft tissue structures on ultrasound. The procedure is then similar to sampling lymph nodes and is especially useful in diagnosing centrally located tumors without any airway involvement. In the demonstration of non-caseating granulomatous inflammation, EBUS-TBNA has a diagnostic yield for sarcoidosis of 85–94% [3]. This has been shown to be more effective than standard TBNA. If bigger tissue specimens are needed for histological analysis in conditions such as lymphoma, it is even possible to insert a 1.15-mm miniforceps through the EBUS scope and push it past the airway wall via a needle puncture [3]. This can potentially obtain real-time forceps biopsies of mediastinal lesions. Furthermore, EBUS-TBNA has been used therapeutically to drain mediastinal, as well as bronchogenic cysts and consequently relieve symptomatic central airway obstruction [3].

Complications have rarely been attributed directly to either radial EBUS or EBUS-TBNA. Radial EBUS-guided lung biopsies have a reported rate of pneumothorax of 0–5% and risk of moderate bleeding of 1% which is in keeping with the complication rates expected from conventional transbronchial lung biopsies [3, 4]. Therefore, these cases are considered complications of forceps biopsy rather than that of EBUS imaging. However, damage to the delicate radial transducer probes and perforation of the EBUS-TBNA bronchoscopes with careless use are complications that need to be avoided with the appropriate training. Radial probes should not be inserted into the working channel when 'active' and spinning. By ensuring that the needle sheath is clearly visible before attempting TBNA, inadvertent perforation of the EBUS-TBNA scope can be prevented.

EBUS can also add to endoscopy time and this has implications for what can be achieved under moderate sedation. However, in expert hands, radial EBUS adds less than 3 min to TBNA and about 60 s to the transbronchial biopsy of peripheral lesions. Targeted EBUS-TBNA of enlarged lymph nodes has been reported to take a mean of 12.5 (range 8–21) min [3]. However, a longer procedure duration is likely to be needed if complete mediastinal staging is attempted with evaluation of non-enlarged lymph nodes as well.

Conclusion

EBUS has the potential to become part of standard bronchoscopy because of negligible complications, improved diagnostic yield and a short learning curve. It enhances histopathological staging of the mediastinum in non-small cell lung cancer, as well as increases the diagnostic yields of both peribronchial and peripheral lung lesions. Ultrasonographic reflections enable the endoscopist to view beyond the surface of the airway walls and identify deeper structures. This ability to 'see through walls' without the need for ionizing radiation remains the premise on which EBUS has been developed. It is also the reason why EBUS continues to gain widespread acceptance.

Recommendations

- Radial EBUS facilitates airway wall assessment, TBNA of paratracheal lymph nodes and biopsies of peripheral lung lesions via a guide sheath.

- Linear EBUS-TBNA improves diagnostic yield compared to conventional 'blind' TBNA of mediastinal and hilar lymph node stations, as well as peribronchial tumors.
- EBUS-TBNA is a recognized modality for the invasive staging of the mediastinum in non-small cell lung cancer and is recommended if the necessary equipment and expertise are available.
- Negative biopsies from EBUS-guided procedures need to have subsequent biopsies from alternative procedures because of the risk of false negative results.

References

1 Herth F, Ernst A, Schulz M, Becker H: Endobronchial ultrasound reliably differentiates between airway infiltration and compression by tumor. Chest 2003;123:458–462.

2 Herth F, Becker HD, Ernst A: Conventional vs. endobronchial ultrasound-guided transbronchial needle aspiration: a randomized trial. Chest 2004;125: 322–325.

3 Anantham D, Koh MS, Ernst A: Endobronchial ultrasound. Respir Med 2009; 103:1406–1414.

4 Paone G, Nicastri E, Lucantoni G, et al: Endobronchial ultrasound-driven biopsy in the diagnosis of peripheral lung lesions. Chest 2005;128:3551–3557.

5 Yamada N, Yamazaki K, Kurimoto N, et al: Factors related to diagnostic yield of transbronchial biopsy using endobronchial ultrasonography with a guide sheath in small peripheral pulmonary lesions. Chest 2007;132:603–608.

6 Lee HS, Lee GK, Lee HS, et al: Real-time endobronchial ultrasound-guided transbronchial needle aspiration in mediastinal staging of non-small cell lung cancer: how many aspirations per target lymph node station? Chest 2008;134: 368–374.

7 Ernst A, Anantham D, Eberhardt R, et al: Diagnosis of mediastinal adenopathy real-time endobronchial ultrasound-guided needle aspiration versus mediastinoscopy. J Thorac Oncol 2008;3:577–582.

8 Detterbeck FC, Jantz MA, Wallace M, et al: American College of Chest Physicians: Invasive Mediastinal Staging of Lung Cancer: ACCP Evidence-Based Clinical Practice Guidelines, ed 2. Chest 2007;132(suppl):202S–220S.

9 Herth FJ, Eberhardt R, Krasnik M, et al: Endobronchial ultrasound-guided transbronchial needle aspiration of lymph nodes in the radiologically and positron emission tomography – normal mediastinum in patients with lung cancer. Chest 2008;133:887–891.

10 Nakajima T, Yasufuku K, Fujiwara T, et al: Endobronchial ultrasound-guided transbronchial needle aspiration for the diagnosis of intrapulmonary lesions. J Thorac Oncol 2008;3:985–988.

Devanand Anantham
Consultant
Department of Respiratory and Critical Care Medicine
Singapore General Hospital
Outram Road, Singapore 169608 (Singapore)
Tel. +65 6321 4700, Fax +65 6227 1736, E-Mail anantham.devanand@sgh.com.sg

Esquinas AM (ed): Applied Technologies in Pulmonary Medicine. Basel, Karger, 2011, pp 89–95

Minimally Invasive Thoracic Surgery for Pulmonary Resections

Michele Salati · Gaetano Rocco

Division of Thoracic Surgery, Department of Thoracic Surgery and Oncology, National Cancer Institute, Pascale Foundation, Naples, Italy

Abbreviations

MITS Minimally invasive thoracic surgery
NSCLC Non-small cell lung cancer
VATS Video-assisted thoracic surgery

The era of MITS began almost 100 years ago when Hans Christian Jacobaeus first introduced a cystoscope through the chest wall to explore the pleural cavity and to cauterize pleural adhesions favoring lung collapse in the treatment of pulmonary tuberculosis [1]. Since then the evolution of technologies with consequent development of more sophisticated and reliable surgical procedures has led to the modern concepts and practice of VATS [2].

In this paper we present the technical aspects of a currently minimally invasive approach in the scenario of modern thoracic surgery, emphasizing its benefits in comparison to conventional open techniques. In addition, considering the fact that the process of technologic improvement is still ongoing and will probably become even more rapid than in the past, we also describe the frontiers that nowadays have been reached by MITS.

Analysis

Traditional Technique to Perform VATS and the Indication of This Approach

VATS emerged as a routine procedure to treat several thoracic diseases after 1990, as it is testified by a multitude of papers inherent to this topic published since this date. Reports from different institutions and the concomitant effort by the industries to improve the efficiency of the surgical instruments gave a contribution to further define in most recent years the precise role of this technique and in treating all those pathologic conditions previously approached via open surgery.

From a practical point of view, VATS is a MITS procedure that usually requires three small incisions (fig. 1) on the chest wall (ports) through which the instruments can be placed to see inside the pleural space (thoracoscope) and to perform a large variety of procedures (operative instruments). As a rule, the VATS technique can be performed only in those patients in whom the placement of an endotracheal double-lumen tube by the anesthesiologist allows the collapse of the affected lung obtaining an effective space within the pleural cavity. However, recent evidence seems to support the feasibility of VATS in the

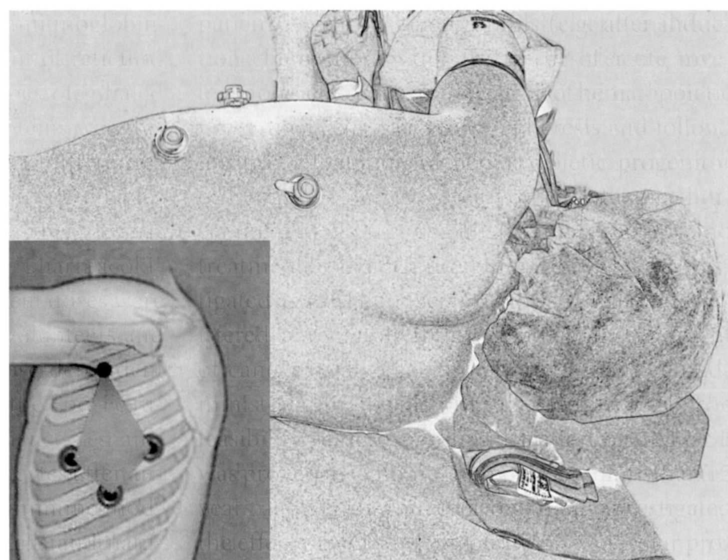

Fig. 1. Usual localization of the ports on the chest wall for conventional VATS technique and the 'baseball diamond'.

Table 1. Absolute and relative contraindication for VATS

Absolute contraindications	Medical contraindication for general anesthesia (i.e. recent cardiac disease, insufficient pulmonary function test, severe coagulopathy)
	Anatomic deformity of the airways or inability to tolerate a single lung ventilation
	Prior decortication or pleurodesis
Relative contraindications	Extensive pleural adhesions or previous intrathoracic procedures
	Target lesion not accessible (i.e. small central tumors)
	Masses with a large involvement of the chest wall
	Thoracic anatomic deformities

awake patient [3]. Table 1 shows the contraindications usually reported in the literature for safely performing this surgical approach.

Technical Aspects. The positions reported of the three incisions can vary depending on the site of the target lesion and it should respect the concept of the so-called 'baseball diamond theory' [4]. Accordingly, the thoracoscope and the other instruments should be positioned in order to obtain a strategic ideal triangulation that allows the maximal visibility and manipulation of the pathologic site (fig. 1). It is also important to take into consideration that during the operation the sites of the scope and of the instruments can be swapped around in order to maximize the visibility and to optimize the operative angles [5].

Over the last two decades the surgical industries have multiplied and refined a multitude of instruments that now make it possible to perform nearly all the procedures traditionally approached with open surgery [6, 7]. Obviously, the introduction of any new technique in thoracic surgery is a challenge that involves not only surgeons, but the entire surgical team (surgeons, anesthesiologists and nurses). Before starting a VATS program the center must have acquired a large and consolidated experience in open thoracic surgery [8].

Applications and Clinical Advantages of the VATS Procedure

The applications of the VATS approach are increasing in modern thoracic surgery as shown and today the VATS approach is the standard of care for many intrathoracic diseases [9–13]. The technical features of VATS lobectomies compared to open surgery have been investigated in several studies [14], although the applied methodology was not always rigorous.

VATS lobectomy as well as minor resections of the lung performed through MITS techniques seem to warrant the same effectiveness of the conventional thoracotomy procedures. Moreover, VATS offers advantages in some clinical aspects when compared to the previous thoracotomy approach. When the results of VATS for minor resections (i.e. wedge resections with curative or diagnostic purposes or for pneumothorax) are compared to open surgery, it is clear that the VATS techniques are associated with a shorter hospital stay and a reduced need for pain medication as a consequence of less postoperative pain [15–18]. At the same time, one randomized controlled trial showed that such advantages were obtained with higher costs in case of lung biopsies for interstitial lung disease [19].

Recently, large case series of patients submitted to VATS lobectomy to treat early-stage NSCLC have been published. Although the information derived from randomized controlled trials is scarce, it appears that VATS lobectomy is associated to less postoperative pain, reduced postoperative complications and mortality rate, shorter chest tube duration and length of stay [13, 20, 21]. In addition, the oncologic results are comparable between traditional surgery and MITS approach to cure patients affected by NSCLC [22, 23].

Recent Evolutions of the MITS

Nowadays the MITS is evolving towards frontiers that in some centers are already the preferred treatment option for specific thoracic diseases. In this scenario the robotically assisted thoracic surgery and the uniportal VATS probably represent the most important evolutions. In, 2008, Melfi and Mussi [24] published a detailed paper about the learning curve and complications related to the robotically assisted lobectomy. Table 2 reports the advantages and disadvantages of VATS compared to robotic surgery as clearly defined in this study. Although some other papers [25, 26] demonstrated the feasibility and safety of this technique for performing several thoracic procedures, this high technologic approach appears to be still in an evolving phase.

At present the most complete device for the robotically assisted surgery is the Da Vinci Robotic System (Surgical Intuitive, Mountain View, Calif., USA) [27]. This high-tech and expensive system is made of a console where the surgeon sits and manipulates two joysticks looking through binoculars that give a three-dimensional view of the operative field. The console is connected to the surgical manipulator which offers two arms directly moved by the surgeon at the console (instrument arms) and another arm to guide the endoscope. Moreover, the instrument is provided with a motion scaling that increases the precision of the surgeon's original movement and at the same time reduces the natural human tremor.

The theoretic and practical phases of the training program should provide the knowledge of a new and extremely technological surgical armamentarium and develop new capabilities inherent to the robotic surgery such as the binocular three-dimensional vision, the sensibility of the joystick and the degrees of the robotic arm movement.

Table 2. Advantages and disadvantages of video-thoracoscopic surgery vs. robotic surgery [from 24, with permission]

	Video-thoracoscopic surgery	Robotic surgery
Advantages	Well-developed technology Affordable and ubiquitous Proved efficacy	Three-dimensional imaging Dexterity Seven degrees of freedom No fulcrum effect No physiologic tremors Scale motions Ergonomic position
Disadvantages	Loss of touch sensation Compromised dexterity Limited degrees of motion Fulcrum effect Amplification of physiologic tremors	No tactile feedback Expensive Unproved benefit

Table 3. Technical recommendations to perform different uniportal VATS procedures [from 28, with permission]

Procedure		Intercostal space	Line	Decubitus
Bullectomy		5th	Posterior-median axillary line	lateral
Lung biopsy or lung resection	upper lobe	5th	Median axillary line	lateral
	middle lobe-lingula	5th–6th	Posterior axillary-scapular line	lateral
	lower lobe	4th	Median-posterior axillary line	lateral
Mediastinal nodes biopsy	middle mediastinum	5th	Scapular line	lateral
	posterior mediastinum	5th	Posterior axillary line	supine
Sympathectomy		3rd	Axillary hair line	lateral
Pericardial window		5th	Axillary line	supine-semilateral

The uniportal VATS represents the evolution of MITS towards the least invasive approach. It can be used to treat several intrathoracic conditions (table 3) with both diagnostic and curative purposes, given its high versatility to reach different targets inside the thoracic cavity [28]. The operative steps and the feasibility of performing lung wedge resection using the uniportal approach were

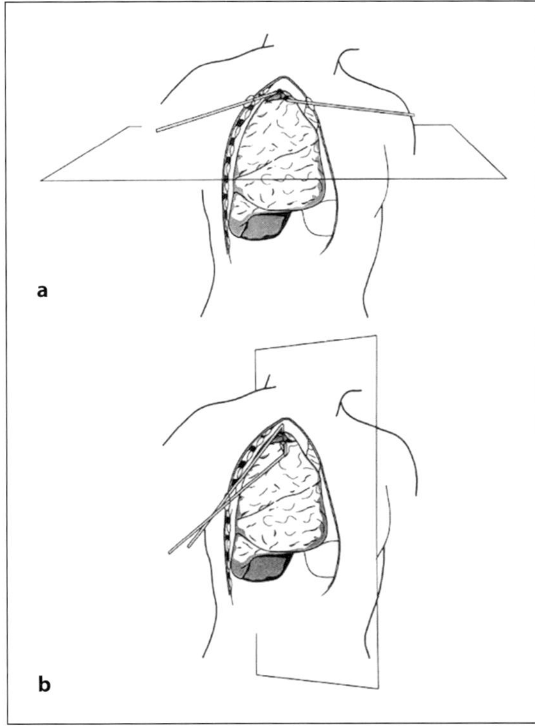

Fig. 2. Diagram representing the different geometric approaches to the pulmonary lesion by (**a**) standard three-port VATS compared with (**b**) uniportal VATS [from 29, with permission].

initially reported in a paper published in 2004 by Rocco et al. [29]. In the uniportal VATS, a single-port incision (about 2.0–2.5 cm long) is used as the unique access to insert the optical source and all the operative instruments. To perform uniportal VATS a radical change of the traditional concepts related to the conventional three-portal VATS is necessary. In fact, in the uniportal VATS technique the geometric approach to reach the target lesion is completely different and it is represented by a sagittal plane where the lesion and the operative instruments should ideally lie (fig. 2).

Taking into consideration this new perspective and the fact that the instruments are inserted through the same port incision, which can be considered the fulcrum for all of them, it is intuitive that the use of roticulating instruments with very small diameter (5.0–3.0 mm) is necessary to reduce at a minimum their mutual interference. Obviously this approach does not allow to mutually change the position of the operative instruments and the optical source during the operation. So it is fundamental to carefully choose the right intercostal space where to place the single incision (table 3).

Considering the clinical benefits of this technique, it seems that the uniportal VATS magnifies the results already obtained with the conventional VATS. In fact, several studies have shown that in comparison to the three-portal VATS, the uniportal VATS can offer clinical advantages for the patient, such as a reduction of pain and paraesthesia, a shorter hospital stay and a shorter time for return to work [29–31]. Interestingly, at least one paper published by Salati et al. [32] that compares the results of uniportal VATS vs. three-portal VATS for treating primary spontaneous pneumothorax demonstrated that the uniportal approach minimizes the global hospital costs.

Discussion

The technical improvements achieved in recent years have made VATS a valuable option for performing minor and major lung resection and a MITS approach has become the first choice to treat many intrathoracic diseases, particularly benign conditions (i.e. primary spontaneous pneumothorax and emphysematous bullae) or lesions without diagnosis (i.e. solitary pulmonary nodule and interstitial lung disease) [9]. The use of VATS is more controversial in case of primary or secondary pulmonary tumors, due to the lack of strong scientific evidence [14].

Although several papers have investigated the benefits of VATS vs. open surgery, demonstrating that the latter is superior in many aspects, we think that the widespread use of VATS would need more prospective randomized trials on several

Table 4. Ideal terms of comparison between the conventional thoracic surgery and VATS

Clinical terms of comparison	Pain quantification Postoperative respiratory function recovery Complication rate reduction Ability to work impairment Chest tube duration Immunocompetence involvement Oncologic benefit Quality of life impact
Cost comparison	Postoperative hospital stay duration Operative cost evaluation Postoperative cost evaluation Recovery to work and social cost

related aspects (table 4). In particular, the potential oncologic benefit of approaching lung cancer by VATS is still not completely known. The demonstration that MITS procedures allow to maintain a high immunocompetence against lung tumors could provide further trust for its use [33]. Undoubtedly, nowadays VATS should be made available in every thoracic surgical unit performing an adequate yearly volume of procedures [34]. Possibly, one or two VATS lobectomists should be part of a surgical team of dedicated thoracic surgeons [35]. Costs of VATS may not necessarily represent an issue when the reduction in length of hospitalization is taken into account [35]. For that reason it seems important to include a VATS training program during the thoracic surgery residency in order to acquire the technical skills to perform a minimally invasive procedure independently and safely [36].

Recommendations

- VATS should be considered the standard of care to treat several lung disease in modern thoracic surgery (diagnosis of pulmonary nodules, surgical lung biopsies for interstitial lung disease, bullectomy for primary spontaneous pneumothorax).
- VATS offers substantial clinical benefits for the patients in comparison to the conventional open approach (reduction of pain and shorter hospital stay).
- A VATS lobectomy program should be developed in every thoracic surgery center given the proved clinical and oncological benefits for treating early-stage NSCLC.

References

1 Jacobaeus HC: The practical importance of thoracoscopy in surgery of the chest. Surg Gynecol Obstet 1922;34: 289–296.
2 Landreneau RJ, Mack MJ, Dowling RD, et al: The role of thoracoscopy in lung cancer management. Chest 1998;113:6S–12S.
3 Pompeo E, Mineo D, Rogliani P, et al: Feasibility and results of awake thoracoscopic resection of solitary pulmonary nodules. Ann Thorac Surg 2004;78:1761–1768.
4 Landreneau RJ, Mack MJ, Hazelrigg SR, et al: Video-assisted thoracic surgery: basic technical concepts and intercostals approach strategies. Ann Thorac Surg 1992;54:800–807.
5 Sasaki M, Hirai S, Kawabe M, et al: Triangle target principle for the placement of trocars during video-assisted thoracic surgery. Eur J Cardiothorac Surg 2005;27:307–312.
6 Ng CSH, Yim APC: Video-assisted thoracoscopic surgery bullectomy for emphysematous/bullous lung disease. MMCTS April 2005:265.
7 Asamura H, Suzuki K, Kondo H, et al: Mechanical vascular division in lung resection. Eur J Cardiothorac Surg 2002; 21:879–882.
8 McKenna RJ: Complications and learning curves for video-assisted thoracic surgery lobectomy. Thorac Surg Clin 2008;18:275–280.
9 Yim APC: VATS major pulmonary resection revisited – controversies, techniques, and results. Ann Thorac Surg 2002;74:615–623.

10 Solli P, Spaggiari L: Indications and developments of video-assisted thoracic surgery in the treatment of lung cancer. Oncologist 2007;12:1205–1214.
11 McKenna RJ Jr, Houck W, Fuller CB: Video-assisted thoracic surgery lobectomy: experience with 1,100 cases. Ann Thorac Surg 2006;81:421–426.
12 Loscertales J, Jimenez-Merchan R, Congregado M, et al: Video-assisted surgery for lung cancer. State of the art and personal experience. Asian Cardiovasc Thorac Ann 2009;17:313–326.
13 Tomaszek SC, Cassivi SD, Shen KR, et al: Clinical outcomes of video-assisted thoracoscopic lobectomy. Mayo Clin Proc. 2009;84:509–513.
14 Sedrakyan A, van der Meulen J, Lewsey J, et al: Video-assisted thoracic surgery for treatment of pneumothorax and lung resections systematic review of randomised clinical trials. BMJ 2004;329: 1008.
15 Waller DA, Forty J, Morritt GN: Video-assisted thoracoscopic surgery versus thoracotomy for spontaneous pneumothorax. Ann Thorac Surg 1994;58: 372–377.
16 Ayed AK, Al-Din HJ: Video-assisted thoracoscopy versus thoracotomy for primary spontaneous pneumothorax: a randomized controlled trial. Med Principles Pract 2000;9:113–118.
17 Santambrogio L, Nosotti M, Bellaviti N, et al: Videothoracoscopy versus thoracotomy for the diagnosis of the indeterminate solitary pulmonary nodule. Ann Thorac Surg 1995;59:868–871.
18 Landreneau RJ, Mack MJ, Dowling RD, et al: The role of thoracoscopy in lung cancer management. Chest 1998;113(suppl):6S-12S.
19 Miller JD, Urschel JD, Cox G, et al: A randomized, controlled trial comparing thoracoscopy and limited thoracotomy for lung biopsy in interstitial lung disease. Ann Thorac Surg 2000;70:1647–1650.
20 Kirby TJ, Mack MJ, Landreneau RJ, et al: Lobectomy – video-assisted thoracic surgery versus muscle-sparing thoracotomy. A randomized trial. J Thorac Cardiovasc Surg 1995;109:997–1002.
21 Flores RM, Park BJ, Dycoco J, et al: Lobectomy by video-assisted thoracic surgery versus thoracotomy for lung cancer. J Thorac Cardiovasc Surg July 2009;138:11–18.
22 Walker WS, Codispoti M, Soon SY, et al: Long-term outcomes following VATS lobectomy for non-small cell bronchogenic carcinoma. Eur J Cardiothorac Surg 2003;23:397–402.
23 Sugi K, Kaneda Y, Esato K: Video-assisted thoracoscopic lobectomy achieves a satisfactory long-term prognosis in patients with clinical stage IA lung cancer. World J Surg 2000;24: 27–31.
24 Melfi FMA, Mussi A: Robotically Assisted Lobectomy: Learning Curve and Complications. Thorac Surg Clin 2008;18:289–295.
25 Bodner J, Wykypiel H, Wetscher G, et al: First experiences with the da Vinci™ operating robot in thoracic surgery. Eur J Cardiothorac Surg 2004;25:844–851.
26 Park BJ, Flores RM, Rusch VW: Robotic assistance for video-assisted thoracic surgical lobectomy: technique and initial results. J Thorac Cardiovasc Surg 2006; 131:54–59.
27 Melfi FMA, Ambrogi MC, Lucchi M, et al: Video robotic lobectomy. MMCTS June 2005:448.
28 Salati M, Brunelli A, Rocco G: Uniportal video-assisted thoracic surgery for diagnosis and treatment of intrathoracic conditions. Thorac Surg Clin 2008;18: 305–310.
29 Rocco G, Martin-Ucar A, Passera E: Uniportal VATS wedge pulmonary resections. Ann Thorac Surg 2004;77:726–728.
30 Rocco G: VATS lung biopsy: the uniportal technique. MMCTS January 2005:356
31 Jutley RS, Khalil MW, Rocco G: Uniportal vs. standard three-port VATS technique for spontaneous pneumothorax: comparison of post-operative pain and residual paraesthesia. Eur J Cardiothorac Surg 2005;28:43–46.
32 Salati M, Brunelli A, Xiume F, et al: Uniportal video-assisted thoracic surgery for primary spontaneous pneumothorax: clinical and economic analysis in comparison to the traditional approach. Interact Cardiovasc Thorac Surg 2008;7: 63–66.
33 Craig SR, Leaver HA, Yap PL, et al: Acute phase responses following minimal access and conventional thoracic surgery. Eur J Cardiothorac Surg 2001;20: 455–463.
34 Klepetko W, Aberg TH, Lerut AE, et al: EACTS/ESTS Working Group on Structures in Thoracic Surgery Structure of General Thoracic Surgery in Europe. Eur J Cardiothorac Surg 2001;20:663–668.
35 Walker WS, Casali G: The VATS lobectomist: analysis of costs and alterations in the traditional surgical working pattern in the modern surgical unit. Thorac Surg Clin 2008;18:281–287.
36 McKenna RJ: Complications and learning curves for video-assisted thoracic surgery lobectomy. Thorac Surg Clin 2008;18:275–280.

Michele Salati, MD
Via A. De Gasperi 17/c
IT–60020 Offagna, Ancona (Italy)
Tel. +39 349 2599 060, Fax +39 071 5964 481
E-Mail michelesalati@hotmail.com

Esquinas AM (ed): Applied Technologies in Pulmonary Medicine. Basel, Karger, 2011, pp 96–101

Acute Lung Collapse during Open-Heart Surgery

Praveen Kumar Neema · S. Manikandan · Ramesh Chandra Rathod

Department of Anaesthesiology, Sree Chitra Tirunal Institute for Medical Sciences and Technology, Trivandrum, Kerala, India

Abbreviations

CPAP	Continuous positive-airway pressure
CPB	Cardiopulmonary bypass
ECMO	Extracorporeal membrane oxygenation
ET	Endotracheal tube
IPPV	Intermittent positive pressure ventilation
OHS	Open-heart surgery
PEEP	Positive end-expiratory pressure
RV	Right ventricle

Patients undergoing OHS invariably suffer either total or partial lung collapse on discontinuation of ventilation during CPB. The collapse of the lung is total if the pleura or chest wall is opened. Acute unyielding lung collapse during OHS is very rare, but if it develops it can seriously compromise respiratory and circulatory functions that may pose life-threatening challenges. This review describes mechanisms of acute lung collapse during OHS, the pathophysiology of cardiovascular and respiratory complications in the presence of acute lung collapse, the measures that help re-expansion of the collapsed lung, the measures that help separation of the patient from CPB in spite of persistent lung collapse and the measures that may prevent acute lung collapse during CPB.

Mechanisms of Acute Lung Collapse

Passive recoil of the lungs occurs when ventilation is discontinued on CPB; passive recoil returns lung volume to its functional residual capacity. The inherent tendency of lungs to collapse is due to fluid lining the alveoli and the presence of elastin fibers in the lung parenchyma; the tendency of collapse is opposed by outward pull by the chest wall, and by the presence of negative intrapleural pressure [1]. The presence of surfactant in the alveolar fluid lining reduces surface tension and decreases the tendency of alveolar collapse; similarly, presence of nitrogen in the alveolar gas delays gaseous absorption, provides stability to the alveoli, and delays alveolar collapse (atelectasis). Despite these opposing forces the lungs gradually collapse on discontinuation of ventilation. The collapsed lungs generally re-expand on manual inflation and resumption of IPPV. Occasionally, because of the obstruction, compression, or collapse of the main airway or its branches or pneumothorax (table 1), it is not possible to achieve complete re-expansion of the lung parenchyma. With extraluminal airway compression, lung collapse occurs only if the obstruction is complete, otherwise it results in air trapping and hyperinflation of the lung supplied by the partially

Table 1. Causes of acute lung collapse during open heart surgery

Intraluminal
Mucous plugs
Inspissations of accumulated secretions
Clotted blood in the airway
Intraluminal lesion
Extraluminal
Left lower lobe bronchus compression due to enlarged left ventricle
Left lower lobe bronchus compression due to aneurysmal left atrium
Left main bronchus compression due to enlarged and tense left pulmonary artery
Left bronchus compression due to transesophageal echocardiography probe
Right middle lobe bronchus compression due to enlarged right pulmonary artery
Right airway compression due to aneurysm of ascending aorta
Direct origin of right upper lobe bronchus from trachea
Vascular ring
Others
Inadvertent advance of the ET tube into the right or left bronchus
Pneumothorax secondary to:
Central venous cannulation
Pleural injury during internal mammary artery dissection
Pleural and lung injury during adhesiolysis in redo open heart surgery
Pleural injury during sternal closure and wiring

compressed airway and compression collapse of the surrounding normal lung parenchyma. The CPB-associated inflammatory responses and loss of surfactant, myocardial dysfunction, and transfusion-related acute lung injury, etc., are other important mechanisms that decrease the lung compliance, increase the inherent tendency of lung collapse and might necessitate application of increased inflation pressures and PEEP to ensure sustained lung expansion.

Pathophysiology of Cardiovascular and Respiratory Complications during Acute Lung Collapse

It is important to understand various aspects of cardiopulmonary interactions between IPPV and the ventricular function. During IPPV the cardiopulmonary interactions depend on cardiac reserve, circulating blood volume, autonomic tone, lung volume, attained intrathoracic pressure and its effects on pulmonary vasculature and juxtacardiac pleural pressure [2]. The cardiopulmonary effects of lung collapse and incomplete lung expansion depend on the magnitude of the lung collapse, the integrity of the pleura, the tidal volume chosen for ventilation, the circulating blood volume, ventricular preload and the contractility of the heart, etc. It should be noted that the small areas of lung collapse are usually of no clinical consequence. Cardiopulmonary interactions manifest as mechanical and physiologic effects. The mechanical effects are due to heterogeneity of airway resistance and lung compliance, and lead to differential ventilation of lung parenchyma including overdistension of compliant alveoli with normal airways, poor ventilation of compliant alveoli with compromised airways and air trapping of alveoli with grossly compromised airways and no ventilation of alveoli with obstructed airways. Additionally, the alveoli are repeatedly subjected to volutrauma as well as barotrauma. The ventilation-perfusion effects vary from no perfusion in overdistended alveoli to absence of ventilation in collapsed alveoli with varying effects on gaseous exchange. The overdistended alveoli act as dead space whereas collapsed alveoli as shunt and others lie within this wide spectrum; this heterogeneity of ventilation-perfusion leads to varying degrees of hypoxemia and hypercapnia. The overdistended alveoli act as Starling's resistor because of collapse of the surrounding capillary network and increased pulmonary vascular resistance. The peak and plateau airway pressures are increased but do not offer a clue to the extent of existing heterogeneity of ventilation and perfusion. The cardiovascular effects are secondary to increased afterload to RV, raised catecholamine levels due to hypoxemia and hypercarbia, and impaired filling of the left ventricle due to decreased RV output and possibly due to a shift of the interventricular septum. The presence of increased peak airway pressure, decreased air entry on auscultation, absent movement of the pleura and presence of visibly collapsed lung confirms the diagnosis. The clinical manifestations during separation from CPB may include raised central venous pressure, visible or echocardiographic demonstration of RV distension with or without interventricular septum shift with or without impaired left ventricular filling, increased pulmonary artery pressure, systemic hypotension, tachycardia, decreased saturation, visible differential ventilation of the lung if the pleura is opened, increasing requirement of inotropes to support the circulation and possible failure to separate the patient from CPB. The afterload to the RV and the possibility of RV failure is greater if the tidal volume and/or the RV preload are increased further in an attempt to improve hemodynamics and arterial blood gases.

Measures That May Help Re-Expansion of the Collapsed Lung

Careful repositioning of the ET tube and/or ET suction generally restores airway integrity. Sustained inflation (up to 45 cm H_2O for approximately 20 s in patients with noncompliant lungs and 40 cm H_2O for approximately 8 s in healthy patients) has been shown to recruit collapsed alveoli [3]. Rarely, it may not be possible to establish a clear airway and in such situations it is not possible to achieve complete re-expansion of the lungs. In the presence of proximal thick airway secretions, the ability to deliver a high inspiratory pressure to recruit collapsed lung units is inhibited. Fiberoptic bronchoscopy offers numerous advantages: it allows the anesthesiologist to visualize the tracheobronchial anatomy, the physical characteristics, the quantity, and the source of the secretions. In addition, extraluminal obstructions can be recognized. The limitation to this technique in the pediatric population is related to the size of the bronchoscope. Pediatric bronchoscopes fit through a 5.0-mm ET tube. However, suctioning through small scopes may be suboptimal, especially when thick secretions are present. The clinical scenario of full CPB can be taken advantage of, however, and allow for temporary removal of the ET tube from the trachea (recognizing that it may be challenging to re-intubate a patient under the surgical drapes). Room for passage of a larger bronchoscope into the trachea and bronchi then becomes available. The larger size scope, with greater suctioning capabilities, will ensure more effective bronchial lavage. Bronchoscopy also assists in repositioning a new ET tube endobronchially for direct ventilation and recruitment of the collapsed lung. An example of this clinical scenario is the cystic fibrosis patient population in whom secretion management, bronchial toilet,

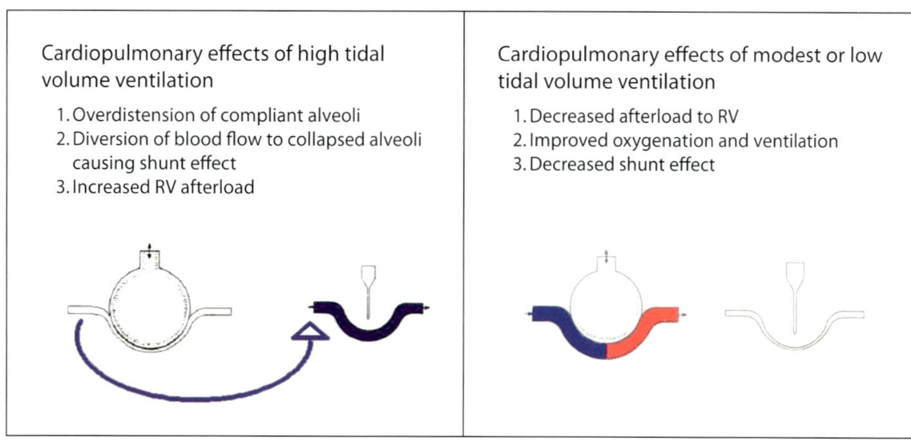

Fig. 1. Schematic diagram explaining the mechanism of improvement in arterial blood gases and decrease in RV afterload with changes in tidal volume in the presence of acute lung collapse.

and lung recruitment are components of the disease treatment [4].

Measures That May Help Separation of the Patient from CPB

It is necessary to have a clear understanding of the underlying pathophysiology. Areas of lung collapse result in asymmetric lung compliance within and between the two lungs and altered respiratory mechanics [5]. In this situation, during IPPV, a greater proportion of the tidal volume distributes to the more compliant areas of the lung. Hypoxic pulmonary vasoconstriction [6] in the areas of lung collapse tends to divert blood flow toward the ventilated areas of the lung and decreases the shunt effect. However, this beneficial effect, diversion of blood flow toward well-ventilated areas of the lung, would be negated if the ventilated areas are hyperinflated (fig. 1). Therefore, in the presence of significant lung collapse, IPPV with normal as well as with larger tidal volume is expected to result in hyperinflation of ventilated areas, increased afterload to the RV, its distention and failure, and failure to wean the patient from CPB [7]. Logically, the appropriate management in such a situation is to facilitate perfusion of the well-ventilated areas of the lung by avoiding hyperinflation of the ventilated areas of the lung (fig. 1). However, how to select an appropriate tidal volume in such a situation is not known. We believe that with modest tidal volume (5–7 ml/kg) ventilation, the compression of the alveolar vessels in the well-ventilated areas is likely to be minimal. Perhaps visual assessment of the effects of chosen tidal volume on airway pressure, lung inflation, and RV volume/distension may provide the key to the appropriateness of the chosen tidal volume. A decreasing peak airway pressure indicates alveolar recruitment and allows further increases in tidal volume and RV preload. An important critical decision in the presence of acute lung collapse is the timing of reversal of anticoagulation. With protamine administration, pulmonary vasoconstriction is known that may result in increased afterload to RV and its failure; therefore, the administration of protamine should be delayed until hemodynamics and pulmonary functions show improvement.

It should also be realized that full hemodynamic support for a certain period of time may be needed; therefore, switching to an ECMO circuit should be considered as an alternative. Femoral vessels accept the cannulae required for full circulatory support, however in small children these vessels are often small. In such situations, use of the carotid artery and internal jugular vein for vascular access provides an alternative access for cannulation and ECMO support. The ECMO is a closed circuit, needs less anticoagulation (activated coagulation times ~160 to 180 s), relies on kinetic drainage, and allows for easy testing for successful weaning.

Measures That May Prevent Acute Lung Collapse during CPB

During CPB the common practice to deflate lungs can contribute to some of the pulmonary dysfunction seen post-CPB; strategies such as mechanical ventilation [8] and CPAP have been tried [9, 10]. However, there has been little proven benefit to these measures. Earlier we use to deflate the lungs during CPB, but of late we routinely apply 2–5 cm of CPAP during CPB depending on the surgeon's comfort; a higher CPAP often forces the lung in the surgical field particularly if the pleura is opened. The value of CPAP lies in easy re-expansion of the partially collapsed lungs on manual inflation. ET suction, particularly in the presence of left heart failure, chronic obstructive and restrictive pulmonary disease, and in potentially infected patients, would ensure a clear airway and is useful. For thoracotomy approaches, Mittnacht et al. [11] describe lung isolation by using a double-lumen endobronchial tube and application of CPAP, during CPB, to the dependent lung. In patients where insertion of a double-lumen endobronchial tube is not possible, use of a bronchial blocker allows lung isolation, allowing for both surgical exposure and dependent lung ventilation.

Besides these mechanical issues that result in pulmonary dysfunction, there are systemic sequelae related to CPB that can have deleterious physiologic effects as well. The inflammatory response includes activation of mediators such as interleukins, leukotrienes, and polymorphonuclear cells that have been implicated in lung injury. Leukocyte depletion, hemofiltration, use of asanguineous prime, preoperative treatment with steroids, and intraoperative aprotinin have all been used to attenuate the inflammatory response. However, attempts to mitigate the inflammatory response or its sequelae have not been successful. In fact, Chaney et al. [12] showed that patients receiving methylprednisolone actually had worsened post-CPB pulmonary function. It was believed that aprotinin had anti-inflammatory properties that might reduce some of the end-organ damage seen, but given the controversies surrounding this drug, its routine use has been questioned.

Recommendations

- Lung collapse during CPB, on discontinuation of ventilation, occurs invariably in patients undergoing OHS. The collapsed lungs generally re-expand on manual inflation and resumption of IPPV. Minor areas of lung collapse are of no clinical significance.
- The clinical manifestations of significant lung collapse during separation from CPB may include raised central venous pressure, visible or echocardiographic demonstration of RV distension with or without interventricular septum shift with or without impaired left ventricular filling, increased pulmonary artery pressure, systemic hypotension, tachycardia, decreased peripheral saturation, visible differential ventilation of the lung if the pleura is opened.
- Careful ET suction and/or repositioning of the ET tube generally resolves the airway

issues. The fiberoptic bronchoscopy allows the anesthesiologist to visualize the ET tube position, tracheobronchial anatomy, the physical characteristics, the quantity, and the source of the secretions. However, suctioning through small scopes may be suboptimal, especially when thick secretions are present. Bronchoscopy also assists in repositioning a new ET tube endobronchially for direct ventilation and recruitment of the collapsed lung.

- Ventilation with modest tidal volume (5–7 ml/kg) and careful preloading of the RV help separation of the patient from CPB. A decreasing peak airway pressure indicates alveolar recruitment and allows further increases in tidal volume and RV preload. In the presence of lung collapse and increased central venous pressures, protamine should be administered carefully.
- Application of CPAP of 2–5 cm during CPB allows easy re-expansion of the collapsed lung on manual inflation.

References

1 West JB: Mechanics of breathing; in West JB (ed): Best and Taylor's Physiological Basis of Medical Practice. New Delhi, B.I. Waverly Pvt Ltd, 1996, pp 560–587.

2 Pinsky MR: Heart-lung interactions; in Grenvik A, Ayres SM, Holbrook PR, Shoemaker WC (eds): Textbook of Critical Care, ed 4. Noida/India, Harcourt Asia Pte Ltd, 2000, pp 1204–1221.

3 Rothen HU, Neumann P, Berglund JE, et al: Dynamics of re-expansion atelectasis during general anesthesia. Br J Anaesth 1999;82:551–556.

4 Slieker MG, Van Gestel JP, Heijerman HG, et al: Outcome of assisted ventilation for acute respiratory failure in cystic fibrosis. Intensive Care Med 2006;32: 754–758.

5 Carlon GC, Ray C Jr, Klein R, et al: Criteria for selecting positive end expiratory pressure and independent synchronized ventilation of each lung. Chest 1978;74: 501–507.

6 Benumof JL: General respiratory physiology and respiratory function during anesthesia, in Benumof JL (ed): Anesthesia for Thoracic Surgery. Philadelphia, Saunders, 1995, pp 43–122.

7 Neema PK, Manikandan S, Ahuja A, et al: Difficult weaning from cardiopulmonary bypass in the lateral position caused by lung collapse. J Cardiothorac Vasc Anesth 2008;22:616–624.

8 Lake C, Booker PD: Pediatric Cardiac Anesthesia, ed 4. Philadelphia, Lippincott Williams & Wilkins, 2005.

9 Altmay E, Karaca P, Yurtseven N, et al: Continuous positive airway pressure does not improve lung function after cardiac surgery. Can J Anesth 2006;53: 919–925.

10 Loeckinger A, Kleinasser A, Linner KH, et al: Continuous positive airway pressure at 10 cm H_2O during cardiopulmonary bypass improves postoperative gas exchange. Anesth Analg 2000;91:522–527.

11 Mittnacht AJ, Jashi U, Nguyen K, et al: Continuous positive airway pressure and lung separation during cardiopulmonary bypass to facilitate congenital heart surgery via the right thorax in children. Pediatr Anesth 2007;17:693–696.

12 Chaney MA, Durazo-Arvizu RA, Nikolov MP, et al: Methylprednisolone does not benefit patients undergoing coronary artery bypass graft surgery. J Thorac Cardiovasc Surg 2001;121:561–569.

Dr. Praveen Kumar Neema
B-9, NFH, Sree Chitra Residential Quarters
Poonthi Road, Kumarpuram, Trivandrum, Kerala 695011 (India)
Tel. +91 471 2557 321, Fax +91 471 2446 433
E-Mail neema@sctimst.ac.in, praveenneema@yahoo.co.in

Esquinas AM (ed): Applied Technologies in Pulmonary Medicine. Basel, Karger, 2011, pp 102–106

Anesthesia in the Intraoperative MRI Environment

Sergio D. Bergese · Erika G. Puente

Department of Anesthesiology, The Ohio State University, Columbus, Ohio, USA

Abbreviations

ASA American Society of Anesthesiologists
ECG Electrocardiography
iMRI Intraoperative magnetic resonance imaging
MR Magnetic resonance
MRI Magnetic resonance imaging
OR Operating room

MRI technology has gradually acquired a prominent role in the iMRI environment. This modern equipment can provide substantial benefits when incorporated as a diagnostic, monitoring and treatment tool in the iMRI setting. At the same time, incorporating the MRI technology can add an extra challenge for the anesthesiologist and healthcare providers involved. Safety, for both the patient and the OR staff, and adequate monitoring are the main concerns for the anesthesia provider when dealing with MRI equipment into the OR. As in many surgical environments, the primary goals of the anesthetic management in the iMRI setting are to avoid heart rate and blood pressure fluctuations, hypoxia, hypercapnia, to prevent increased venous pressure, and to allow for a rapid recovery, which in turn allows for an early neurological assessment [1].

In order to accomplish optimal anesthesia management in the iMRI setting, there are several special considerations that need to be addressed, including the OR design, whether the equipment is MRI-compatible or not, patient monitoring, safety and personnel.

The design of the OR requires special considerations in terms of size, logistics, and distribution of space and equipment. The room must be larger than the standard ORs in order to allow enough space for the equipment and allow proper access to the patient. The challenge of being able to balance the requirements of access to the patient and the magnetic field strength in and around the room must be taken into consideration. A larger room will allow enough space to install an MRI machine, a portable shield, if required, and to move the patient in and out of the MRI core. A larger room can also facilitate the transit of an increased number of hospital personnel, who are required in the iMRI suite to provide adequate care of the patient. The size of the room should also allow for the incorporation of special 'MR-safe' equipment, designed to minimize interference from the magnetic field, and to ensure an adequate distance from the location where this field is the strongest. Since these devices have some ferromagnetic properties, maintaining a specific distance from the magnet is required in order to avoid attraction of these objects into the magnet.

The specific room design will be determined according to the use of the scanner and the types of procedures to be conducted in that OR. MRI in the OR may be used for solely monitoring purposes or for surgical guidance during a procedure.

These applications need to be taken into consideration for the final design. Monitoring surgical progress and tissue changes, and confirming the accomplishment of the surgical goal can be achieved with intermittent imaging performed at predetermined points during the operation. Conversely, in the case of continuous real-time MR guidance of surgical tools such as biopsy needles, endoscopes, or laser fibers, throughout the procedure demands a more sophisticated MRI system [2].

Currently, there are two types of ORs that have been designed which incorporate the MRI technology. In the first, the MRI is incorporated into the permanent construction of the OR. This is more frequently used with high-field MRI technology. This structure is permanent and allocates the OR entirely for iMRI use. The second is a mobile design, which is compatible with most models of low-field MRI scanners. This design requires the use of a portable shield or portable Faraday cage. This design renders the OR suitable for two different uses, with the iMRI and without, the latter allows its use as a regular OR. The unique design of the portable cage requires a closed shield so that it collapses into the shape of an accordion when not in use. The bottom of the cage is a permanent stainless steel shield, which is located under the OR table. The shiny finish of the stainless steel plate below the OR table can reflect onto the images causing artifacts and corruption on image appearance. Therefore, a matte finish is recommended for the floor shield of the Faraday cage.

Additionally, the bottom of the accordion-shaped shield must have an aluminum foil type wrapping that when making contact with the floor will act as an impermeable shield. It is critical to ensure that the bottom of the Faraday cage surrounding the stainless steel plate is properly positioned to provide adequate sealing of the cage. Devices, such as infusion pumps, plasma and liquid crystal displays, physiologic monitors, and computers can generate a detectable electric noise trace. The Faraday cage has been specially designed to minimize the impact of this low-energy electric noise on the magnetic field and therefore the quality of the images [3].

In order to decrease the interference with the magnetic field as much as possible and achieve high-quality interpretation, the set-up of the OR in preparation for the scanning is crucial. The set-up usually involves a multi-step process from patient positioning, to portable shield preparation, to monitoring equipment placement. The anesthesiologist must take into consideration that the use of tubing extension is required in order to adequately reach the patient. It is also necessary to have more than one intravenous access, telemetry ECG monitoring, fiberoptic temperature skin probes, pulse oximeter, blood pressure cuff, and vital signs monitors. All of these must be arranged properly so as to minimize the possibility of moving, interrupting, or disconnecting the breathing circuit, infusion lines, or monitoring cables with the Faraday cage. This preparation requires the involvement of numerous trained hospital staff in order to have the patient safely ready for the magnet to be positioned and be able to initiate the scanning. Barua et al. [4] described a learning curve effect in the set-up time that significantly decreased the set-up time with increased training of the staff.

There are also certain constraints and hazards to consider when incorporating MRI technology into the OR environment. These are mainly related to the monitoring equipment, anesthesia machine, and infusion devices. According to the ASA, monitoring standards of the patient's ventilation, circulation, temperature, and oxygenation should be continuously evaluated throughout the entire procedure. A restriction of the portable iMRI setting is that during the time the patient is inside the Faraday cage, within the bore of the scanner, they are not under direct supervision or visibility of the anesthesiologist for the duration of the scan. During this period, it is essential to assure adequate temperature control, continuous ventilatory support, intravenous drugs or contrast media infusions, and inhalation anesthetics, in compliance with the ASA guidelines [5]. The anesthesiologist must also be certain that the appropriate drugs and equipment are readily available in case of encountering unexpected airway or cardiovascular complications [1].

The role of the anesthesiologist is most important when promoting safety in order to minimize accidents associated with the iMRI technology. To ensure adequate patient monitoring and supervision, the anesthesiologist must perform a detailed MRI compatibility preoperative examination. This exam should include exploring for history of acquired or implanted metallic devices in the patient, such as cerebrovascular clips, cardiac pacemakers, stents, bullets, braces, dentures, or even extensive tattoos. These metallic devices may generate imaging artifacts, may move from their place and cause trauma, or may even heat up and produce severe burns.

The anesthesiologist must be hasty to request MR-compatible medical supplies to avoid such complications. For instance, a specific detail to remember when fastening the endotracheal tube by inflating the safety balloon, the balloon needs to be drawn away from the patient's face. The safety balloon from the endotracheal tube has a metallic component that can cause serious burns to the patient's skin. In some institutions the use of temperature Foley catheters is very common. The anesthesiologist must be aware that for iMRI these catheters must not be used and instead, replaced with a standard Foley catheter without a temperature probe. The temperature probe is also metallic and can produce severe local burns in the bladder and proximal urethra. For temperature monitoring, a MRI-compatible probe is recommended.

During the scan, the magnet will generate a strong magnetic field that can interfere with monitoring and anesthetic equipment. This may affect or cause failure of electrical, electronic, or mechanical life support and monitoring equipment [6]. At the same time, the monitoring equipment can interfere with the nuclear magnetic signals, leading to poor-quality images [1]. Special non-ferromagnetic equipment has been designed over time to decrease interference as much as possible with the iMRI system, and in turn obtaining the highest quality imaging as possible. Unfortunately, this results in considerable cost increments.

Non-magnetic MRI equipment available includes continuous infusion pumps and vital signs monitors. There are also non-magnetic MRI laryngoscope handles and blades that function with non-magnetic MRI lithium laryngoscope batteries. It is important to point out that the rechargeable batteries should never be recharged in the presence of the electromagnetic field.

Other important aspects to take into consideration when providing anesthesia in the iMRI setting is the length of the different tubing systems required. In order for the intravenous tubing to reach the patient within the Faraday cage, it is necessary to use extension tubing. Adequately long breathing tubes are also required due to the remote location of the anesthesia machine. This extended anesthesia circuit may pose additional challenges for the anesthesia provider to maintain adequate ventilation and administration of drugs. The dead space from the extensions creates a time delay upon the administration of volatile anesthetics and drugs before the expected onset of effects can be observed [3].

One of the most vulnerable signals affected by the high-energy radiofrequency pulses and electric noise generated by the iMRI technology is the ECG signaling. This can be decreased by the use of safeguarded cables, telemetry, or fiberoptic machinery [1]. The use of telemetry for ECG eliminates the use of wires. The ECG electrodes must be non-magnetic or 'MR-safe' to protect the patient from potential injuries and should be placed carefully to minimize MRI-related artifacts [7]. The use of special shielded non-magnetic MRI pulse oximeters is also recommended.

Equipment can be modified so that it can be used within a range from the MRI scanner and therefore can be designated as either 'MR-safe', 'MR-unsafe' or 'MR-conditional'. Equipment that is 'MR-compatible' not only is proven safe but does not interfere with the quality of the scanner. Some special equipment considerations when monitoring a patient during iMRI [8–10] include the following: (1) *Blood pressure:* utilize MRI-safe or MRI-compatible blood pressure monitors. (2) *ECG:* only MRI-compatible ECG pads should be used and the use of special MRI-compatible electrocardiographic leads is recommended in order to minimize interference with the readings. (3) *Ventilation:* consider visibility impairment of chest movements. We recommend the use of respiratory capnography that is usually available in MR-compatible systems. (4) *Oxygenation:* to prevent severe burns from the pulse oximeter cables we recommend the use of MR-specific fiberoptic pulse oximeters which do not overheat. (5) *Temperature:* the magnet may produce overheating during the scan or the temperature may decrease from the air conditioning required to protect the superconductors.

Finally, patients should be educated on this procedure prior to undergoing their surgery under iMRI techniques, as well as the hospital staff should be adequately trained and requested to complete a detailed MRI compatibility exam, when required to ambulate within the iMRI setting.

Recommendations

- Ensure adequate patient safety by performing a detailed MRI compatibility preoperative examination (verify if the patient does not have acquired or implanted metallic device, such as cerebrovascular clips, cardiac pacemakers, stents, bullets, braces, dentures, or even extensive tattoos).
- Ensure that the patients are aware of the procedure and know what to expect from the use of the scanner during such procedure, e.g. use of additional tubing, loud noise of the magnet during the scanning periods, colder room temperature setting.
- Ensure that the anesthesia and monitoring equipment is MR-safe before being utilized and introduced into the iMRI setting.
- Ensure that during the time the patient is not under the direct visual supervision of the anesthesiologist there is reliable and accurate monitoring of pulse oximetry, electroencephalographic signaling, blood pressure and temperature control, and continuous ventilatory support in compliance with the ASA standard.
- Ensure that intravenous drug administration, contrast media infusions, inhalation anesthetics, and supplemental oxygen availability and delivery follow ASA guidelines.
- Ensure that the appropriate drugs and equipment are readily available in case of encountering unexpected airway or cardiovascular complication.

References

1 Kraayenbrink M, McAnulty G: Neuroanesthesia; in Moore JA, Newell DW (eds): Neurosurgery: Principles and Practice. London, Springer, 2005.

2 Scott A: Interventional and Intraoperative Magnetic Resonance Imaging. Copyright Alberta Heritage Foundation for Medical Research (2004). Available at http://www.ihe.ca/documents/ip17.pdf (accessed March 2010).

3 Bergese SD, Puente EG: Anesthesia in the intraoperative MRI environment. Neurosurg Clin N Am 2009;20:155–162.

4 Barua E, Johnston J, Fujii J, et al: Anesthesia for brain tumor resection using intraoperative magnetic resonance with the polestar N-20 system: experience and challenges. J Clin Anesth 2009;21: 371–376.
5 Standards for Basic Anesthetic Monitoring Committee of Origin: Standards and practice parameters. Approved by the House of Delegates of October 21, 1986, and last amended on October 25, 2005. Available at http://www.asahq.org/publicationsAndServices/sgstoc.htm (accessed September 2009).
6 Bendo AA, Kass IS, Hartung J, et al: Anesthesia for neurosurgery; in Barash PG, Cullen BF, Stoelting RK (eds): Clinical Anesthesia, ed 5. Philadelphia, Lippincott-Raven, 2006.
7 Trankina MF: Neurodiagnostic procedures; in Cucchiara RF, Black S, Michenfelder JD (eds): Clinical Neuroanesthesia, ed 2. New York, Churchill Livingstone, 1998.
8 Stoelting RK, Miller RD: Basics of Anesthesia, ed 5. Philadelphia, Churchill Livingstone, 2007.
9 Dorsch JA, Dorsch SE (eds): Equipment for the Magnetic Resonance Imaging Environment; in Understanding Anesthesia Equipment, ed 5. Philadelphia, Lippincott Williams & Wilkins, 2008.
10 American Society of Anesthesiologists: Practice advisory on anesthetic care for magnetic resonance imaging. A report by the ASA task force on anesthetic care for magnetic resonance Imaging. Anesthesiology 2009;110:459–479.

Erika G. Puente, MD
Department of Anesthesiology, The Ohio State University
410 W 10th Ave, N411 Doan Hall, Columbus, OH 43210 (USA)
Tel. +1 614 293 8487, Fax +1 614 293 8153
E-Mail Erika.puente@osumc.edu

Esquinas AM (ed): Applied Technologies in Pulmonary Medicine. Basel, Karger, 2011, pp 107–113

Awake Thoracic Epidural Anesthesia Pulmonary Resections

Eugenio Pompeo · Federico Tacconi · Tommaso Claudio Mineo

Cattedra di Chirurgia Toracica, Policlinico Università Tor Vergata, Rome, Italy

Abbreviations

TEA Thoracic epidural anesthesia
VATS Video-assisted thoracoscopic surgery

VATS is now routinely employed to perform non-anatomical pulmonary resections in a number of neoplastic and non-neoplastic conditions. In these instances, general anesthesia with one-lung ventilation is considered mandatory to accomplish a safe operation. However, the use of this type of anesthesia can induce several adverse effects [1] that increase the overall invasiveness of the procedure with a potentially negative impact on morbidity and hospitalization time.

In order to avoid these detrimental effects, we have started in 2001 a clinical research program of VATS pulmonary resections performed by sole TEA in spontaneously ventilating, awake patients [2–4]. So far, awake VATS resection of undetermined nodules [2], solitary metastases [3], and even non-small cell lung cancer have been reported [4]. In these early series, results have been encouraging although awake VATS pulmonary resections must be still considered investigational procedures since indications, comparative results with standard surgical approaches and many pathophysiological aspects remain to be elucidated. Moreover, currently, few surgeons do perform awake thoracic surgery procedures and some skepticism still survives regarding their feasibility and potential advantages.

In this article we sought to review the current state of the art of this fascinating, newly available surgical option.

Background

Videothoracoscopy

The first thoracoscopy probably dates back to 1865 when the Irish physician Francis Richard Cruise employed a modified Désormeaux's cystoscope to perform a binocular thoracoscopy in an 11-year-old girl with empyema. Nonetheless, the Swedish internist Hans Jacobaeus contributed to disseminate this minimally invasive technique that he initially employed to sever pleural adhesions and thus help lung collapse during the Forlanini's artificial pneumothorax [5]. Following this pioneering work, thoracoscopy remained underused for decades being relegated to a minor role in management of undetermined pleural diseases and effusions.

The eclipse of thoracoscopy lasted until the early 1990s when the introduction of video technology and magnified imaging led to the explosive birth of the modern videothoracoscopic surgery. This minimally invasive surgical approach was immediately thought to mandate general anesthesia and one-lung ventilation to allow adequate surgical manipulation of the lung and easy accomplishment of several types of surgical procedures including lung resections.

Awake Thoracic Surgery

As far as the use of regional anesthesia in thoracic surgery is concerned, in 1950, Buckingham et al. [6] reported on 617 thoracic surgical operations including thoracoplasties, pneumonectomies, plumbage with acrylate pack, lobectomies, and open pneumolysis, performed through sole epidural anesthesia. More recently, use of regional anesthesia in thoracoscopy was advocated in 1984 by Boutin et al. [7] in France and in 1987 by Rusch and Mountain [8] in the USA to diagnose and manage pleural diseases. Reports of awake VATS pulmonary resection are much more recent and scant; wedge resection was first reported in 1997 by Nezu et al. [9] to resect blebs in patients with spontaneous pneumothorax, whereas more recently our group reported on videothoracoscopic resection of undetermined pulmonary nodules [2].

Anesthesia

Adverse Effects of General Anesthesia

The birth of modern thoracic surgery coincided with the development of double-lumen endobronchial tubes permitting single-lung ventilation that were adapted for surgery by Björk and Carlens [10] in 1950. Unfortunately, despite some indisputable advantages, general anesthesia with single-lung ventilation can cause several adverse effects including hemodynamic disturbances and a multifactorial mechanical-ventilation-related injury [1].

Tekinbas et al. [11] have recently shown that biochemical and histopathologic injury occur in collapsed lung during one-lung ventilation possibly due to generation of oxygen-derived free radicals as a consequence of a sort of ischemia reperfusion tissue injury caused by intraoperative-atelectasis-postoperative-reventilation of lung tissue. Moreover, Hemmerling et al. [12] have recently shown that 70% of patients undergoing thoracic surgery with one-lung ventilation longer than 1 h suffered from cerebral desaturation >20% from their baseline. This level of deoxygenation is accepted as the threshold of cerebral ischemia and can be associated with a high incidence of postoperative cognitive and major cerebral dysfunction.

Physiologic disturbances associated with single-lung ventilation in the lateral position include hypoxic pulmonary vasoconstriction in the nondependent lung, an overall increase in venous admixture from about 10% to more than 27% [13], a decrease in oxygen partial pressure, and a change in alveolar-arterial oxygen tension gradient [14]. In addition, one-lung ventilation has shown to enhance the hypothalamus-pituitary-adrenal axis response to surgical stress [15], which eventually impairs activity of natural killer cells. Yet, a complex series of compartmental changes in both the ventilated and the non-ventilated lung can stimulate local release of pro-inflammatory mediators and oxidative stress products [1].

The rationale for performing videothoracoscopic operations in awake patients through regional anesthesia is to avoid the adverse effects of general anesthesia and mechanical ventilation, maintain more physiologic muscular, neurologic and cardiopulmonary conditions, and create a satisfactory environment for surgical maneuvering while providing optimal thoracic analgesia. Nonetheless, some theoretical concerns arise in this regard since the need of operating on a ventilating lung may reveal more technically demanding and the idea still survives that surgical pneumothorax in a spontaneously ventilating patient is poorly tolerated and increases operative risk.

Physiologic Effects of Epidural Anesthesia

In awake patients under local or epidural anesthesia, we can attain the best type of monitoring, namely neurologic vigilance. The net effect of TEA on lung function is mainly determined by the extension of the motor blockade depending on the height of the insertion of the catheter, the choice of local anesthetic and its concentration. Evidence exists that TEA may potentially impair to some extent dynamic lung volumes. It has been suggested that following limited sensory block from dermatome T1 to T5, vital capacity is decreased by 5.6% and FEV_1 by 4.9% [16], an effect which can be explained by a direct motor blockade of intercostal muscles. Yet, the effect of sympathicolysis could result in an unopposed vagal tone leading to increased bronchial tone and reactivity. Nevertheless, we did not find any remarkable change in small airway flows and Tiffeneau index during spirometric examinations performed during awake VATS. This seems to suggest that TEA had no significant detrimental effects on bronchial tone in these patients.

TEA improves diaphragmatic contractility [17] and breathing pattern, and provides better postoperative analgesia than patient-controlled intravenous administration of opioids. In fact, we have reasoned that one of the effects that contribute to keep respiratory function satisfactory throughout awake VATS, is the maintained diaphragmatic motion that might decrease the detrimental effect of the abdominal pressure leading the paralyzed diaphragm to compress the dependent lung during general anesthesia.

Following general anesthesia, early postoperative lung function is influenced by residual muscular relaxation, the time of extubation, pain therapy, and vigilance. In particular, immediately after an operation, the ability to cough seems to be one of the most important factors affecting lung function and depends in great part on the efficacy of diaphragmatic contraction and pain relief.

Conversely, in awake VATS, the absence of diaphragmatic relaxation, better synchronization of rib-cage-abdominal motion, and preserved ability to cough are all contributing factors that justify the better ventilation observed in these patients when compared to those operated on through general anesthesia.

Cardiovascular effects of epidural anesthesia include decreased determinants of myocardial oxygen demand, improved myocardial blood flow and left ventricular function, and reduced thrombotic-related complications. Furthermore, it has been shown that epidural anesthesia can reduce heart rate and occurrence of arrhythmias in pulmonary resections [16, 18].

Epidural Anesthesia in Awake VATS

TEA is carried out to achieve somatosensory and motor block from T1 to T8 level, while preserving diaphragmatic motion. The epidural catheter is inserted at the T4 level to achieve an optimal analgesia to the targeted hemithorax. Analgesia is induced with a 20-cc bolus of 2% ropivacaine + sufentanil 5 μg/ml and the patient is placed in lateral decubitus position for about 15–20 min with the side targeted for surgery in a dependent position to help gravity distribution of anesthetics. Sensory level is tested every 5 min with warm-cold discrimination and/or pinprick tests. Care is taken to avoid extending sympathetic block over T1 level, which can be disclosed by the development of a Bernard-Horner syndrome.

Oral or intravenous premedication with benzodiazepines is useful in anxious patients. We recommend usage of short-acting sedatives at minimum dosage to assure a light sedation while maintaining adequate patient's vigilance and awakeness. Intravenous opioids are preferably avoided due to their recently described potential depression of cortical centers controlling voluntary respiration [19].

Intraoperatively, continuous infusion of ropivacaine 0.5% with sufentanil 1.66 μg/ml is delivered into the epidural space at a rate of 5–7 ml/h via an elastomeric device. Peripheral oxygen saturation is continuously monitored and additional

O_2 is given through a Venturi mask only if room air ventilation leads to a drop of saturation below 90%. A potential intraoperative adverse effect is the development of a panic attack, which can be triggered by either an unsatisfactory analgesia or by dyspnea that may occur following induction of the surgical pneumothorax, particularly in patients with poor pulmonary function and hypercapnia. Although the exact etiology of panic attacks is still unknown, it has been suggested that an abnormal sensitivity to CO_2 and disturbances of acid-base balance in brainstem could trigger an erroneous 'suffocation alarm' by the locus coeruleus neurons [20].

During wound closure, the epidural anesthetic regimen is changed to ropivacaine 0.16% and sufentanil 1 μg/ml at 2–5 ml/h for postoperative analgesia. The epidural catheter is removed 24–48 h after surgery. Postoperatively, liquids infusion is stopped immediately and drinking, meal intake, ambulation and physiotherapy can be started on the same day of surgery [4].

Surgery

Physiolologic Effects of Surgical Pneumothorax

In physiologic conditions, intrapleural pressures are negative throughout most of the respiratory cycle. Instead, during awake videothoracoscopic surgery procedures, atmospheric air enters the pleural cavity and induces an immediate collapse of the non-dependent lung, the degree of which is related to a series of factors including absence of pleural adhesions anchoring the lung to the chest wall, the elastic properties of the lung and resistances of the airways.

Regarding the effect of an open pneumothorax on oxygenation, some human and animal investigations suggested that changes in ventilation/perfusion ratio are more relevant that impairment in ventilation. Anthonisen [21] found that a pneumothorax of 25–40% in extent is associated with an even redistribution of ventilation in the collapsed lung, which alters the physiologic regional ventilation/perfusion ratios within the lung and seems to play a major role in determining the degree of intraoperative hypoxia. However, in our clinical experience, we have found that following the surgical pneumothorax, the decrease in arterial oxygenation is usually of limited extent and can be corrected by oxygen administration through a Venturi mask. A hypothetical explanation of this effect might be that a certain ventilatory excursion is still maintained in the collapsed lung despite the presence of intrapleural atmospheric pressure [22]. In addition, it is likely that in most instances a sufficient degree of compensatory ventilation is assured by the dependent lung whose efficiency is increased by the maintained diaphragmatic function.

A frequent finding in awake VATS is the development of intraoperative hypercarbia [23]. In this respect, although the reduced tidal ventilation may be regarded as the major causative mechanism, this fails to explain why sometimes hypercarbia is not paralleled by a relevant decrease in oxygenation. We hypothesize that perioperatively, a certain degree of rebreathing effect may occur due to the existence of inter-pleural pressure gradients. Nonetheless, the increase in $PaCO_2$ is usually well tolerated even in patients with severe emphysema [23] and rarely requires conversion to general anesthesia and mechanical ventilation. Yet, we have shown that it resolves within 1 h after the completion of the awake surgical procedure [24] (fig. 1).

Awake VATS Resection of Undetermined Pulmonary Nodules

Overall, all candidates suitable of videothoracoscopic resection of a pulmonary nodule and who have no contraindications for TEA are theoretically eligible for an awake approach. In a randomized comparison of 60 patients with undetermined solitary pulmonary nodules who underwent thoracoscopic wedge resection through either sole TEA or general anesthesia with double-lumen

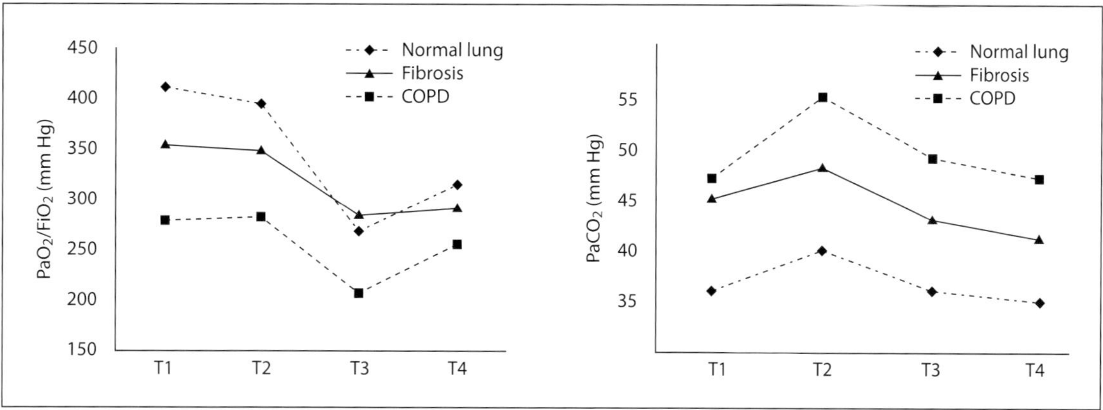

Fig. 1. Perioperative behavior of PaO_2/FiO_2 ratio and $PaCO_2$ assessed at four fixed time intervals: T1 = closed chest in lateral decubitus; T2 = after creation of the surgical pneumothorax; T3 = end of the surgical procedure; T4 = 1 h after the operation.

intubation plus TEA [11], we had found no difference in technical feasibility although 2 patients in each group required conversion due to unexpected lung cancer requiring lobectomy. Comparative results amongst study groups showed that anesthesia satisfaction score, changes in arterial oxygenation, need of nursing care and median hospital stay were significantly better in the awake group [2].

It is likely that in spontaneously ventilating awake patients, avoidance of general anesthesia- and single-lung-ventilation-related adverse effects resulted in a more physiologic lung reexpansion and a faster recovery with immediate resumption of normal daily life activities. As a result, 47% of the patients in the awake group could be discharged within the second postoperative day whereas this was possible only in 17% of patients in the control group.

Awake VATS Pulmonary Metastasectomy

Videothoracoscopic pulmonary metastasectomy is advocated in patients with single peripheral lung lesions although the accuracy of digital and instrumental lung palpation by VATS has been questioned.

Our surgical strategy in patients with pulmonary metastases is based on the assumption that since iterative operations can be required to prolong survival, it might be better to employ a less invasive surgical approach initially, while deserving more aggressive ones for eventual reexplorations in case of relapse. For this reason, in 1999 we had developed the transxiphoid approach [25] that allowed to accomplish bimanual palpation of the lung during VATS metastasectomy to help identify all lung lesions that might have been missed by sole instrumental palpation.

More recently, we have proposed a new surgical approach entailing awake VATS metastasectomy through TEA [3] in order to minimize surgical and immunological stress that has been hypothesized as a potential cause of further cancer metastasization.

Eligibility criteria include complete control of the primary tumor and absence of extrapulmonary metastases, a newly discovered solitary pulmonary nodule localized in the peripheral one third of the lung and measuring <3 cm at the helical computed tomography. Exclusion criteria included the presence of multiple metastases, radiologic evidence of pleural scarring and/or a history of previous thoracic surgery on side targeted for metastasectomy.

In a 14-patient cohort undergoing awake VATS metastasectomy at our institution, the procedure was easily and safely accomplished in all patients under sole TEA with no operative mortality or major morbidity. Awake pulmonary metastasectomy resulted in optimal patient acceptance and satisfaction which was rated as excellent to good in 12 patients (86%). Hospital stay was significantly shorter than in a control group operated through general anesthesia, while oncologic results and survival were similar [3].

Awake VATS Resection of Lung Cancer

Resection of lung cancer represents the most provocative indication for awake VATS pulmonary resection although it is worth noting that in a recent series even awake anatomic lung resections through thoracotomy have been reported by Al-Abdullatief et al. [26].

Proposed inclusion criteria for awake resection of lung cancer include peripheral stage I lesions, poor pulmonary function or other important comorbidity leading to consider the patient high-risk for anatomical resection and/or even sole general anesthesia [4]. A further indication for this approach might entail the resection of peripheral tumors in medically inoperable patients already treated with non-surgical local therapies such as percutaneous radiofrequency ablation or stereotactic radioablation.

Our initial results have been encouraging and in the first patients operated on there was no mortality or major morbidity with satisfactory 2-year survival.

Conclusions

Awake VATS pulmonary resections have now been successfully performed in many patients and in several pathologic conditions. Early series have suggested that these procedures can assure a new patient-friendly approach that minimizes operative risks and permits short hospitalizations and immediate resumption of daily life activities.

TEA has been preferred by our group as well as by other surgeons and allowed to achieve optimal thoracic analgesia and few adverse effects. The main concern raised against awake VATS procedures is the fear that surgical pneumothorax is poorly tolerated by spontaneously ventilating awake patients. However, data that is progressively accumulating seems to contradict this empiric thought showing that adequate ventilation is assured in most of patients whereas satisfactory oxygenation can be easily maintained throughout these procedures. Nonetheless, this fascinating surgical option has opened several new doors that need light to be shed through. Many physiopathology aspects need to be better elucidated and real advantages, disadvantages and cost-effectiveness still require further investigation to be definitively indicated. Surgery is changing and several valid surgical procedures are likely to become obsolete within few years. Innovative non-surgical options are being actively investigated to cure diseases avoiding surgical trauma and even the need for hospitalization. Thoracic surgeons of the third millennium have to pick up the gauntlet and jump on board of new less and less invasive surgical options. Awake thoracic surgery is expected to represent one strong answer to this challenge.

References

1 Gothart J: Lung injury after thoracic surgery and one-lung ventilation. Curr Opin Anaesthsiol 2006;19:5–10.

2 Pompeo E, Mineo D, Rogliani P, et al: Feasibility and results of awake thoracoscopic resection of solitary pulmonary nodules. Ann Thorac Surg 2004;78:1761–1768.

3 Pompeo E, Mineo TC: Awake pulmonary metastasectomy. J Thorac Cardiovasc Surg 2007;133:960–966.

4 Pompeo E, Mineo TC: Awake operative videothoracoscopic pulmonary resections. Thorac Surg Clin 2008;18:311–320.
5 Hoksch B, Birken-Bertsch H, Muller JM: Thoracoscopy before Jacobaeus. Ann Thorac Surg 2002;74:1288–1290.
6 Buckingham WW, Beatty AJ, Brasher GA, Ottosen P: The technique of administering epidural anesthesia in thoracic surgery. Dis Chest 1950;17:561–568.
7 Boutin C, Velardocchio JM, Prud'homme A: Value of thoracoscopy. Presse Med 1984;13:2635–2639.
8 Rusch VW, Mountain C: Thoracoscopy under regional anesthesia for the diagnosis and management of pleural disease. Am J Surg 1987;154:274–278.
9 Nezu K, Kushibe K, Tojo T, et al: Thoracoscopic wedge resection of blebs under local anesthesia with sedation for treatment of a spontaneous pneumothorax. Chest 1997;111:230–235.
10 Björk VO, Carlens E: The prevention of spread during pulmonary resection by use of a double-lumen catheter. J Thorac Surg 1950;20:151–157.
11 Tekinbas C, Ulusoy H, Yulug E, et al: One-lung ventilation: for how long? J Thorac Cardiovasc Surg 2007;134:405–410.
12 Hemmerling TM, Bluteau MC, Kazan R, Bracco D: Significant decrease of cerebral oxygen saturation during single-lung ventilation measured using absolute oximetry. Br J Anaesth 2008;101:870–875.
13 Bardoczky GI, Szegedi LL, d'Hollander AA, et al: Two-lung and one-lung ventilation in patients with chronic obstructive pulmonary disease: the effects of position and FiO_2. Anesth Analg 2000;90:35–41.
14 Karzai W, Schwarzkopf K: Hypoxemia during one-lung ventilation. Prediction, prevention, and treatment. Anesthesiology 2009;110:1402–1411.
15 Tonnesen E, Hohndorf K, Lerbjerg G, Christensen NJ, Huttel S, Andersen K: Immunological and hormonal response to lung surgery during one-lung ventilation. Eur J Anaesth 1993;10:189–195.
16 Groeben H: Epidural anesthesia and pulmonary function. J Anesth 2006;20:290–299.
17 Pansard JL, Mankikian B, Bertrand M, et al: Effects of thoracic extradural block on diaphragmatic electrical activity and contractility after upper abdominal surgery. Anesthesiology 1993;78:63–71.
18 Oka T, Ozawa Y, Ohkubo Y: Thoracic epidural bupivacaine attenuates supraventricular tachyarrhythmias after pulmonary resection. Anesth Analg 2001;93:253–259.
19 Pattinson KT, Governo RJ, MacIntosh BJ, et al: Opioids depress cortical centers responsible for the volitional control of respiration. J Neurosci 2009;29:8177–8186.
20 Harvey H, Hayashi J, Speigel DR: Chronic obstructive pulmonary disease and panic disorder: their interrelationships and a unique utilization of beta-receptor agonists. Psychosomatics 2008;49:546.
21 Anthonisen NR: Regional lung function in spontaneous pneumothorax. Am Rev Respir Dis 1977;115:873–876.
22 Subotic D, Mandaric D, Gajic M, Vukcevic M: Uncertainties in the current understanding of gas exchange in spontaneous pneumothorax: effective lung ventilation may persist in smaller-sized pneumothorax. Med Hypoth 2005;64:1144–1149.
23 Mineo TC, Pompeo E, Mineo D, et al: Awake non-resectional lung volume reduction surgery. Ann Surg 2006;243:131–136.
24 Mineo TC: Epidural anesthesia in awake thoracic surgery. Eur J Cardiothorac Surg 2007;32:13–19.
25 Mineo TC, Pompeo E, Ambrogi V, et al: Transxiphoid video-assisted approach for bilateral pulmonary metastasectomy. Ann Thorac Surg 1999;67:1808–1810.
26 Al-Abdullatief M, Wahood A, Al-Shirawi N, et al: Awake anaesthesia for major thoracic surgical procedures: an observational study. Eur J Cardiothorac Surg 2007;32:346–350.

Prof. Eugenio Pompeo
Cattedra di Chirurgia Toracica, Policlinico Università Tor Vergata
Viale Oxford, 81, IT–00133 Rome (Italy)
Tel. +39 06 2090 2877, Fax +39 06 2090 2881
E-Mail pompeo@med.uniroma2.it

Esquinas AM (ed): Applied Technologies in Pulmonary Medicine. Basel, Karger, 2011, pp 114–118

Preservation of Organs from Brain-Dead Donors with Hyperbaric Oxygen

Benan Bayrakci

Pediatric Intensive Care Unit, Hacettepe University School of Medicine, Ankara, Turkey

Abbreviations

eNOS Endothelial nitric oxide synthase
iNOS Inducible nitric oxide synthase

Organ transplantation is an established therapeutic modality for the end-stage organ failures. It has been used as a life-saving treatment modality for decades. As a matter of fact, the incremental application of organ transplantation increased the demand for donor organs. The main limitation of its wider application is the availability of suitable donor organs. This limitation put forwards the use of marginal donor organs in order to increase the donor pool. Especially brain-dead donors constitute an alternative organ pool. However, the irreversible loss of the brain functions inevitably leads to a progressive deterioration in function of the donor organs. The various described mechanisms of organ injury and cellular death are predominantly related to ischemia and reperfusion which account for the majority of graft loss, although the importance of a well-functioning organ in the recipient is of utmost importance for the success of transplantation. The present methods of preventing ischemia are regional or total body perfusion with chemicals and application of hypothermia. However, the beneficial effects of these techniques are limited. Organ preservation is a field of increasing importance due to the advances in transplantation medicine but unfortunately an excellent system for the preservation of harvested organs has not yet been defined. Hopefully, hyperbaric oxygen seems to be a promising candidate as a bridge to transplantation by keeping the donated organs viable. A number of studies have demonstrated that hyperbaric oxygen therapy influences reperfusion injury and consequential acute cellular rejection. Hyperbaric oxygen therapy is a technology that involves oxygen treatment at supra-atmospheric pressures in high concentrations, generating increased levels of physically dissolved oxygen in plasma. This form of transported oxygen, compared with oxygen chemically bound to hemoglobin, is able to enter tissues with almost no blood flow. Recent evidence also suggests a correlation between the severity of reperfusion injury and acute cellular rejection which further causes organ damage. Acute cellular rejection affects approximately 30–40% of patients after transplantation and adds significantly to the postoperative morbidity and overall cost of transplantation. Hyperbaric oxygen therapy has been shown to reduce the severity of reperfusion injury as well as modulate both humoral and cellular immune response. Organs procured from brain-dead hyperbaric oxygen-treated donors have less cellular injury from ischemia, reperfusion, and the no-reflow phenomenon, thus yielding organs in an optimized state for transplantation. Treating the harvested organs with hyperbaric oxygen carries the potential benefit of better preservation prior to reimplantation.

Main Topics

Brain Death. The death of the brain is associated to an autonomic storm causing the massive release of circulating endogenous catecholamines. Light and electron microscopy of organs procured from experimental animals and human brain-dead organ donors shows typical catecholamine-calcium-induced injury, which results from the tissue ischemia-reperfusion [1]. Brain death leads to a series of pathophysiological changes referred to as the autonomic storm (an initial period of excessive parasympathetic activity followed by a significant adrenergic activity) which cause a significant impact on major organs used for transplantation [2]. The catecholamines activate lipases, proteases, and endonucleases, while nitric oxide synthase leads to further decay in membrane channel integrity and increased oxygen free radical production. Oxygen free radicals participate in the peroxidation of lipids and injure the endothelium and cell membranes, resulting in a net loss of cellular integrity. Membrane permeability causes excess Ca^{2+} influx to the cell which results in further injury. Cellular aerobic oxidative respiration collapses and the cellular oxygen lack results in intracellular inhibition of cellular energy, although ion gradients require constant energy at cellular channels. The failure of the Ca^{2+} channels precipitate the Ca^{2+}-induced injury [2].

Reperfusion Injury. After reimplantation of the organ the re-establishment of blood flow causes oxygenation of the ischemic tissues which adds a new injury related to toxic oxygen free radicals. The amount of tissue injury caused by reperfusion seems to be proportional to the ischemic time and particularly nitric oxide appears to play a role in this event. The cumulative effect of warm ischemia and cold preservation is an energy deficiency within the endothelial cells leading to intracellular edema and exacerbating the hypoxic injury to the donor organ [3]. These detrimental events are of paramount relevance in the global understanding of tissue injury, as transplanted organs undergo this process prior to, during and following brain death, cold storage and finally at the time of reperfusion in the recipient [1]. Hyperbaric oxygen treatment gives the tissues the opportunity to be kept oxygenated throughout all entire process so neither a hypoxic nor a reperfusion state can occur.

Acute Cellular Rejection. Acute cellular rejection is an additional effect of reperfusion injury due to its potential to stimulate the host response. The pathophysiology of acute cellular rejection is complex and has not been fully understood yet. Many antigens that are not normally present are expressed in response to reperfusion injury. This exposure results in an innate immune response that involves humoral components such as cytokines, complement and coagulation proteases as well as cellular components made up of macrophages and neutrophils. This initial response is followed by an adaptive immune response which leads to the activation of T and B cells acting specifically against exposed alloantigens. The host response to donor alloantigens is centered on the major histocompatibility complex antigens [4]. Activation of cytokines leads to the transformation of the T cells to take on immunoregulation and cytotoxicity [5]. Hyperbaric oxygen therapy has previously been shown to alter cell surface major histocompatibility complex class I antigen expression and ultimately inhibit the transcription of immunomodulatory cytokines, especially IL-2 along with its ability to reduce the expression of MHC class I antigens [6].

Hyperbaric Oxygen Therapy. Hyperbaric oxygen therapy has been used since 1662 for a wide spectrum of applications including diabetes mellitus, atherosclerosis, microangiopathy and blood clotting disturbances, decompression sickness, carbon monoxide poisoning, gas embolism and radionecrosis. Hyperbaric oxygen therapy increases the oxygen supply to the target tissue. Recent experimental studies have suggested that hyperoxemia provided by hyperbaric oxygen may be beneficial in the treatment of reperfusion injury. Hyperbaric oxygen was found to limit infarct size in the reperfused rabbit heart and further evidence that hyperbaric oxygen plays a role in restoration of oxidative enzyme activity was shown in a dog model [3, 7]. Hyperbaric oxygen therapy has been used in enhancing the survival of the skin grafts with approximately 50% less graft failures [8]. Delivery of oxygen at high partial pressures in the plasma may attenuate endothelial cell hypoxia and reverse a potentially self-propagating cycle, ischemia and response to ischemia that compromises microvascular flow [9].

Discussion

Organs used for transplantation undergo a series of injuries starting from the period before the event of brain death, although relevance of a well-functioning transplanted organ is clearly crucial for the success of organs requiring immediate function. The viability of any organ will depend on how soon it depletes its oxygen and finally its energy stores. Currently harvested organ preservation consists of using preservation solutions and cooling the organ to slow down metabolism but these only allow a limited time before transplantation. Time of survival for the stored organ is limited (maximum 48 h for kidneys and 12 h for liver). One other concern following a prolonged anaerobic tissue state is reperfusion injury where oxygen radicals and superoxides destroy cellular components and compromise the success of transplantation. A hyperbaric preservation technique facilitates that the organ remains in an aerobic state thus preventing reperfusion and related injury, but it is still doubtful whether or not the addition of hyperbaric oxygen to organ preservation algorithms might greatly prolong the storage period.

Hyperbaric oxygen therapy has recently been shown to be a useful adjunct in several models of ischemic reperfusion injury, but its mechanism of action remains mysterious. Oxygen is a critical substrate in the alleviation of hypoxia, anoxia and ischemia, but paradoxically it also functions as a deleterious metabolite during the reperfusion of previously ischemic tissues. In addition to this controversy, a hyperoxygenation and its metabolites demonstrate cellular and clinical benefit, particularly in the field of ischemic reperfusion injury. Hyperbaric oxygen has been used with a beneficial therapeutic effect in a wide variety of models of reperfusion injury including myocardium, skeletal muscle, small intestine and the liver. The majority of in vivo studies have shown a reduction in the tissue injury when reperfusion is performed in the presence of hyperbaric oxygen. Hyperbaric oxygen interacts with the effects of reperfusion injury at numerous interfaces, which include the endothelium, neutrophils, mediators of inflammation, microvascular blood flow, lipid peroxidation and cellular energy levels. A number of studies have confirmed the ability of hyperbaric oxygen to selectively induce eNOS while inhibiting iNOS production and the reduction of lipid peroxidation [6].

Another important role of hyperbaric treatment is immunomodulation. The effect of minimizing reperfusion injury is also known to reduce immune activation as it prevents the upregulation of major histocompatibility antigen class II molecules in the donor organ [6]. The mainstay of controlling acute cellular rejection remains with immunosuppressive therapies. If the laboratory studies were proven in the clinical situation, it may provide the opportunity to minimize drug-based immunosuppression.

Organs procured from brain-dead, hyperbaric oxygen-treated donors have less cellular injury from ischemia, reperfusion and the no-reflow phenomenon, thus yielding organs in an optimized state for transplantation. Our clinical observation in 2 brain-dead donors supports the fact that hyperbaric oxygen improves transplantation success. Both of the donors were CO intoxication cases who had received hyperbaric oxygen treatment and had to wait 72 h in brain-dead state before the harvesting process took place because of the toxic etiology. Due to the prolonged process they suffered multiple cardiac arrest episodes causing additional ischemia-reperfusion injury to the donor organs. Abundant organ functioning after transplantation suggests a possible therapeutic effect of hyperbaric oxygen treatment limiting the ischemic insult generated from brain death and repetitive cardiac arrests. The frozen biopsy obtained from the liver during transplantation surgery, showing no evidence of necrosis and inflammation, also gives a countenance to this suggestion [10]. Hyperbaric oxygen is a promising treatment as a bridge to transplantation, keeping the donated organs viable until the harvesting procedure take place for potential brain-dead donors.

Hyperbaric oxygen therapy seems to reduce the effect of reperfusion injury by various mechanisms depending on where it is applied, including exposure to the donor organ prior to reimplantation as well as the recipient both before and after transplantation [6]. Hyperbaric oxygen chambers are both cumbersome and expensive. The difficulty of moving critically ill patients in and out of the chambers and the high infrastructure requirements have been major obstacles to the delivery of hyperbaric oxygen therapy in the clinical setting. Today, mini-hyperbaric oxygen chambers are available for biological materials. Such chambers may help us overcome these current obstacles. Treating the donor organ itself with hyperbaric oxygen has the potential to carry the good effects of hyperbaric oxygen described above to the transplantation process. These mini organ chambers have the ability to be mobile giving donor organs the opportunity to receive hyperbaric oxygen throughout the whole harvesting to implantation process compromising the transport time as well.

Conclusions

Based on the available scientific evidence, hyperbaric oxygen application seems to have the capacity to influence the outcomes of transplantation at multiple levels. Adding hyperbaric oxygen therapy into the organ preservation algorithm may be of considerable benefit, not only by keeping the organs oxygenated but also impairing the inevitable reperfusion injury. Keeping organs in a more optimal condition for transplantation is crucial for the success of transplantation. Hyperbaric oxygen greatly increases the viability of the organ while awaiting a host either applied to the donor prior to the harvesting process or to the recipients after reimplantation. Nevertheless, the most promising type of application seems to be the hyperbaric treatment of the isolated donor organ because of its ease of use, being handy for transport and of relatively low cost.

References

1 Novitzky D: Donor management: state of the art. Transplant Proc 1997;29:3773–3775.

2 Novitzky D: Detrimental effects of brain death on the potential organ donor. Transplant Proc 1997;29:3770–3772.

3 Thomas MP, Brown LA, Sponseller DR, et al: Myocardial infarct size reduction by the synergistic effect of hyperbaric oxygen and recombinant tissue plasminogen activator. Am Heart J 1990;120:791–800.

4 Pober JS, Orosz CG, Rose ML, Savage CO: Can graft endothelial cells initiate a host anti-graft immune response? Transplantation 1996;61:343–349.

5 Lipman ML, Stevens AC, Strom TB: Heightened intragraft CTL gene expression in acutely rejecting renal allografts. J Immunol 1994;152:5120–5127.
6 Muralidharan V, Christophi C: Hyperbaric oxygen therapy and liver transplantation. HPB (Oxford) 2007;9:174–182.
7 Sterling DL, Thornton JD, Swafford A, et al: Hyperbaric oxygen limits infarct size in ischemic rabbit myocardium in vivo. Circulation 1993;88:1931–1936.
8 Svehlik J Jr, Zábavniková M, Guzanin S, et al: Hyperbaric oxygenotherapy as a possible means of preventing ischemic changes in skin grafts used for soft tissue defect closure. Acta Chir Plast 2007;49: 31–35.
9 Glazier JJ: Attenuation of reperfusion microvascular ischemia by aqueous oxygen: experimental and clinical observations. Am Heart J 2005;149:580–584.
10 Bayrakci B: Preservation of organs from brain-dead donors with hyperbaric oxygen. Pediatr Transplant 2008;12:506–509.

Benan Bayrakci, MD
Pediatric Intensive Care Unit, Hacettepe University School of Medicine
Yeni Ladin Sitesi No: 19, Angora Caddesi
TR–06532 Beytepe, Çankaya, Ankara (Turkey)
Tel. +90 533 749 33 99, Fax +90 312 311 23 98
E-Mail benan@hacettepe.edu.tr

Esquinas AM (ed): Applied Technologies in Pulmonary Medicine. Basel, Karger, 2011, pp 119–125

Teleassistance in Chronic Respiratory Failure Patients

Michele Vitacca

Divisione di Pneumologia Riabilitativa, Fondazione Salvatore Maugeri, IRCCS, Lumezzane, Italy

Abbreviations

COPD	Chronic obstructive pulmonary disease
e-health	Electronic health
GP	General practitioner
HMV	Home mechanical ventilation
MV	Mechanical ventilation
TA	Teleassistance

Socioeconomic trends have led to a markedly increased interest in improving society's ability to deliver effective care to older and chronically ill patients at home [1]. Challenges in the care of frail elders include the organization and sustainability of the continuum of services, resource allocation and cultural competence in service delivery as case management programs and partnerships with families [1]. In patients submitted under HMV, underlying disease, level of their dependency, hours spent under MV, presence of tracheotomy, distance from home to hospital, and hospital accesses are the causes of the major care burden [2] for the family and healthcare system. The time spent by caregivers to provide assistance for patients with poor daily life activities has been described as enormous [3]. At the same time, the additional time required for caregivers to provide transportation to physician visits is usually not included in the cost analysis [3]. The family burden of HMV patients has been described to be particularly high with regard to money, which was reported to be excessive in 17.3% of the cases [3].

Homecare Systems

Homecare for respiratory patients is a complex array of services delivered in an uncontrolled setting in which patients and families are integral members of the healthcare team [4]. Complexity, lack of direct control, and acute exacerbations on chronic conditions all likely contribute to the difficulty in organizing homecare assistance [4]. Among homecare programs, HMV shows a great prevalence in European countries. A recent American Thoracic Society statement [4] has emphasized the need for a strict follow-up of these frail patients. In particular, homecare should focus on a patient-centered perspective and patient and family satisfaction: reduction of complications resulting from hospitalization, maintaining

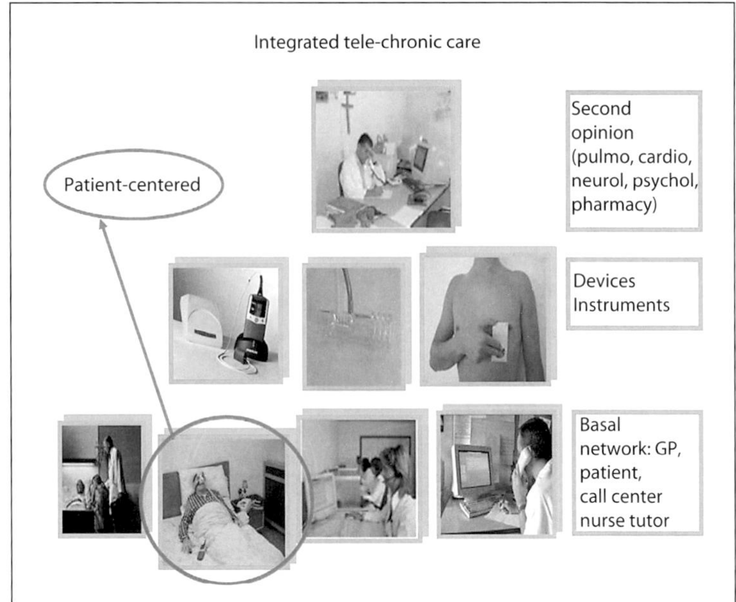

Fig. 1. Operative chain for the tele-chronic care program from our group, with permission. The integrated tele-chronic care program offers a network between the GP, patient, family, call center and nurse tutor. According to different diseases and level of severity, devices are prescribed and inserted into the program. A multidisciplinary sanitary staff is available for a second opinion 24 hours a day.

an acceptable quality of life, and enabling a comfortable and dignified death have been proposed as major endpoints [4].

Telemedicine – Telesupport – Teleassistance

Recent advances in technology make it possible to reach patients in their homes through e-health or telemedicine. Telemedicine is a very useful and critical application of information and communication technologies, and may deliver high-quality healthcare services regionally, nationally, or globally. Telemedicine is a combination of medical expertise, medical equipment, computer hardware and software, and communication technology, by which a patient can be examined, investigated, monitored and treated by a medical expert in a distant place [5]. 'Tele' is a Greek word meaning 'distance' and 'mederi' is a Latin word meaning 'to heal'. Hence, telemedicine is 'medicine practiced at a distance' [5]. Temedicine enables remote, isolated and rural areas to have clinical support from those hospitals and medical systems with a higher level of medical expertise [5–7]. Telemedicine can be classified on the basis of the mode of operation or on the basis of application [5]. According to the mode of operation it can be divided into two groups: real-time (interactive) mode and store-and-forward mode. In the real-time interactive mode, the patient is present with an attending physician or paramedical personnel, and a specialist is present at a remote medical center. In the store-and-forward mode, all relevant information (data, graphics, images, etc.) is transmitted electronically to the specialist. It is possible to distinguish two similar methods: one in which telemedicine is an aid for helping the nurse in the management of patients with chronic diseases (telenursing), and the other, completely automated, in which a computerized voice-answering system and a computer algorithm checked the patient's vital signs with an acceptable range previously set by the physician

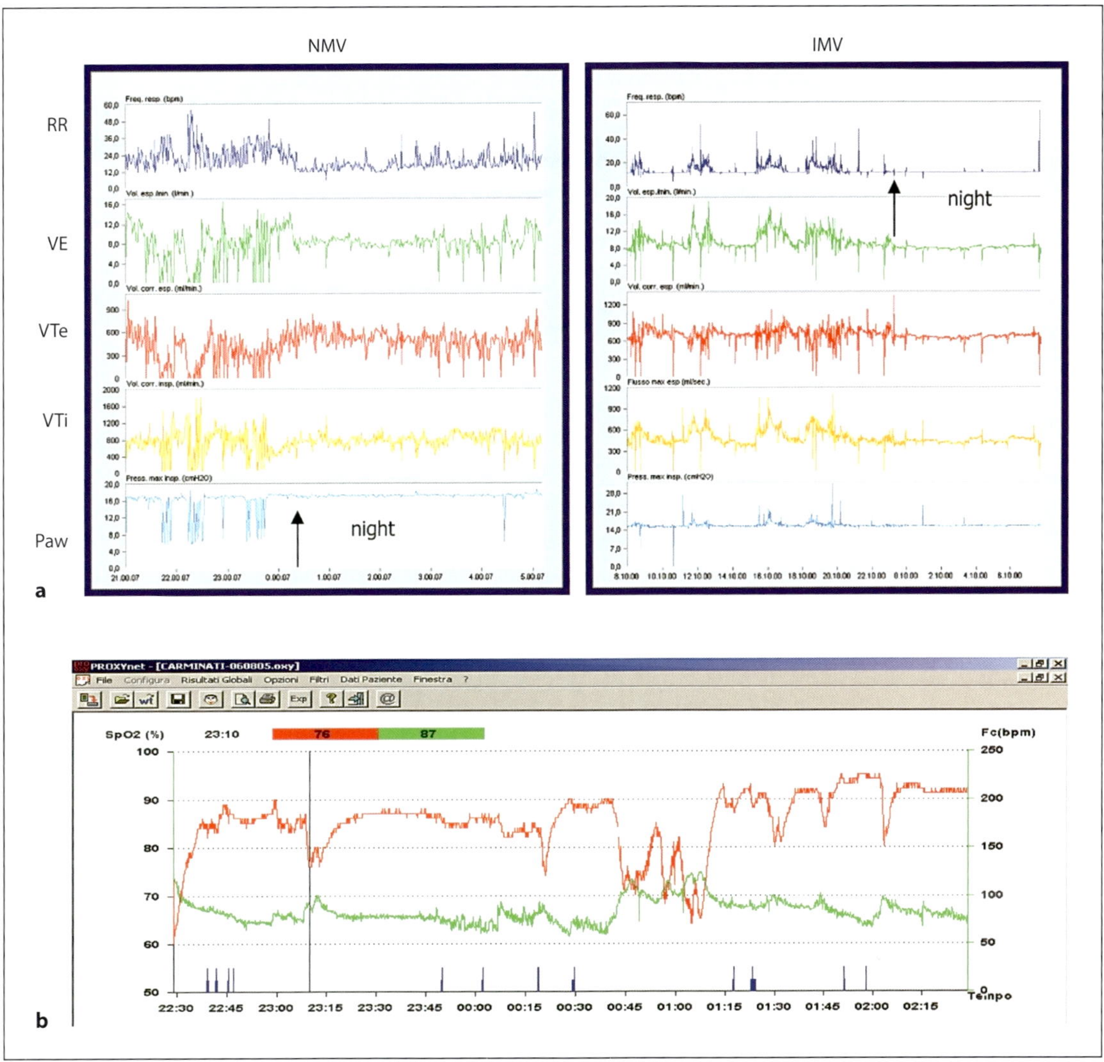

Fig. 2. From top to bottom: representative tracings sent by phone to call center of respiratory rate, minute ventilation, expiratory tidal volume, inspiratory tidal volume, airway pressure, pSat O_2 and heart rate trends during non-invasive mechanical ventilation (NMV) (**a** left, **b** bottom) and during invasive mechanical ventilation (IMV) (**a** right).

(telemanagement). Nurse-telephone triage lines have been running for over 10 years. The nurses who answer the phones are specially trained and use algorithms on computers to steer the conversation to a particular conclusion. Figure 1 shows an example of an operative chain for a telemedicine program, while figure 2 shows representative tracings of biological signs transmitted by means of TA. The three main types of benefit arising from the e-health investment are quality, access and efficiency. Table 1 summarizes the main benefits and opportunities of e-health.

Table 1. Main benefits and opportunities of e-health

Supporting the delivery of care tailored to individual patients
Improving transparency and accountability of care processes and facilitating shared care across boundaries
Aiding evidence-based practice and error reduction
Improving diagnostic accuracy and treatment appropriateness
Improving access to effective healthcare by reducing barriers created
Facilitating patient empowerment for self-care and health decision-making
Improving cost efficiency by streamlining processes, reducing waiting times and waste
More responsibility of referral center
More information among actors
Educational model
'Self-responsibility' of patient and caregiver
Transmission of data and real-time consultation
Complimentary to classical models
Reducing omission of care
Increasing continuity
Increasing effectiveness
Prompt attention to emergencies
Improving patient satisfaction
Improving effectiveness
Reducing costs
Reducing communication errors

Results from the Literature

The Kaiser Permanente Organization study [8] reported the first formal randomized controlled trial of home videophones. Patients in the intervention group were equipped with home videophones, an electronic stethoscope and a digital blood pressure monitor; over 18 months, patients in the telemedicine group received 17% fewer home visits by nurses than the control group and the average cost of care in this group was 27% less than in the control group [8]. In an intervention group of 46 patients, Farrero et al. [9] studied monthly telephone calls, home visits every 3 months, and home or hospital visits on a demand basis. 48 patients as control group completed the 1-year follow-up period. The authors found a decrease in the mean number of emergency department visits, decrease in hospital admissions and days of hospital stay. Young et al. [10] described the general application of telephone-linked communication systems in the healthcare setting for COPD patients discussing the rationale for expected improvements in disease control and quality of life, and for a reduction in acute healthcare utilization. Cost and effectiveness data from the Milwaukee and Iron Mountain Veterans Affairs Medical Centers telepulmonary program [11] were collected for a period of 1 year. Telemedicine was found to be more cost effective (USD 335 per patient/year) compared to routine care (USD 585 per patient/year) and on-site care (USD 1,166 per patient/year). Hernandez et al. [12] tested a home vs. conventional hospitalization with a randomized study of 8 weeks. 222 COPD patients admitted to the emergency room received an integrated care with a specialized nurse, a home visit within 24 h and patient free phone access. Rehospitalization, emergency room visits, days of hospitalization and quality of life were significantly in favor of the homecare group. Bourbeau et al. [13] compared a treated group with an education program, nurse weekly visit, monthly telephone follow-up with a control group with usual care. Maiolo et al. [14] for 12 months followed 23 patients with chronic respiratory failure with a fixed twice-a-week transmission of pSat and heart rate. Comparing the healthcare utilization in the year before the study they demonstrated a reduction in hospital admission and home relapses of 50 and 55% respectively. Patients were satisfied with the quality of the personal telemonitoring process in 96% of cases. Eighteen [15] well-motivated patients with advanced COPD, who had had at least four hospitalizations during the previous 2 years, were included in a home-based telemedicine program including nurse visits, a laptop computer, an electrocardiogram, spirometer, oximeter and blood pressure monitor, and a videoconference camera. After 9 months there was a decrease in hospitalizations, emergency department visits and use of health services. Casas at al. [16] demonstrated with a randomized controlled trial on 155 exacerbated COPD patients that a standardized integrated care intervention, based on shared care arrangements among different levels of the system with support of information technologies, effectively prevents hospitalizations for exacerbations in COPD patients. In their study [16], only 24% of patients were on long-term oxygen therapy while none was mechanically ventilated. In this study, periodic phone calls were scheduled every 3 months as 'store-and-forward necessity'. We [17] have recently demonstrated that the TA program is effective in preventing hospitalizations, home acute exacerbations, and urgent GP calls, and may be cost-effective in severe chronic respiratory failure patients needing home oxygen therapy and/or MV. The COPD group seems to take the greater advantage from TA [17]. In this perspective, we [17] should first ask whether a TA program could be effective also in severe patients on long-term oxygen therapy and HMV. In line with Casas et al. [16] and Maiolo et al. [14], our study confirms that an integrated multidisciplinary monitoring and care with the aid of information technologies can reduce hospitalizations by about 36%, GP urgent calls by 65%, home relapses by 71%, even in more severe patients. According to our primary endpoint (reduction of hospitalizations), this study also confirmed that patients affected with COPD seem to take a greater advantage from TA. We [17] have confirmed the key role of nurses as a specialized figure able to educate patients and their families/caregivers before discharge, to screen all requests and to coordinate all actors involved in the follow-up.

Conclusion

The real 'technology' includes human resources available in hospitals and home and social health organizations; TM models need to respond to criteria of equity, simplicity, efficiency, efficacy, and have to be patient-centered and safe. The challenge that telemedicine will become part of the standard of care remains open.

Recommendations

- Hospitalization of chronically ill patients is a 'failure' for the health system and chronic diseases are becoming the case for the large-scale deployment of e-health.
- e-Health may be an opportunity for health organization, new strategic politician vision and clinical reorganization. Table 2 summarizes the recommendations and limitations for telecare.
- The future of homecare and telemedicine will depend on (i) human factors, (ii) economics,

and (iii) technology. Patients need healthcare and they want to remain at home for as long as possible.

- While intervention trials have utilized different designs, the nurse practitioner is common to all the trials and appears to have a key role in the management of chronic disease.
- Results on long-term effect, cost-effective analysis, quality of life, and public health burden reduction remain to be demonstrated.
- Nowadays a lot of applications of homecare and telemedicine are possible and operative. Home telemedicine is not strictly 'technology' but an innovative instrument (based on health figures more than high-tech instruments) which will help the daily job of doctors with patients and their families: telemedicine changes the way we deliver care to patients by changing the space and time in the relations between patients and health professionals.

Table 2. Recommendations and limitations for telecare

Recommendations
Clearly and articulated mission
Specific goals to be achieved
Accountable governance structure
Well-defined service
Well-defined target population
Well-structured service providers
Detailed procedures and protocols (scheduled quality controls)
Correct choice of technology adequate for each situation
Well-structured outcomes perspective
Self-sustaining programs
Limitations
Many different software, hardware and telecommunication options
Poor specification design for each condition
Poor uniformity for standards
No clear strategies for promoting wide utilization
Limited technological and clinical research
Legal problems between subjects involved
Costs
Poor knowledge and culture
Skepticism of doctors
Absence of reimbursements

References

1 Young HM: Challenges and solutions for care of frail older adults. Online J Issues Nurs 2003;8:5. WHO Global Observatory for e-Health. Global e-Health Survey, Geneva, July 2005.

2 Vitacca M, Escarrabill J, Galavotti G, Vianello A, Prats E, Scala R, Peratoner A, Guffanti E, Maggi L, Barbano L, Balbi B: Home mechanical ventilation patients: a retrospective survey to identify level of burden in real life. Monaldi Arch Chest Dis 2007;67:142–147.

3 Langa KM, Fendrick AM, Flaherty KR, Martinez FJ, Kabeto MU, Saint S: Informal caregiving for chronic lung disease among older Americans. Chest 2002; 122:2197–2203.

4 American Thoracic Society Documents: Statement on home care for patients with respiratory disorders. Am J Respir Crit Care Med 2005;171,1443–1464.

5 Scalvini S, Vitacca M, Paletta L, Giordano A, Balbi B: 'Telemedicine: a new frontier for effective healthcare services. Monaldi Arch Chest Disease 2004;61:226–233.

6 Wootton R: Telemedicine: clinical review. BMJ 2001;323:557–560.

7 Wooton R, Dimmick SL, Kvedar JC (eds): Home Telehealth: Connecting Care within the Community. London, The Royal Society Medicine Press, 2006.

8 Johnston B, Wheeler L, Deuser J, Sousa KH: Outcomes of the Kaiser Permanente Tele-Home Health Research Project. Arch Fam Med 2000;9:40–45.

9 Farrero E, Escarrabill J, Prats E, Maderal M, Manresa F: Impact of a hospital-based homecare program on the management of COPD patients receiving long-term oxygen therapy. Chest 2001; 19:364–369.

10 Young M, Sparrow D, Gottlieb D, Selim A, Friedman R: A telephone-linked computer system for COPD care. Chest 2001; 119:1565–1575.

11 Agha Z, Schapira RM, Maker AH: Cost-effectiveness of telemedicine for the delivery of outpatient pulmonary care to a rural population. Telemed J E Health 2002;8:281–291.

12 Hernandez C, Casas A, Escarrabill J, Alonso J, Puig-Junoy J, Farrero E, Vilagut G, Collvinent B, Rodriguez-Roisin R, Roca J: Home hospitalisation of exacerbated chronic obstructive pulmonary disease patients. Eur Respir J 2003; 21:58–67.

13 Bourbeau J, Julien M, Maltais F, Rouleau M, Beaupré A, Bégin R, Renzi P, Nault D, Borycki E, Schwartzman K, Singh R, Collet JP: Chronic Obstructive Pulmonary Disease Axis of the Respiratory Network Fonds de la Recherche en Santé du Québec: Reduction of hospital utilization in patients with chronic obstructive pulmonary disease a disease-specific self-management intervention. Arch Intern Med 2003;163:585–591.

14 Maiolo C, Mohamed EI, Fiorani CM, De Lorenzo A: Home tele-monitoring for patients with severe respiratory illnesses: the Italian experience. J Telemed Telecare 2003;9:67–71.

15 Vontetsianos T, Giovas P, Katsara T, Rigopoulou A, Mpirmpa G, Giaboudakis P, Koyrelea S, Kontopyrgias G, Tsoulkas B: Telemedicine-assisted home support for patients with advanced chronic obstructive pulmonary disease: preliminary results after a nine-month follow-up. J Telemed Telecare 2005;11(suppl 1): 86–88.

16 Casas A, Troosters T, Garcia-Aymerich J, Roca J, Hernández C, Alonso A, del Pozo F, de Toledo P, Antó JM, Rodríguez-Roisín R, Decramer M: Integrated care prevents hospitalizations for exacerbations in COPD patients. Eur Respir J 2006; 28:123–130.

17 Vitacca M, Bianchi L, Guerra A, Fracchia C, Spanevello A, Balbi B, Scalvini S: Teleassistance in chronic respiratory failure patients: a randomised clinical trial Eur Respir J 2009;33:411–418.

Michele Vitacca, MD
Divisione di Pneumologia Riabilitativa, Fondazione Salvatore Maugeri
IRCCS, Via Mazzini 129, IT–25066 Lumezzane/BS (Italy)
Tel. +39 030 825 3168, Fax +39 030 825 3188
E-Mail michele.vitacca@fsm.it

Esquinas AM (ed): Applied Technologies in Pulmonary Medicine. Basel, Karger, 2011, pp 126–131

Capnography: Gradient $PACO_2$ and $PETCO_2$

Michael E. Donnellan

Oridion Capnography Inc., Needham, Mass., USA

Abbreviations

ARDS	Adult respiratory distress syndrome
CO_2	Carbon dioxide
FRC	Functional residual capacity
$PaCO_2$	Partial pressure arterial carbon dioxide
$P(a\text{-}ET)CO_2$	Gradient
PaO_2	Partial pressure of oxygen
PEEP	Positive end-expiratory pressure
$PETCO_2$	End-tidal carbon dioxide
Q_{sp}/QT	Physiological shunt
VD/VT	Dead-space tidal volume ratio
V/Q ratio	Ventilation-perfusion ratio

Capnography provides a numeric and graphic wave display of measured fractional CO_2 in real time with breath-to-breath feedback known as $PETCO_2$ monitoring providing feedback on patient's clinical standing by determining and tracking the baseline ventilatory status over time [1, 2]. A capnometer displays a number ($PETCO_2$) whereas a capnograph displays a number and a waveform (capnogram) (fig. 1), both monitoring changes in CO_2 concentration during the respiratory cycle [3].

The difference between the $PETCO_2$ and $PaCO_2$ is referred to as the gradient which is a result of the relationship between V (ventilation) airflow to the alveoli and Q (perfusion) blood flow to the capillaries. This is the V/Q ratio which in a normal healthy individual can be closely correlated suggesting the $PETCO_2$ may be able to predict the $PaCO_2$.

The gradient is largely dependent upon the physiological dead space and the slope of the alveolar plateau displayed in phase lll of the graphic waveform in figure 1. An increase in dead space can result in a corresponding increase in the $PaCO_2$-$PETCO_2$ gradient. However, a negative relationship can also exist between the $PaCO_2$-$PETCO_2$ and the slope in phase lll where an increase can indicate a reduction in the gradient. Subsequently, it may be stated that the net change in the $PaCO_2$-$PETCO_2$ is the result of changes in dead space and the patterns of the various V/Q alveoli [4–6].

$P(a\text{-}ET)CO_2$ is dependent and influenced upon underlying pulmonary disease in patients where the $PETCO_2$ can differ from the $PaCO_2$ because of V/Q mismatching. There also may be wide variations in gradients when a patient's condition does not remain constant over time [7, 8].

Trending

A constant $PETCO_2$ does not insure a constant $PaCO_2$, especially in pre-hospital ventilatory management where fluctuations in the gradient

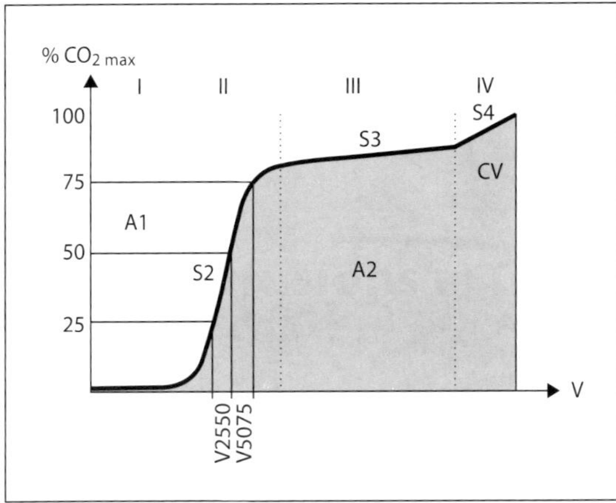

Fig. 1. Capnogram displaying a number and a waveform.

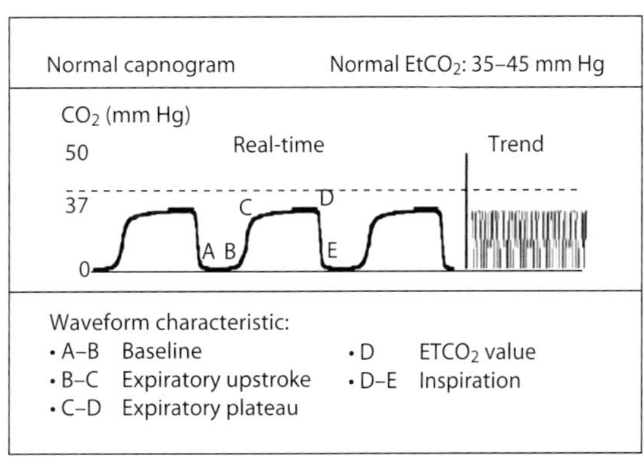

Fig. 2. A 'normal' capnogram is a waveform representing the varying CO_2 level throughout the breath cycle.

are common over time. In mechanically ventilated patients, changes in the individual parameters such as rate and tidal volumes can contribute to the variability in the $PaCO_2$-$PETCO_2$ gradient [8]. However, although these variations in the gradient may not be used to predict the $PaCO_2$, it remains useful in documenting changes in V/Q mismatches and can alert the clinician to changing physiological conditions [9].

There are other reviews and opinions claiming the $PETCO_2$ will closely approximate the $PaCO_2$ or may differ by an acceptable constant or range, especially in intubated patients where a closed ventilatory system exists. In these scenarios, the $PaCO_2$ may no longer require as frequent monitoring and comparisons [9] (fig. 2). It is generally accepted that a sizeable difference in the gradient does not diminish or preclude the value of the $PETCO_2$ and that a rise in the $PETCO_2$ indicates a rise in the $PaCO_2$. However, equating the exact numeric values is not advised and at least two comparisons should be obtained between the $PaCO_2$-$PETCO_2$ before completely relying upon the $PETCO_2$, especially in patients that are clinically stable [10].

Case Reviews

Chronic Obstructive Pulmonary Disease

Figure 3 is the breath-to-breath tracing of a severe tachypneic chronic obstructive pulmonary disease patient. The breaths appear compressed displaying a slight variation in $PETCO_2$. The $PaCO_2$ was 74 mm Hg resulting in a gradient difference of 24 mm Hg. This is an example where the diseased alveoli are not emptying evenly resulting in the end-tidal sample containing considerable dead-space air. While the 24 mm Hg difference in this gradient is considered high (a normal value being between 2 and 6 mm Hg), it renders the $PETCO_2$ useful in determining the $PaCO_2$ when subject to occasional validation in light of the complete clinical picture in real time. Given the assumption that a verified $PETCO_2$ can act as a proxy for $PaCO_2$, it can be a valuable tool in intensive care and will reduce arterial blood sampling [10].

ARDS PEEP Titration

V/Q mismatching is considered a primary cause for hypoxemia in the ARDS patient where the distribution of V/Q ratios are altered as shown by

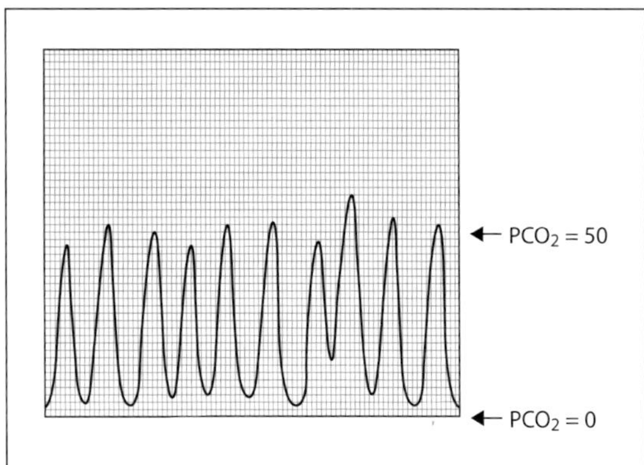

Fig. 3. Breath-to-breath tracing of a severe tachypneic chronic obstructive pulmonary disease.

multiple inert elimination techniques [11]. PEEP has been shown to increase FRC and directly effect intrapulmonary shunting Q_{sp}/QT (physiological shunt) while improving oxygenation in ARDS patients when applying various levels of PEEP [12]. However, determining the level of PEEP where the beneficial effects supersede harmful ones is important when titrating the PEEP, improving the PaO_2 and minimizing the effect upon the cardiac output, dead-space volume, and barotraumas [13].

It has been observed that the $PaCO_2$-$PETCO_2$ gradient decreases when PEEP is applied and minimized at 15 cm H_2O, but increased again at 20 cm H_2O. The VD/VT value had a direct and corresponding cause of action with the $PaCO_2$-$PETCO_2$ gradient. The PaO_2 is correspondingly at its highest when the $PaCO_2$-$PETCO_2$ gradient is minimal and intrapulmonary shunts decrease with increasing levels of PEEP and was minimal at 20 cm H_2O [14]. The values are easily monitored and a trend can be seen with simple arterial blood gas analysis and simple capnograms. The $PaCO_2$-$PETCO_2$ gradient is a useful and simple value too.

Respiratory Distress Non-Intubated Patient

In a study conducted in the outpatient emergency unit of a French University Hospital, 5 mobile ICU patients with respiratory distress, not requiring immediate tracheal intubation, were managed in a standard manner to include arterial blood gas monitoring (i-Stat® Analyzer; Abbott Laboratories, Ill., USA) and the $PETCO_2$ by a cannula (Microstream Smart Capnoline Plus®; Oridion Inc., Needham, Mass., USA) in order to determine and monitor the $PaCO_2$-$PETCO_2$ gradient [15]. Of the 49 patients reviewed, the gradient between the $PaCO_2$-$PETCO_2$ was >5 mm Hg in 41 of the patients and >10 mm Hg in 25 of the patients. The maximum gradient was 34 mm Hg. It was determined that although capnography monitoring in this non-intubated patient population with respiratory distress presented minimal problems, the $PETCO_2$ poorly reflected the $PaCO_2$ and the $PaCO_2$-$PETCO_2$ experienced the largest gradient in the hypersonic and tachypneic patients. The accuracy was incompatible with routine clinical use of $PETCO_2$ and as a predictor of the $PaCO_2$ [16].

Massive Pulmonary Emboli

Six patients with hypertension undergoing thrombolysis for massive pulmonary emboli were evaluated by $PaCO_2$-$PETCO_2$ gradient monitoring for several hours after the treatment. Two of the patients experienced a large decrease in the $PaCO_2$-$PETCO_2$ gradient (from 17 mm Hg before treatment to 1.5 mm Hg) at 2–4 h and 12–24 h respectively. In the initial attempt to evaluate the use of capnography and a gradient during the treatment of massive pulmonary emboli, it was suggested that the decrease in the gradient suggests the efficacy of the thrombolysis and the elevated persistent $PaCO_2$-$PETCO_2$ gradient may question the efficacy of the treatment. However, capnography shows promise as a non-invasive bedside monitoring application in this treatment [17].

Newborns

Two groups of mechanically ventilated newborns at Children's Hospital Boston, Mass., were separated into two sections: group A with pulmonary disease and group B without pulmonary disease. 20 infants were selected and gas sampling performed using a sidestream hand-held device (Microcap®; Oridion Inc.) with microstream sampling technology [18].

$PaCO_2$-$PETCO_2$ gradients were collected from 13 of the patients with pulmonary disease and 7 without. The patients in group A were diagnosed with persistent pulmonary hypertension, respiratory distress syndrome and pneumonia, while group B was free of pulmonary disease. Birth weight, gestational age, postnatal age and mode of ventilation were similar. The mean $PaCO_2$-$PETCO_2$ gradients were significantly different between groups A and B, demonstrating wide gradients in group A with pulmonary disease. However, it is noted that because tidal volumes are small and respiratory rates are high in this patient population, $PaCO_2$ was diluted with dead-space gas from the ventilator circuit. As a result, sidestream technology that continuously samples exhaled gases from a side port on the proximal endotracheal tube before entry into the breathing circuit lowered dead-space gas dilution and is preferred over mainstream monitoring devices because of positioning and increased dead space in the system which competes with the already small tidal volumes of this patient population [19].

Analysis
Four independent VD/VT ranges and the corresponding relationship between the $PaCO_2$ and $PETCO_2$ using Pearson's correlation coefficient were assessed. The mean $PaCO_2$-$PETCO_2$ difference in each VD/VT range was also calculated using multivariable linear regression models to review the relationships between all dependent and independent variables to appraise the concurrence between $PaCO_2$ and $PETCO_2$. StataCorp (College Station, Tex., USA) statistics software was used in the evaluation of the data presented [20].

A homogeneous lung model that generated five non-linear first-order differential equations and two equations for gas exchange implemented mathematical modeling describing variations in CO_2 and O_2 compartmental fractions and alveolar volumes to include pulmonary capillary gas exchange. The $PaCO_2$-$PETCO_2$ between adjusted experimental and sinusoidal ventilatory flow rates while at rest and during exercise indicated similar values in $PaCO_2$ and $PETCO_2$ for different flow dynamics. The model studies regarding the effects of metabolic, circulatory and cardiac output and respiratory parameters indicated a significant difference in the $PaCO_2$-$PETCO_2$ during exercise [21].

Discussion

Monitoring the physiological dead space is a critical value in determining a pathway of clinical care for the patient. Specific numeric determinations of the VD/VT, and other formulas, are interrelated as dead-space determinants project direct correlations to the status and effectiveness of ventilatory efforts to include ventilator management.

Capnography is accepted by many as a useful parameter by continuously monitoring the $PETCO_2$ which can be used as an indicator of the $PaCO_2$ even in patients with significant pulmonary disease. However, many studies have indicated that the $PaCO_2$-$PETCO_2$ gradient will increase as the VD/VT ratios increase, therefore the strength of the correlation between the two may decrease as the VD/VT increases [20].

There are other opinions based on studies that maintain that there is no way of knowing how large the $PaCO_2$-$PETCO_2$ will be in a given patient and what conditions may exist at any particular time to impact the gradient on rapid intervals [10]. For instance, in a severe ARDS patient, the homodynamic and pulmonary status can create consistent and rapid V/Q shifts which do not allow for consistent or constant correlation between

$PaCO_2$-$PETCO_2$ monitoring [12]. There are also physiological circumstances where negative values of the $PaCO_2$-$PETCO_2$ gradient are present which affects its ability in assessing dead-space ventilation, for example in the terminal part of the expiration phase, PCO_2 can rise rapidly and may exceed $PaCO_2$. The slope of phase III (fig. 1) increases and the likelihood of sampling a $PETCO_2$ greater than the $PaCO_2$ exists. Wide ranges of V/Q mismatching and reduced FRC in patients after cardiopulmonary bypass surgery for example may result in a negative $P(a\text{-}ET)CO_2$ value and reduced FRC, and increased CO_2 production may cause a negative $P(a\text{-}ET)CO_2$ value in infants [22, 23].

A non-related dead-space issue that will directly affect the accuracy of the $PaCO_2$-$PETCO_2$ monitoring and gradient is the level of secretions being produced by the patient and the amount of suctioning required. Accumulation of thick secretions in the CO_2 sensor is not unusual and will require sensor cleaning, removal and in many cases result in inaccurate $PETCO_2$ if any reading can be taken. Reliance of the $PaCO_2$-$PETCO_2$ gradient with acute or chronic, intubated or non-intubated patients as a definitive diagnostic parameter is controversial requiring more analysis, especially in the pulmonary acute patient population.

Conclusions

Physiological dead-space ventilation is a major factor in determining the relationship of the $PaCO_2$-$PETCO_2$ gradient. The difference between the $PaCO_2$-$PETCO_2$ gradient is directly proportional to the degree of physiological dead space and maintains a direct relationship or constant as the VD/VT ratio increases. It remains a useful indicator of $PaCO_2$ within the stable patient as well as with those with substantial lung disease with elevated VD/VT ratios, or under controlled anesthesia, as long as the elevations in the gradient remain predictable or correlate with the increase in physiological dead space. However, as the clinical status of the patient deteriorates, the gradient become less predictable, especially in that patient population experiencing extremely elevated physiological dead space from severe lung disease, hemodynamic instability and/or multisystem failure. At this point, the $PETCO_2$ becomes the predictor only when verified by periodic arterial blood gases which is the denominator and as such will be less required as $PaCO_2$-$PETCO_2$ gradients are utilized.

References

1 Breen PH: Carbon dioxide kinetics during anesthesia: pathophysiology and monitoring; in Breen PH (ed): Respiration in Anesthesia: Pathophysiology and Clinical Update. Anesthesiology Clinics of North America. Philadelphia, Saunders, 1998, vol 16, pp 259–293.

2 Swedlow DB: Capnometry and capnography. The anesthesia disaster early warning system. Semin Anesth 1986;3: 194–205.

3 Krauss B, Hess DR: Capnography for procedural sedation and analgesia in the emergency department. Ann Emerg Med 2007;50:172–181.

4 Tyburski J, Carlin AM, Harvey EH, et al: End-tidal CO_2 and arterial CO_2 differences: a useful intraoperative mortality marketing trauma surgery. J Trauma 2003;55:892–897

5 Shankar KB, Moseley H, Kumar Y: Negative arterial to end-tidal gradients. Can J Anesth 1991;38:260–261.

6 Fletcher R, Janson B, Cumming G, Brew J: The concept of dead space with special reference to the single breath test for carbon dioxide. Br J Anaesth 1981;53: 77–88.

7 Yamanaka MK, Sue DY: Comparison of arterial end-tidal PCO_2 difference and EAD space/tidal volume ration in respiratory failure. Chest 1987;92:832–835.

8 Belpomme V, Ricard-Hibon A, Devoir C, et al: Correlation of arterial PCO_2-$PETCO_2$ in prehospital controlled ventilation. Am J Emerg Med 2005;23:852–859.

9 Anderson CT, Breen PH: Carbon dioxide kinetics and capnography during critical care. Crit Care 2000;4:207–215.

10 Lawrence MM: All You Really Need to Know to Interpret Arterial Blood Gases – Non-Invasive Blood Gas Interpretation, ed 2. Philadelphia, Lippincott, 1999.

11 Rodriguez-Roisen R, Wagner PD: Clinical relevance of ventilation-perfusion inequality determined by inert gas elimination. Eur Respir J 1998;3:469–482.
12 Dall'ava-Santucci J, Armaganidis A, Brunet F, et al: Mechanical effects of PEEP in adult respiratory distress syndrome. J Appl Physiol 1990;3:843–848.
13 Petty TI: The use, abuse and mystique of positive and emergency pressure. Am Rev Respir Dis 1998;138:875–878.
14 Coffey RL, Albert RK, Robertson HT: Mechanism of physiological dead-space response to PEEP after oleic acid induced lung injury. J Appl Physiol 1983; 55:1550–1557.
15 Yosefy C, Hay E, Nasri Y, Magen E, Reisin L: End-tidal carbon dioxide as a predictor of the arterial PCO2 in the emergency department setting. Emerg Med J 2004;21:557–559.
16 Plewa MC, Sikora S, Engoren M, et al: Evaluation of capnography in non-intubated emergency department, patients with respiratory distress. Acad Emerg Med 1995;2:901–908.
17 Clause D, Liistro G, Thys F, et al: Arterial to end-tidal CO2 (PaCO2-EtCO2) gradient as a monitoring parameter of efficacy during thrombolytic therapy for massive pulmonary embolism in spontaneously breathing patients. 23rd Int Symp Intensive Care & Emergency Medicine, Brussels, March 2003. Critical Care 2003(suppl 12):P114.
18 Hagerty JJ, Kleinman ME, Zurakowski D, Lyons AC, Krauss B: Accuracy of a new low-flow sidestream capnography technology in newborns: a pilot study. J Perinatol 2002;22:219–225.
19 Badgwell JM, McLead ME, Lerman J, Creighton RE: End-tidal PCO2 measurements sampled at the distal and proximal ends of the endotrachael tube in infants and children. Anesth Analg 1987;66:959–664.
20 McSwain SD, Hamel DS, Smith PB, Gentile MA, Srinivasan S, Meliones JN, Cheifetz IM: End-tidal and arterial carbon dioxide measurements correlated across all levels of physiologic dead space. Respir Care 2010;55;350–352.
21 Benallal H, Busso T: Analysis of end-tidal and arterial PCO2 using a breathing model. Eur J Appl Physiol 2000;83:402–408.
22 Russell GB, Graybeal JM, Strout JC: Stability of arterial to end-tidal carbon dioxide gradients during postoperative cardiorespiratory support. Can J Anaesth 1990;37:560–566.
23 Rich GF, Sconzo JM: Continuous end-tidal CO2 difference sampling within proximal end tracheal tube estimates arterial CO2 tension in infants. Can J Anaesth 1991;38:201–203.

Michael E. Donnellan, MBA
Oridion Capnography Inc.
160 Gould Street, Suite 205
Needham, MA 02494 (USA)
Tel. +1 707 422 8538, Fax +1 707 435 9231
E-Mail michael_resp@yahoo.com

Esquinas AM (ed): Applied Technologies in Pulmonary Medicine. Basel, Karger, 2011, pp 132–135

Problems of Air Travel for Patients with Lung Disease

Andrew G. Robson

Respiratory Function Service, Western General Hospital, Edinburgh, UK

Abbreviations

COPD Chronic obstructive pulmonary disease
FEV_1 Forced expiratory volume in one second
FiO_2 Inspired fraction of oxygen
PaO_2 Arterial partial pressure of oxygen
PO_2 Partial pressure of oxygen

Air travel is a rapidly expanding mode of travel worldwide. By analogy, many more passengers with chronic respiratory disease will be flying as a result of this increase.

At normal cruising altitudes (9,000–12,500 m for commercial traffic) most aircraft are designed to maintain a reduced cabin pressure which is the equivalent to an altitude of not greater than 2,438 m (8,000 ft) above sea level [1]. At this altitude, PO_2 is ~14.4 kPa and FiO_2 is the equivalent of 15.1% at sea level. Because of the sigmoid shape of the oxygen dissociation curve, most passengers can tolerate this reduction in PO_2 without experiencing any respiratory distress, but patients with chronic respiratory disease may develop clinically significant hypoxia.

The accurate prediction of symptoms at altitude is not currently possible, so most studies have focused on attempts to predict the possibility of hypoxia at altitude and a number of different assessment protocols have been developed. These protocols either expose patients to the conditions they are likely to encounter during air travel or use sea level arterial blood gas analysis to estimate altitude PO_2.

High Altitude Physiology

The sigmoid shape of the oxygen dissociation curve allows individuals with no respiratory disease to ascend to moderate altitude without any appreciable hypoxaemia. Beyond this altitude the fall in alveolar PO_2 is steep and significant hypoxia can quickly develop. Patients with respiratory disease may have a rightward shift in the oxygen dissociation curve due to chronic respiratory acidosis which will result in a decreased affinity of haemoglobin for oxygen, increasing the possibility for the development of desaturation.

The normal response to increasing altitude is an increase in cardiac output and minute ventilation, which will compensate for the reduced PO_2. However, passengers with either cardiac or respiratory limitation may experience difficulty in increasing either of these parameters sufficiently to compensate for the increased altitude. Patients with chronic respiratory disease may also have a blunted ventilatory response to hypoxia and this may lead to alveolar and tissue hypoxia, which is of considerable clinical significance.

Existing Guidelines

Two comprehensive guides giving advice on the management of patients with chronic lung disease have been published [2, 3]. These publications aim to provide guidance for physicians who are involved in assessing patients who are considering commercial air travel. Both publications stress that they are not intended to provide inflexible rules for air travel but should be used as a basis for advising each patient on an individual basis.

There are very few absolute contraindications to commercial air travel, but they include infectious tuberculosis and unresolved pneumothorax, the latter because air trapped in the pleural space will expand at altitude. Following thoracic surgery some airlines will accept patients after 2 weeks of recovery but individual assessment is required. All patients in these categories will require individual assessment.

The British Thoracic Society guidelines suggest that anybody with a resting ground level O_2 saturation >95% will be able to fly without the risk of developing significant hypoxia. The Society's guidelines also recommend that anybody with a resting O_2 saturation <92% should fly with supplemental O_2. Patients already receiving supplemental O_2 (i.e. patients on long-term oxygen therapy) should have their usual flow rate increased by 2 l/min for the duration of the flight to compensate for the reduction in PO_2.

Preflight Assessment of Patients with Respiratory Disease Considering Air Travel

In order to assess a patient's risk of hypoxia during air travel, a number of different assessment protocols have been developed. The easiest method is for the patient to breathe a hypoxic gas mixture (commonly referred to as a hypoxic challenge) which will replicate the PO_2 experienced in a pressurised commercial airliner. Ideally the patient's FiO_2 should be 15.1% as this replicates the PO_2 likely to be experienced at 2,438 m (8,000 ft). Most commercial flights actually have a simulated cabin altitude lower than this figure (~2,000 m), but it is prudent to assess a patient for the 'worst-case' scenario.

Hypoxic challenge can be carried out using a specially prepared gas mixture either from a gas cylinder or by utilising a Douglas bag, which acts as a reservoir for the hypoxic gas mixture which a patient breathes from using a non-rebreathing valve [4]. A simplification of the hypoxic inhalation challenge method was described by Vohra and Klocke [5], who used a 40% Venturi-type oxygen mask driven by 100% nitrogen, which lowers the FiO_2 to 15.1%. This method has the advantage that very little specialist equipment is required to perform the challenge and this method is being used in a number of respiratory function laboratories within Europe.

The ideal method to assess a patient's fitness to fly is to take them to a hypobaric chamber, where simulated altitude can be reproduced, but these chambers are uncommon and the author is not aware of any chambers which are used for the routine clinical assessment of patients considering commercial air travel.

Cramer et al. [6] have used a modified body plethysmograph as an exposure chamber, a method which has the advantage of eliminating the need for the patient to breathe through a mask which some patients find uncomfortable or inhibiting. The FiO_2 within the exposure chamber needs to be closely monitored to ensure that it remains with the desired range.

A number of authors have developed prediction equations, which use a patient's sea-level PaO_2 and FEV_1 to estimate PaO_2 at altitude. Although the prediction equations described will predict hypoxia in groups of patients, their accuracy in individual patients has been questioned. For example, Christensen et al. [7] found that despite adequate sea level PaO_2, significant hypoxia occurred in simulated flight in 33% of patients at rest and 66% during light exercise. These and other data support the view that the most precise way to predict hypoxia in individuals is by hypoxic challenge of the individual patient.

Oxygen Supplementation during Air Travel

Most of the studies described above have not only used hypoxic challenge or hypobaric chamber exposure to investigate the development of hypoxia, but have also explored the use of oxygen supplementation to reverse the hypoxia induced. In most cases the use of supplemental oxygen at low flow rates (2–4 l/min) has proved effective in restoring PaO_2 to ground level values. It is important to remember that not all airlines will agree to carry passengers requiring supplemental oxygen and some airlines will not provide supplemental oxygen at a flow rate >4 l/min.

Discussion

Because very few flights are diverted because of in-flight respiratory emergencies, we can assume that commercial air travel is a safe method of transport for the vast majority of patients with respiratory disease. Not all patients require in-depth assessment before flying.

Are long flights more hazardous? Most hypoxic challenges used for the clinical assessment of a patient's fitness to fly are of 20–30 min duration. The assumption has always been made that this is long enough for any physiological changes to have taken place. Akerø et al. [8] have investigated hypoxia in group of patients with COPD during a 6-hour commercial flight who found that there was an initial fall in PaO_2 once the flight had reached cruising altitude which was maintained throughout the flight.

Most published data have been concerned with investigating the response of patients with COPD. This is perhaps understandable as COPD is probably the most common condition amongst airline passengers but research has been published in other patient groups as well. Oades et al. [9] have assessed flight fitness in children with cystic fibrosis and found the hypoxic challenge to be a good predictor of which patients were at risk of significant desaturation during flight. Christensen et al. [10] have studied patients with restrictive lung disease from a variety of different causes in a hypobaric chamber and have demonstrated that these patients may become hypoxic when exposed to 2,438 m of simulated altitude. Further research on the effects of commercial air travel in a range of different respiratory diseases is required.

In summary, a number of methods to predict hypoxia have been developed to assess patient with chronic respiratory disease who wish to fly. Further research is required to answer the harder question of how to predict which patients will develop symptoms or come to actual harm through hypoxia during flight. Fortunately, for patients it is clear that commercial air travel is safe for the great majority of passengers and with adequate planning for in-flight oxygen even patients with more advanced disease can now safely enjoy the benefits of air travel.

Recommendations

- Assess each patient individually – not all patients will require hypoxic challenge.
- Where hypoxic challenge is indicated, the patients FiO_2 should ideally be 15.1%.
- Supplemental oxygen can be titrated to keep patient's PaO_2 within the desired range.

References

1 Cottrell JJ: Altitude exposures during aircraft flight. Flying higher. Chest 1988; 92:81–84.

2 British Thoracic Society: Managing passengers with respiratory disease planning air travel: BTS recommendations. Thorax 2002;57:289–304 (2004 update available at www.brit-thoracic.org.uk).

3 Aerospace Medical Association: Medical Guidelines for Airline Travel, ed 2. Aviat Space Environ Med 2003;74:A1–A19.

4 Gong H, Tashkin DP, Lee EY, et al: Hypoxia-altitude simulation test: evaluation of patients with chronic airway obstruction. Am Rev Respir Dis 1984; 130:980–986.

5 Vohra KP, Klocke RA: Detection and correction of hypoxaemia associated with air travel. Am Rev Respir Dis 1993; 148:1215–1219.

6 Cramer D, Ward S, Geddes D: Assessment of oxygen supplementation during air travel. Thorax 1996;51:202–203.

7 Christensen CC, Ryg M, Refvem OK, et al: Development of severe hypoxaemia in chronic obstructive pulmonary disease patients at 2,438 m (8,000 ft) altitude. Eur Respir J 2000;15:635–639.

8 Akerø A, Christensen CC, Edvardsen A, et al: Hypoxaemia in chronic obstructive pulmonary disease patients during a commercial flight. Eur Respir J 2005; 25:725–730.

9 Oades PJ, Buchdahl RM, Bush A: Prediction of hypoxaemia at high altitude in children with cystic fibrosis. BMJ 1994; 308:15–18.

10 Christensen CC, Ryg M, Refvem OK, et al: Effect of hypobaric hypoxia on blood gases in patients with restrictive lung disease. Eur Respir J 2002;20:300–305.

Andrew G. Robson
Senior Clinical Scientist
Respiratory Function Service, Western General Hospital
Crewe Road South, Edinburgh EH4 2XU (UK)
Tel. +44 131 537 2575, Fax +44 131 537 2351
E-Mail Andy.Robson@luht.scot.nhs.uk

Esquinas AM (ed): Applied Technologies in Pulmonary Medicine. Basel, Karger, 2011, pp 136–144

Intra-Abdominal Hypertension and Abdominal Compartment Syndrome: Measuring Techniques and the Effects on Lung Mechanics

Bart L. De Keulenaer

Intensive Care Unit, Fremantle Hospital, Fremantle, W.A., Australia

Abbreviations

ACS	Abdominal compartment syndrome
ALI	Acute lung injury
APP	Abdominal perfusion pressure
ARDS	Acute respiratory distress syndrome
CW	Chest wall
FRC	Functional residual capacity
HOB	Head of bed angle
IAH	Intra-abdominal hypertension
IAP	Intra-abdominal pressure
MV	Mechanical ventilation
PEEP	Positive end-expiratory pressure
PVR	Pulmonary vascular resistance
V-P curve	Volume-pressure curve
WSACS	World Society of Abdominal Compartment Syndrome

This overview will give an insight into the effects raised IAP can have on respiratory mechanics, its implications and what treatment strategies should be used when faced with IAH or ACS. IAH/ACS is associated with increased morbidity and mortality [1, 2] but despite this good evidence, clinicians are still reluctant to accept the importance of measuring IAP in patients at risk of developing IAH/ACS. Studies have shown that clinical examination alone has a poor sensitivity in detecting raised IAP [3, 4]. Recently, Cheatham [5] showed a significant increased patient survival to hospital discharge from 50 to 72% in 478 consecutive patients requiring an open abdomen when a continued revised IAH/ACS management algorithm was used.

The WSACS (www.wsacs.org) has published definitions, guidelines and recommendations for patients at risk for IAH/ACS. IAH is defined as a sustained pathologic elevation of IAP of 12 mm Hg, whereas ACS is defined as a sustained IAP >20 mm Hg with or without an APP (APP = MAP-IAP) of <60 mm Hg that is associated with new organ dysfunction or organ failure [6, 7]. Keeping this in mind, the application of an IAH/ACS algorithm (see WSACS website) is recommended which includes a non-surgical and surgical approach in patients at risk.

Measuring Techniques

The golden standard to measure IAP is still via the bladder where the pressure is measured in the supine position, along the mid-axillary line at the level of the superior iliac crest at end-expiration and is expressed in mm Hg [6]. There

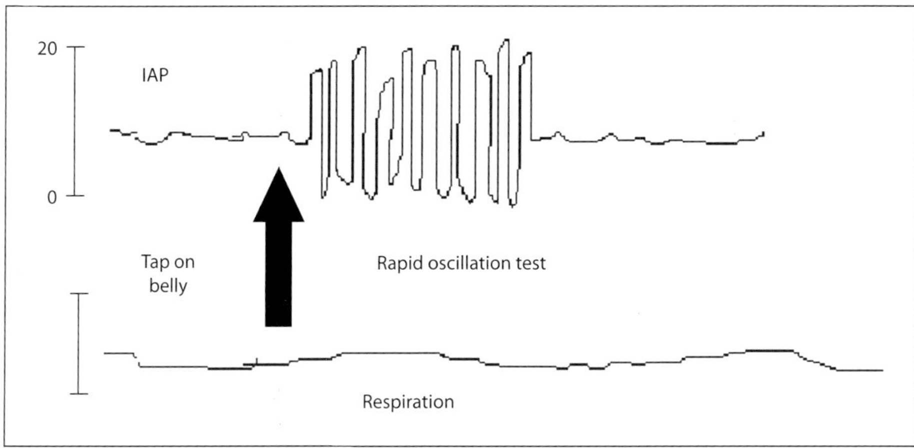

Fig. 1. Rapid oscillation flush test.

are several commercial sets available for intermittent IAP measurement like the AbViser (Wolfe-Tory Medical, Salt Lake City, Utah, USA) or the Foley manometer technique (Holtech Medical, Charlottenlund, Denmark). Some departments will have their own in-house set-up.

It is quite easy to measure the IAP once it is all set up and ready to go. It is simple and easy to familiarize the nursing staff with this technique. However, problems can arise when using a hydrostatic fluid column including changes with positioning, over- or underdamping of the system, and clinicians should be aware of these pitfalls. It is therefore recommended for correct measurement of the IAP to look for respiratory variations during measurement and the presence of oscillations when gently tapping the abdomen. In case of a damped signal the rapid flush test should be instigated (fig. 1).

Measuring IAP via AbViser Kit (fig. 2)

- First connect the AbViser kit to the patient's urinary catheter (fig. 3), then place the patient in the supine position and make sure the patient's abdominal contractions are absent.
- Zero transducer at the level of the iliac crest along the mid-axillary line (mark with a ruler).
- Instill 20 ml of sterile saline into the bladder (green diaphragm will automatically inflate to prevent the sterile saline to drain into the urine bag).
- Wait 30 s and record the IAP in mm Hg at end-expiration.
- Normally after approximately 1 min the diaphragm (green) will deflate automatically to allow urine and saline to drain again into the urine bag.
- Repeat procedure for every IAP measurement.

Measuring IAP Step-by-Step Foley Manometer (fig. 4)

Initial set-up and preparations (use aseptic technique):

- Open the Foley manometer pouch and close the tube clamp.
- Place the urine collection device under the patient's bladder and tape the drainage tube to the bed sheet as shown in figure 3.

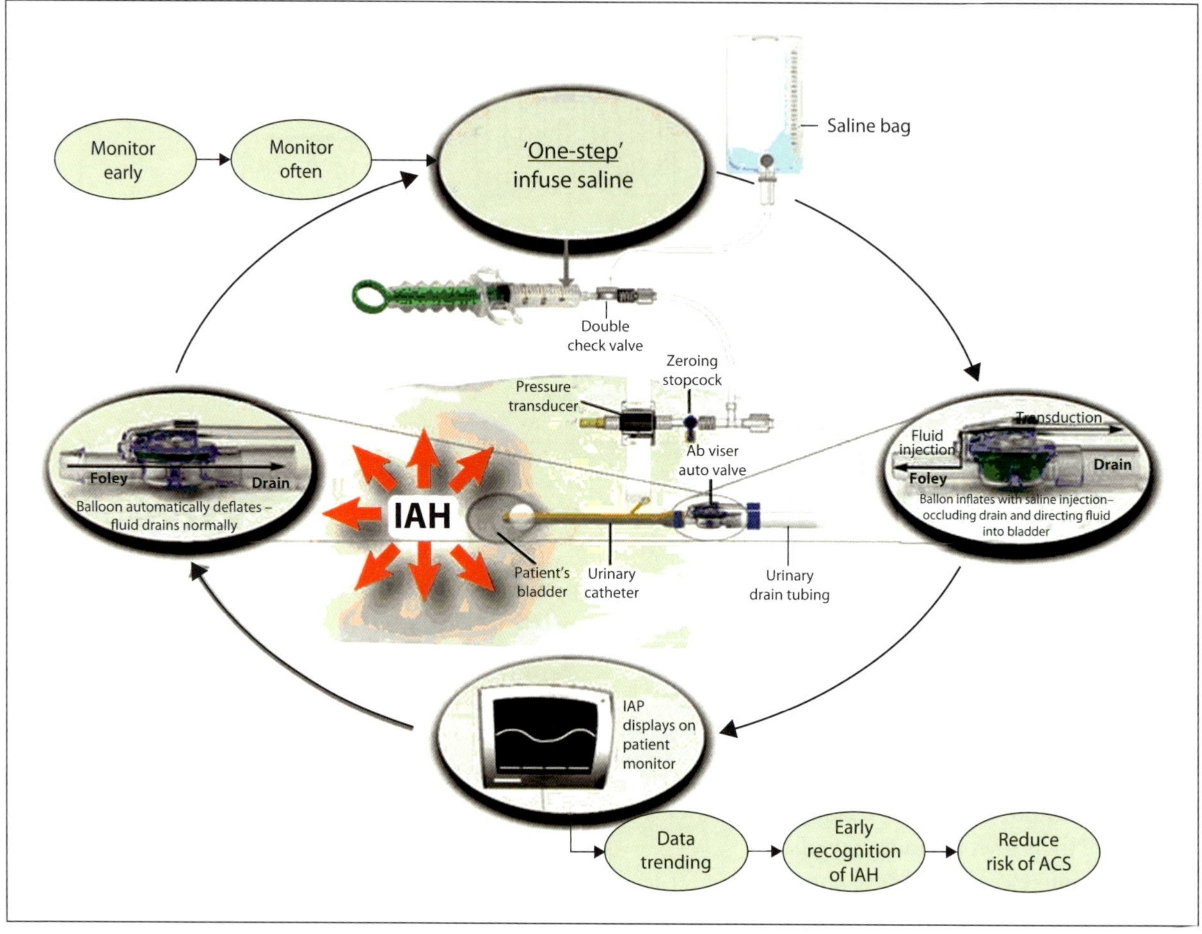

Fig. 2. AbViser diagram on how to measure IAP via the bladder technique and the AbViser kit.

- Insert the Foley manometer between the catheter and drainage device.
- Prime the Foley manometer with 20 ml of sterile saline through its needle-free injection/sampling port. Prime only once, i.e. at initial set-up, or subsequently to remove any air in the manometer tube.

IAP Monitoring

- Place the '0 mm Hg' mark of the manometer tube at the symphysis pubis level and elevate the filter vertically above the patient.
- Open clamp, and read IAP (end-expiration) when the meniscus has stabilized.
- Close clamp and place the Foley manometer in its drainage position.
- Slow descent (>20–30 s) of the meniscus during an IAP determination suggests a blocked or kinked Foley catheter.

Remember that a surgical or non-surgical intervention based on one absolute value of IAP should be avoided, it is the trend over time that is important.

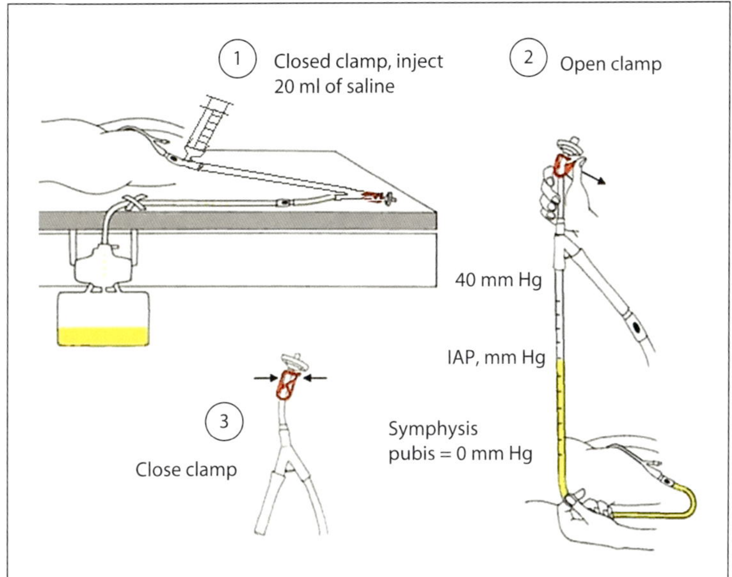

Fig. 3. Foley manometer (Holtech) showing three easy steps to measure IAP.

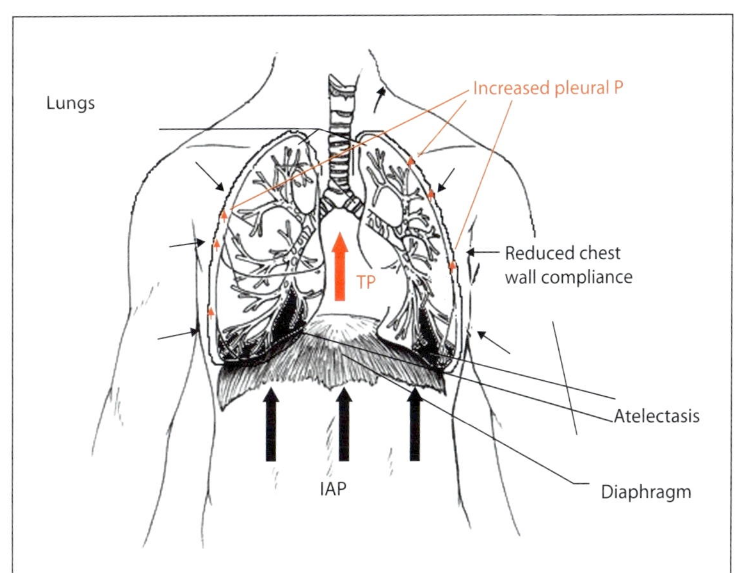

Fig. 4. Effects of raised IAP on respiratory function. TP = Intrathoracic pressure.

Table 1. Effect of body positioning on IAP measurements

	Number (observations)	Supine	HOB 15°	HOB 30°	HOB 45°	Lateral	Reverse Trendelenberg
Malbrain [11]	37 (79)	8.8±3.9	NA	NA	17.1±6.1	6.6±2.9	13.3±4.8
Chionh [12][1]	58 (174)	7 (0.7–13.2)	NA	8.5 (2.2–14)	10.3 (2.9–16.2)	NA	NA
McBeth [13]	37 (300)	13.4±4.2	NA	18.4±4.8	21.5±5.0	NA	NA
Vasquez [14][2,3]	45 (675)	10.2 (8.7–11.8)	12.4 (10.7–14.1)	14.0 (12.3–15.8)	16.7 (14.8–18.5)	NA	19.3 (16.8–21.8)
Cheatham [15][4]	132 (396)	11.8 (11.4–12.2)	13.3 (12.8–13.8)	15.4 (14.9–15.9)	NA	NA	NA
De Keulenaer [16]	10 (60)	6.6±2.9	NA	NA	NA	11.2±3.3	NA
Cobb [17]	20 (180)	1.8±2.0	NA	NA	16.7	NA	NA

Data expressed as: [1] Means ± SD, [2] Median ± range, [3] Means with 95% CI, [4] Means ± range.

Raised IAP and Respiratory Mechanics

Does the Abdomen Behave as a Hydraulic System? First we have to establish if the abdomen behaves as a hydraulic system.

Pressures in the abdomen were recognized to be atmospheric or positive when Rushmer [8] showed that the magnitude of pressure at various levels in the abdomen were related to the height of the hydrostatic column of abdominal contents above the point of measurement. In other words, it was recognized that the abdomen behaved as a hydraulic system and the pressures within were hydrostatic in nature.

Most patients in the ICU are nursed with a HOB elevation of 30–45° to reduce the risk of venous arterial pressure. IAH and ACS, as mentioned before, are associated with increased morbidity and mortality. Therefore, patients at risk of developing IAH or ACS should have their IAP measured every 4 h. It is common practice to measure IAP in the supine position via the bladder (see above) but several authors have shown that body position significantly affects IAP (table 1). This is an important observation as most ICU patients will be nursed in a semirecumbent to lateral position rather than supine causing an underestimation of the measured IAP that could be significant in the critically ill patient. Based on the available literature, IAP in the semirecumbent position at HOB 30° and 45° is on average 4 and 9 mm Hg respectively higher than the standard bladder pressure measurement in the supine position and that in patients with impending ACS or grade 3–4 IAH, this should be taken into account [9].

Table 2. Pulmonary effects of increased IAP

Properties lung/CW	Ventilation values	Bloods	Lung volumes	Others
Diaphragm elevation ↑	Auto-PEEP ↑	Hypercarbia	FRC ↓	Alveolar edema ↑
Intrathoracic pressure ↑	Peak airway pressure ↑	PaO_2 ↓ and PaO_2/FiO_2 ↓	All lung volumes (TLC, TV, ...) ↓	Activated lung neutrophils ↑
Pleural pressure ↑	Mean airway pressure ↑	A-a gradient ↓	Dynamic compliance ↓	Pulmonary inflammatory infiltration ↑
Upper inflection point on V-P curve ↓	Plateau pressure ↑		Static respiratory system compliance ↓	Pulmonary infection rate ↑
Lower inflection point on V-P curve ↑	PVR ↑		Static CW compliance ↓↓	Metabolic cost and work of breathing ↑
	Extravascular lung water ↑		Dead space ventilation ↑	

IAP and Respiratory Physiology

Atelectasis

An increased IAP results in a cephalad displacement of the diaphragm leading to *compression atelectasis* in the dependent lung fields. Such atelectasis and subsequently arterial hypoxemia (increase in physiologic shunt) are common findings in mechanically ventilated or postoperative patients in the ICU. The incidence of these complications has been reported to be as high as 70% after abdominal surgery and much lower after extra-abdominal non-thoracic procedures. In fact, after anesthesia with muscular paralysis, crest-shaped changes of increased densities in the dependent regions of both lungs on CT have been found. As a result of the cephalad displacement of the diaphragm, there will be a *decrease in functional residual capacity, increased alveolar dead space* and an *increase in physiological shunt* all leading to hypoxemia and hypercarbia. These changes can be reduced or prevented when PEEP is applied. Increased IAP are also superimposed onto the chest cavity, subsequently increasing the *intrathoracic pressure* and pulmonary vasculature eventually leading to *pulmonary hypertension* (table 2).

Clinical implications: Raised IAP leads to hypoxia and hypercarbia and can be prevented by PEEP.

Patient Population

We know from previous data that the occurrence of increased IAP and IAH is not limited to surgery or trauma cases alone (45.6%). The incidence of IAH in critically ill medical patients is even higher (54.4%). Therefore, it affects the entire ICU population which makes it quite a challenge in terms of MV when raised IAP and their effects are not accounted for. We have published a case report of a patient on non-invasive positive pressure ventilation experiencing a cardiac arrest whilst he was put into the semirecumbent position, which instantly increased his IAP and led to ACS [10]. High IAP will lead to increased intrathoracic pressures, reduced venous return, increased afterload, increased PVR, reduced cardiac contractility and eventually cardiac arrest. We identified the problem early being severe ACS with an IAP >30 mm Hg due to massive gastric insufflation causing hypercarbia and asystole. As soon as a nasogastric tube was inserted, the dramatic events were reversed almost instantly.

Clinical implications: Raised IAP can affect the entire ICU population and early intervention (surgical or non-surgical) should be instigated.

High IAP and Increased edema Formation

High IAP in oleic acid lung injury in pigs significantly *increased the amount of edema.* In their animal study they investigated the impact of an IAP of 0 and 20 mm Hg on respiration and hemodynamics [18]. They found that after applying 20 mm Hg IAP to healthy lungs the gas content significantly decreased but lung tissue mass was unaffected. In oleic acid-injured lungs, not only was there a further decrease in the gas content, but there was also a significant further increase in tissue weight. This is probably due to increased edema formation and decreased fluid clearance. The former, due to increased thoracic central venous and pulmonary artery pressures in injured lungs with increased permeability, the latter due to increased intrathoracic pressure and its effects on the lymphatic flow.

Clinical Implications: In patients with ALI/ARDS, raised IAP can promote edema formation. Management includes improving abdominal wall compliance, evacuating intraluminal contents, evacuating abdominal fluid collections and correcting positive fluid balance when IAP is raised. An adequate PEEP level to counteract raised IAP is warranted and subsequently will improve hypoxia.

IAP and the Effects in ARDS and ALI?

ARDS has become a well-recognized entity and results from a number of different initiating insults with the final common pathway damage to the alveolar epithelium and endothelium leading to high permeability edema. MV can result in end-inspiratory alveolar overstretching and/or repeated alveolar collapse subsequently disturbing the normal fluid balance across the alveolo-capillary membrane. The effects (disturbance of the integrity of the endothelium, epithelium and impairment of the surfactant system) of MV are similar to those seen in ARDS. There is some evidence that MV may result in translocation of bacteria from the lungs into the bloodstream and the release of inflammatory mediators from the lung tissue into the systemic circulation. Therefore, MV may contribute to the development of multiple organ failure. Recent animal studies have shown that abdominal compression followed by abdominal decompression significantly increased the neutrophils in the lungs. Histopathological findings showed dense pulmonary inflammatory infiltration including atelectasis and alveolar edema.

Clinical implications: Increased IAP can provoke the release of proinflammatory cytokines leading to multiple organ failure.

IAP and Decreased CW Compliance

ARDS is characterized by a reduction in FRC and a decrease in static compliance of the respiratory system. Given the underlying pulmonary injury that is present in patients with ARDS, the decrease in static compliance is thought to reflect mainly alterations of the mechanical properties of the lung rather than those of the CW. However, a number of studies have reported a decrease in CW compliance in mechanically ventilated patients with ALI. Mutoh et al. [19] demonstrated in an animal model that abdominal distension markedly altered respiratory mechanics by its effect on the mechanical properties of the CW. On the basis of these results, the *decrease in CW compliance* found in patients with ARDS was ascribed to abdominal distension. It also seems that alterations in the mechanics of the respiratory system are based on the underlying disease process for ARDS. In patients with medical ARDS, the inspiratory V-P curve of the respiratory system and lung showed a progressive reduction in elastance with inflating volume because of alveolar recruitment (upward concavity) [20]. In patients in whom ARDS followed major abdominal surgery, abdominal distension with increased values of CW elastance was observed (upward convexity indicating a progressive increase in elastance with inflating volume caused by alveolar overdistension). When abdominal pressure was normalized by surgical re-exploration, improvement of the mechanical properties of the respiratory system, lung, and CW was observed. These data suggest that the flattening of the V-P curve at high pressures observed in some patients with ARDS may be due to increase in CW elastance related to abdominal distension. These results may also have importance for the optimal ventilatory management of critically ill patients with ARDS with respect to the selection of optimal PEEP and V_T levels to minimize ventilator-induced lung injury.

The key point is that for a given applied pressure, the transpulmonary pressure falls when the pleural pressure rises. The diaphragm is mechanically coupled to the abdominal wall and contents. If IAP increases, FRC decreases, which will shift the V-P curve of the respiratory system/CW/lung to a lower volume (downward) and rightward. Abdominal distension causes flattening of the inspiratory V-P curve of the respiratory system due to increased CW elastance and or further atelectasis. Decompression of the abdomen shows an upward displacement along the volume axis of V-P curves which reflects recruited volume. Those findings are important with regard to PEEP.

In the early stages of ARDS, PEEP regionally overstretches the pulmonary units that are already open, increasing the elastance. PEEP keeps the alveoli open at expiration (preventing them to collapse), thereby decreasing compliance of the respiratory system. In extrapulmonary ARDS data have shown that PEEP opens collapsed alveoli and induces recruitment, whereas in pulmonary ARDS, PEEP leads more to overstretch and increase in elastance (improvement of gas exchange is more likely to be via regional diversion of ventilation or perfusion). Therefore, in extrapulmonary ARDS, some have suggested best PEEP equals IAP.

Clinical implications: Raised IAP decreases CW compliance. In ARDS secondary to abdominal surgery, reduced CW compliance results in flattening of V-P curve at high pressures, whereas in medical ARDS due to lung recruitment the opposite occurs.

Conclusion

Raised IAP can have a significant impact on the respiratory function and hemodynamic parameters in the critically ill patient and when not accounted for can increase morbidity and mortality. Future studies should focus on outcome and mortality trials and the WSACS has successfully endorsed many multicenter trials in an attempt to promote research in this particular area in the critically ill patient.

References

1 Malbrain ML, Chiumello D, Pelosi P, et al: Prevalence of intra-abdominal hypertension in critically ill patients: a multi-centre epidemiological study. Intensive Care Med 2004;30:822–829.

2 Malbrain ML, Chiumello D, Pelosi P, et al: Incidence and prognosis of intra-abdominal hypertension in a mixed population of critically ill patients: a multiple-center epidemiological study. Crit Care Med 2005;33:315–322.

3 Sugrue M, Bauman A, Jones F, et al: Clinical examination is an inaccurate predictor of intra-abdominal pressure. World J Surg 2002;26:1428–1431.

4 Kirkpatrick AW, Brenneman FD, McLean RF, et al: Is clinical examination an accurate indicator of raised intra-abdominal pressure in critically injured patients? Can J Surg 2000;43:207–211.

5 Cheatham ML: Is the evolving management of intra-abdominal hypertension and abdominal compartment syndrome improving survival? Crit Care Med 2010; 38:402–407.

6 Cheatham ML, Malbrain ML, Kirkpatrick A, et al: Results from the International Conference of Experts on Intra-Abdominal Hypertension and Abdominal Compartment Syndrome. II. Recommendations. Intensive Care Med 2007;33:951–962.

7 Malbrain ML, Cheatham ML, Kirkpatrick A, et al: Results from the International Conference of Experts on Intra-Abdominal Hypertension and Abdominal Compartment Syndrome. I. Definitions. Intensive Care Med 2006;32: 1722–1732.

8 Rushmer R: The nature of intraperitoneal and intrarectal pressure Am J Physiol 1946:242–249.

9 De Keulenaer BL, De Waele JJ, Powell B, et al: What is normal intra-abdominal pressure and how is it affected by positioning, body mass and positive end-expiratory pressure? Intensive Care Med 2009;35:969–976.

10 De Keulenaer BL, De Backer A, Schepens DR, et al: Abdominal compartment syndrome related to noninvasive ventilation. Intensive Care Med 2003;29:1177–1181.

11 Malbrain ML: Different techniques to measure intra-abdominal pressure: time for a critical re-appraisal. Intensive Care Med 2003;30:357–371.

12 Chionh JJ, Wei BP, Martin JA, et al: Determining normal values for intra-abdominal pressure. ANZ J Surg 2006; 76:1106–1109.

13 McBeth PB Zygun D, Widder S, Cheatham M, et al: Effect of patient positioning on intra-abdominal pressure monitoring. Am J Surg 2007;193:644–647.

14 Vasquez DG, Berg-Copas GM, Wetta-Hall R, et al: Influence of semi-recumbent position on intra-abdominal pressure as measured by bladder pressure. J Surg Res 2007;139:280–285.

15 Cheatham ML DWJ, De Keulenaer B, Widder S, et al: Effect of body position on intra-abdominal pressure measurement: A multicenter analysis. Acta Clin Belg 2007;62:246

16 De Keulenaer BL CG, Maddox I, Powell B, et al: Intra-abdominal pressure measurements in lateral decubitus and supine position. Acta Clin Belg Suppl 2007;62:269.

17 Cobb WS, Burns JM, Kercher KW, et al: Normal intra-abdominal pressure in healthy adults. J Surg Res 2005;129:231–235.

18 Quintel M, Pelosi P, Caironi P, et al: An increase of abdominal pressure increases pulmonary edema in oleic acid-induced lung injury. Am J Respir Crit Care Med 2004;169:534–541.

19 Mutoh T, Lamm WJ, Embree LJ, et al: Volume infusion produces abdominal distension, lung compression, and chest wall stiffening in pigs. J Appl Physiol 1992;72:575–582.

20 Chiumello D, Carlesso E, Aliverti A, et al: Effects of volume shift on the pressure-volume curve of the respiratory system in ALI/ARDS patients. Minerva Anesthesiol 2007;73:109–118.

Bart L. De Keulenaer, MD, FJFICM
Intensive Care Unit, Fremantle Hospital
Alma Street, East Fremantle, WA 6160 (Australia)
Tel. +61 8 9431 3333, Fax +61 8 9431 3009
E-Mail bdekeul@hotmail.com

Esquinas AM (ed): Applied Technologies in Pulmonary Medicine. Basel, Karger, 2011, pp 145–150

Pleural Effusions in Critically Ill Patients

Vasilios Papaioannou · Ioannis Pneumatikos

Intensive Care Unit, Alexandroupolis University Hospital, Democritus University of Thrace, Alexandroupolis, Greece

Abbreviations

C_L	Lung compliance
CT	Computed tomography
C_W	Chest wall compliance
CXRs	Chest x-rays
LDH	Lactate dehydrogenase
LUS	Lung ultrasound
PEEP	Positive end-expiratory pressure
PE(s)	Pleural effusion(s)
SCXR	Semirecumbent position chest x-ray

PEs are defined as the excessive accumulation of fluid in the pleural space indicating an imbalance between pleural fluid formation and removal. The incidence of PEs in the ICU seems to be common and varies with screening methods, from approximately 8% for physical examination to more than 60% for routine LUS [1]. Patients in the ICU may develop PEs due to either their primary disease or as a result of several supportive and therapeutic interventions. In particular, hypotension and hemodynamic compromise requiring aggressive hydration may lead to fluid overload and interstitial edema formation with subsequent pleural transudation. The current review focuses on the PE pathophysiology, diagnosis and management in the ICU, based on recent findings from clinical studies. Hemothorax and chylothorax will not be discussed in this article.

Pathophysiology

The pleura space is normally filled with a very small amount of colorless alkaline fluid witch serves as a coupling system between the chest wall and the lung. In cases of both hydrostatic and high-permeability pulmonary edema, fluid can enter the pleural cavity from the interstitial spaces of the lung via the visceral pleura. The lymphatics have the capacity to absorb 20 times more fluid than is normally formed [2]. Accordingly, a PE may occur when excessive formation of fluid can overwhelm absorptive mechanisms or when there is decreased fluid absorption by the lymphatics.

Lung collapse associated with PEs may lead to hypoxemia due to ventilation-perfusion mismatch or true shunt. However, different studies have failed to demonstrate severe oxygenation impairment due to PEs, whereas unilateral drainage of large effusions had mild effects on gas exchange [3]. Furthermore, even if pleural fluid accumulation may reduce lung volumes, it has been demonstrated that the effects of both fluid accumulation and removal upon respiratory mechanics depend on the ratio of lung/C_W [4]. The more compliant the lung, the greater the change in lung functional residual capacity; the more compliant the chest wall, the greater the thoracic cage adjustment with smaller effect upon lung volumes.

Etiology

PEs are traditionally classified as either transudates or exudates. A transudative PE develops when the systemic factors influencing the formation or absorption of pleural fluid are altered. Examples of conditions producing transudative PE are left ventricular failure, pulmonary embolism and cirrhosis. On the contrary, an exudative PE develops due to mismatch between local factors influencing the formation and absorption of pleural fluid [5]. Examples of conditions producing exudative PEs are bacterial or viral pneumonia, malignancy and pulmonary embolism. Only three studies have prospectively referred to the frequency and etiology of PEs in the ICU [1, 6, 7]. Table 1 describes the most common causes of PEs in critically ill patients.

Diagnosis

Chest X-Ray Imaging

Nearly all CXRs taken in the ICU are obtained with patients lying in a semirecumbent position – SCXR. This technique is limited by the fact that the film cassette is placed posterior to the thorax, so the x-ray beam originates anterior, at a shorter distance than recommended and quite often not tangentially to the diaphragmatic dome, thereby making difficult the correct interpretation of the silhouette sign. The most common radiographic finding of a PE in a SCXR is increased homogeneous density over the lower lung field without obliterating normal bronchovascular markings, whereas air bronchogram, and hilar or mediastinal displacement are missing until the effusion is massive. Other common signs are blunted of costophrenic angle and loss of hemidiaphragm silhouette. A normal SCXR does not exclude the presence of a PE. The overall accuracy of a SCXR for detecting a PE with reference to decubitus view has been estimated to 0.67–0.95. A more recent study using the LUS as gold standard estimated the accuracy of SCXR to 82% [8].

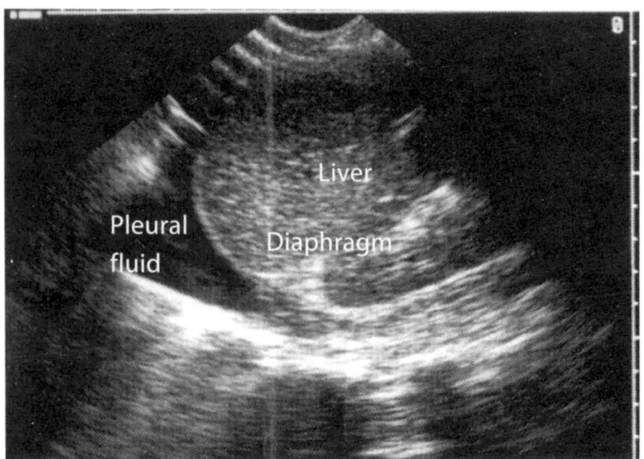

Fig. 1. LUS in an ICU patient showing a PE. Its appearance is anechoic, implying rather a transudate.

Lung Ultrasound

LUS shows better sensitivity and reliability for diagnosis of PEs than bedside SCXR, it rules out other etiologies such as atelectasis or consolidation, takes less time than SCXR and can be repeated serially at the bedside. In addition, the skills required to detect PEs are easy to acquire. A PE is described as an anechoic or hypoechoic layer between two pleural layers (fig. 1). PEs can be easily distinguished from spleen and liver by visualization of the so-called 'sinusoid sign' which indicates the centrifugal shifting of the lung towards the chest wall during inspiration. LUS evaluation of PEs in mechanically ventilated patients is very important because it allows the quantification of pleural fluid, supporting the decision

Table 1. Causes of PEs in ICU patients reported in three studies.

Ca uses of PEs	Mattison et al. [1] (n = 62)	Fartoukh et al. [6] (n = 113)	Chih-Yen et al. [7] (n = 94)
Congestive heart failure	22 (35.5%)	28 (24.8%)	9 (10%)
Atelectasis	14 (23%)	2 (1.7%)	–
Cirrhosis	5 (8%)	6 (5.3%)	2 (2.1%)
Hypoalbuminemia	5 (8%)	–	7 (7.4%)
Nephrotic syndrome	–	1 (0.8%)	–
Parapneumonic effusions	7 (11%)	29 (25.6%)	36 (38.3%)
Pulmonary embolism	–	5 (4.4%)	–
Empyema	1 (2%)	12 (10.6%)	15 (16%)
Malignancies	2 (3%)	11 (9.7%)	1 (1%)
Tuberculosis	–	2 (1.7%)	–
Pancreatitis	1 (2%)	2 (1.7%)	2 (2%)
Postsurgical effusions	–	–	1 (1%)
Collagen vascular disease	–	–	1 (1%)
Uremic pleurisy	1(2)%	–	–
Hemothorax	–	4 (3.4%)	–
Trauma	–	–	–
Sepsis	–	–	10 (10.6%)
Other	1 (2%)	–	–
Unknown	3 (5%)	6 (5.3%)	8 (9%)

whether or not thoracocentesis should be performed and providing visual guidance for pleural fluid evacuation [9]. In the supine position, a maximum interpleural distance at the lung base in end-expiration (S_{ep}) ≥50 mm is highly predictive of a PE ≥500 ml [10]. Another important contribution of LUS is to provide non-invasive information about the nature of PEs. Transudates are always anechoic whereas a liquid with mobile particles or septa is suggestive of exudates or hemothorax.

Chest CT Scan

CT scan is the 'gold standard' examination for detecting and characterizing PEs. CT scan has the advantage over LUS in that it can evaluate the pleural surface better, and it is ideal to assess the lung parenchyma and tracheobronchial tree. In simple uncomplicated PEs, it shows crescent-shaped opacities in the posterior and basal portions of the hemithorax. Moreover, chest CT can aid in differential diagnosis between empyema and lung abscess [1].

Pleural Fluid Examination

Transudates are generally clear with a slightly yellow tint. Exudates are usually cloudy with large numbers of cells. If pus is aspirated, an empyema is established. Pus is determined by its gross appearance, which is a thick, viscous and opaque fluid.

Exudative PEs meet at least one of the Light's criteria, whereas transudative PEs meet none: (1) pleural fluid protein/serum protein >0.5; (2) pleural fluid LDH/serum LDH >0.6; (3) pleural fluid LDH more than two-thirds of the normal upper limit for serum. Light's criteria may label approximately 25% of transudates as exudates [5]. In

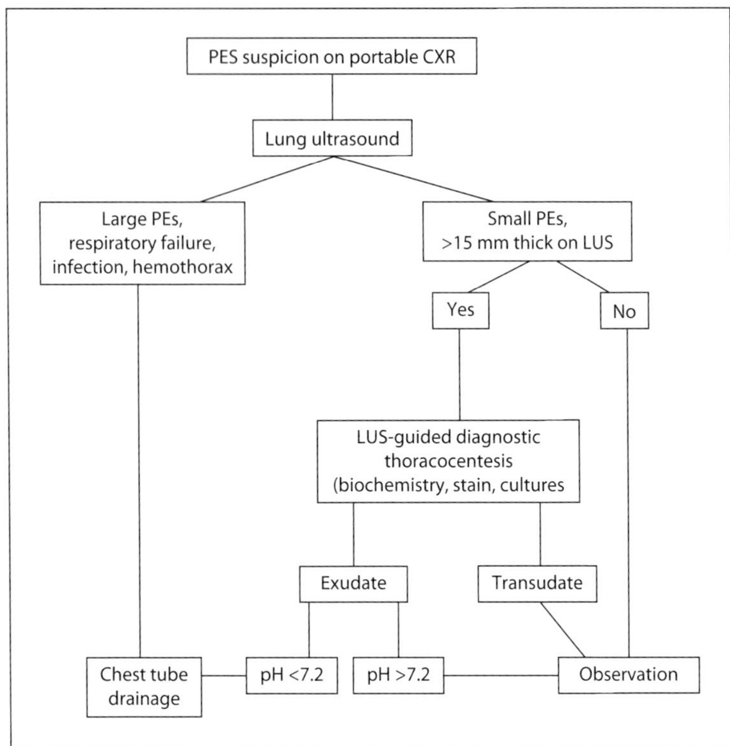

Fig. 2. Flowchart for the management of PE in critically ill patients based on LUS and pleural fluid biochemistry findings.

these conditions, a serum to pleural fluid albumin gradient >1.2 g/dl indicates a transudative PE. A combination of PE cholesterol (criterion for exudates: PE-CHOL >60 mg/dl) and PE LDH concentrations (criterion for exudates: PE-LDH >280 UI/l) seems to have the same or highest discriminatory potential than Light's criteria [11]. The pH of normal pleural fluid is approximately 7.62 owing to active transport of HCO_3^- into the pleural space. A low pH is seen in inflammatory and infiltrative disorders such as infected parapneumonic effusions, empyema, malignancies, and collagen vascular disease. A parapneumonic pleural fluid with pH <7.2 is an indication for pleural drainage. The glucose concentration in transudates and in most exudates is similar to that in the serum, as glucose is of low molecular weight and moves from blood to pleural fluid by simple diffusion. Diseases with low pleural fluid pH may also have a low pleural fluid glucose concentration, defined as <60 mg/dl or a pleural fluid/serum glucose ratio of <0.5 [5].

Management of PEs in the ICU

Pleural fluid characteristics remain the major reliable diagnostic test for guiding management in critically ill patients. Diagnostic sampling (diagnostic thoracocentesis) is recommended in all cases with PEs associated with a lung disease or recent chest trauma or surgery. Figure 2 depicts different steps for the management of PEs in the ICU setting, based on LUS and pleural fluid analysis findings. LUS is especially valuable in guiding drainage of loculated or very small effusions. With the patient adequately positioned on his back or in supine position, one must check for an inspiratory distance of at least 15 mm with the effusion visible at the adjacent upper and lower intercostals spaces. Optimally, the puncture should be done within seconds to minutes of the marking.

The main indications of therapeutic thoracentesis in critically ill patients include drainage of empyema or hemothorax, and improvement of ventilatory compromise in cases of massive effusions. Small PEs do not usually require therapeutic thoracocentesis and typically will resolve with conservative management (i.e., aggressive fluid removal). However, in patients with acute respiratory failure, catheter drainage of even a small PE can improve oxygenation significantly [12].

In a recent review, Graf [13] proposed a therapeutic algorithm based on respiratory mechanics. In cases of low C_W, the same PEs will compress more the adjacent lung, inducing significant collapse that has been shown to be resistant to increasing levels of PEEP. Drainage is likely beneficial in these cases. If chest wall is normal related to reduced C_L PEEP or any recruitment maneuver can reduce the impact of PEs on lung volume and improve oxygenation. Conversely, if C_W is normal and no benefit results from recruitment maneuver, lung collapse from PEs is minor and drainage is not warranted.

Recommendations

- PEs are common in ICU patients but they can easily go unrecognized due to technical and diagnostic limitations of supine portable CXRs. They are usually small, uncomplicated and postoperative, and resolve with conservative management. However, if infection is considered, a thoracocentesis should be done without delay.
- Thoracocentesis in critically ill patients should be performed with the help of LUS or CT scan guidance to decrease the risk of complications.
- Oxygenation effects of PE drainage may vary from lack of response to significant amelioration during mechanical ventilation. In these patients, the ratio of C_W/C_L has a major role on lung volume and gas exchange response to pleural fluid drainage.

References

1 Mattison LE, Coppage L, Alderman DF, et al: Pleural effusions in the medical ICU: prevalence, causes, and clinical implications. Chest 1997;111:1018–1023.

2 Miserocchi G: Physiology and pathophysiology of pleural fluid turnover. Eur Respir J 1997;10:219–225.

3 Nishida O, Arellano R, Cheng DC, et al: Gas exchange and hemodynamics in experimental pleural effusion. Crit Care Med 1999;27:583–587.

4 Brown NE, Zamel N, Aberman A: Changes in pulmonary mechanics and gas exchange following thoracocentesis. Chest 1978;74:540–542.

5 Light RW, MacGregor MI, Luschsinger PC, et al: Pleural effusions: the diagnostic separation of transudates and exudates. Ann Intern Med 1972;62:57–63.

6 Fartoukh M, Azoulay E, Galliot R, et al: Clinically documented pleural effusions in medical ICU patients: how useful is routine thoracentesis? Chest 2002;121:178–184.

7 Tu CY, Hsu WH, Hsia TC, et al: Pleural effusions in febrile medical ICU patients. Chest ultrasound study. Chest 2004;126:1274–1280.

8 Emamian SA, Kaasbol MA, Olsen JF, et al: Accuracy of the diagnosis of pleural effusion on supine chest x-ray. Eur Radiol 1997;7:57–60.

9 Eibenberger KL, Dock WI, Ammann ME, et al: Quantification of pleural effusions: sonography versus radiography. Radiology 1994;191:681–684.

10 Roch A, Bojan M, Michelet P, et al: Usefulness of ultrasonography in predicting pleural effusions >500 ml in patients receiving mechanical ventilation. Chest 2005;127:224–232.

11 Romero S, Martinez A, Hernandez L, et al: Light's criteria revisited: consistency and comparison with new proposed alternative criteria for separating pleural transudates from exudates. Respiration 2000;67:18–23.

12 Miller KS, Sahn SA: Chest tubes. Indications, technique, management and complications. Chest 1987;91:258–264.

13 Graf J: Pleural effusion in the mechanically ventilated patient. Curr Opin Crit Care 2009;15:10–17.

Ioannis Pneumatikos, MD
Intensive Care Unit, Alexandroupolis University Hospital
Democritus University of Thrace
GR–68000 Dragana, Alexandroupolis (Greece)
Tel. +30 25 5107 5081, Fax +30 25 5103 0423, E-Mail ipnevmat@med.duth.gr

Esquinas AM (ed): Applied Technologies in Pulmonary Medicine. Basel, Karger, 2011, pp 151–155

Gravitational Force and Respiratory Colonization in Mechanical Ventilation

Hany Aly[a] · Lorenzo Berra[b] · Theodor Kolobow[c]

[a]Division of Newborn Services, The George Washington University and Children's National Medical Center, Washington, D.C.; [b]Massachusetts General Hospital, Boston, Mass., and [c]Pulmonary and Critical Care Medicine Branch, Heart Lung and Blood Institute, National Institute of Health, Bethesda, Md., USA

Abbreviations

CASS Continuous aspiration of subglottic secretions
ETT Endotracheal tube
VAP Ventilation-associated pneumonia

VAP that develops in patients receiving mechanical ventilation is the most common nosocomial infection in patients with acute respiratory failure, and is associated with prolonged hospitalization, increase in healthcare costs and with a 20–70% mortality [1]. The aerodigestive tract above the vocal cords is always heavily colonized by several species of bacteria. However, in the healthy human, the lower respiratory tract remains free of pathogenic bacteria. The major defense mechanisms in preventing colonization of the lower airways and the development of pneumonia center on the cough reflex and mucociliary clearance. All such mechanisms are greatly impaired in the intubated and mechanically ventilated patient. The ETT itself allows direct access to the lower respiratory tract and thwarts the cough reflex. The inflated ETT cuff blocks the normal flow of mucous clearance which is necessary to remove particles and microbes from the bronchial tree. When the ETT cuff inflates within the trachea, folds on the ETT cuff always form, allowing passage of bacteria-colonized secretions from the oropharynx or by gastric reflux from the stomach, into the lower airways [2]. Leakage of secretions around the ETT cuff has been observed in more than 80% of intubated patients undergoing surgery [2, 3]. It is likely that the semirecumbent position increases the pooling of oral secretions in the oropharynx. The hydrostatic pressure of secretions that collect in the subglottic space (area above the ETT cuff) may facilitate the leakage across the ETT cuff into the lower airways.

Aspiration of a large inoculum of pathogenic bacteria is the primary cause in the development of VAP [1–3]. The stomach of critically ill patients often becomes colonized with Gram-negative bacteria. With aspiration of gastric contents into the oropharynx, these organisms can overgrow the normal oropharynx flora, and through aspiration across the ETT cuff colonize the lower airways and lead to lung infection. Furthermore, during mechanical ventilation, formation of water droplets on the inner surface of the ETT, due to moisture condensation, is unavoidable. A biofilm rapidly develops that covers the inner lumen of the ETT. The biofilm is a potential reservoir of bacteria [4] that will flow into the lungs when the

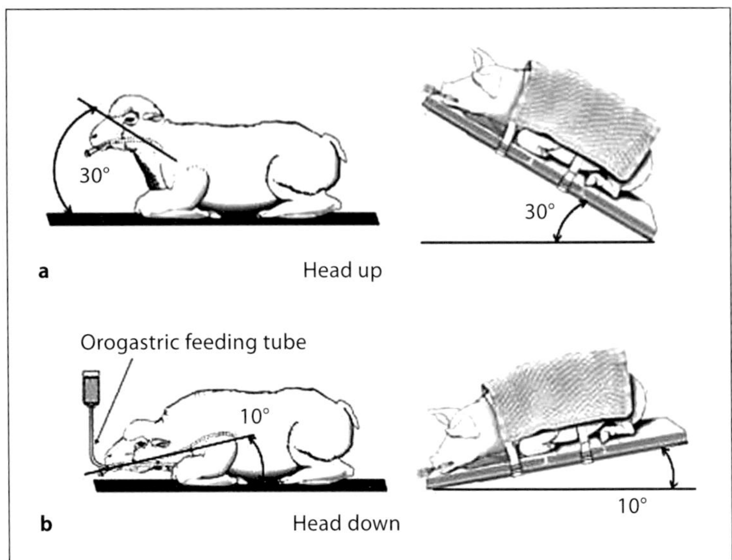

Fig. 1. Illustration of the two study positions: (**a**) the 'head-up' position with orientation of the trachea/ETT upward against gravity (to mimic the semirecumbent position), and (**b**) the 'head-down' position, with the orientation of the trachea/ETT downward [7].

patient is in the semirecumbent position or out of the ETT when the patient is in the Trendelenburg-lateral body position.

Despite these concerns, the US Center for Disease Control recommends positioning the patient in semirecumbent position with the head elevated 30–45° to decrease aspiration of gastric content and colonization of the upper aerodigestive tract by pathogens from the stomach [5, 6]. The level of evidence of this recommendation to prevent VAP is supposedly category II: 'recommendation suggested for implementation and supported by suggestive clinical or epidemiologic studies or by strong theoretical rationale.' However, no animal or human studies were carried out to understand role pathogenic mechanisms of VAP related to gravity until recently.

Animal Studies

The study conducted by Panigada et al. [7] was the first VAP animal model to provide a comprehensive assessment of the effect of gravity on development of VAP. In this experiment, sheep were randomized either to the 'head-up' position to mimic the semirecumbent position, or the 'head-down' position, with the orientation of the trachea/ETT respectively above, or below the horizontal (fig. 1). All sheep in the 'head-down' position were placed in a rotational system that allowed turning sheep from one side to the other in a timed manner. Half of the sheep with the head down received enteral feeding and half did not. Animals were ventilated for 72 h and then sacrificed. No antibiotics were administered at any time. All sheep in the 'head-up' position had a significant decrease in PaO_2/FiO_2 and heavy bacterial colonization of the lungs. All sheep in the 'head-down' rotating position retained excellent lung function with normal PaO_2/FiO_2 and no evidence of VAP or bacterial lung colonization.

In a subsequent study, Berra et al. [8] examined the effects of body position when the ETT is coupled with a side channel just above the cuff for CASS on the development of VAP. Twenty-two sheep were randomized into three groups. Eight sheep were kept prone, with the head

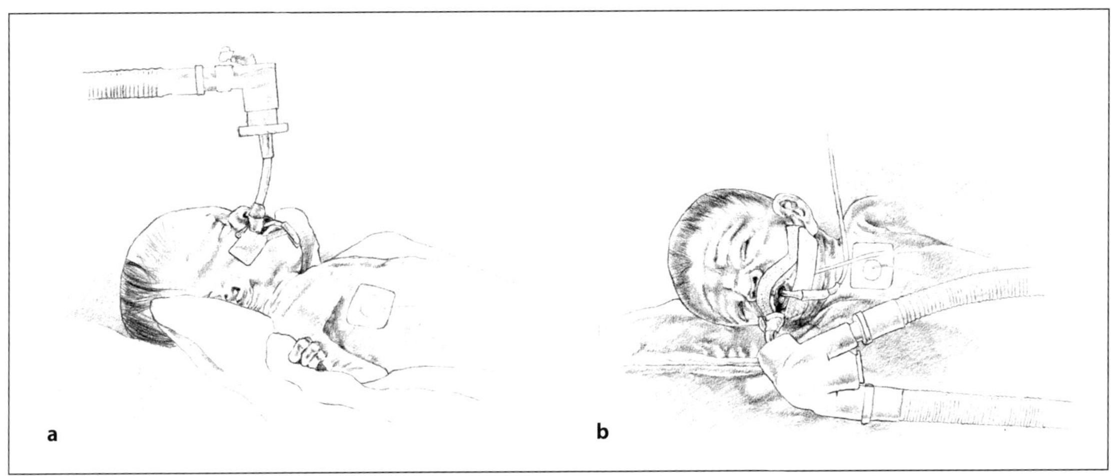

Fig. 2. Illustrations of the two study positions: (**a**) supine position: the infant is maintained on his/her back while the ETT is held upright in the vertical position and the bed is kept horizontal, and (**b**) lateral position: the infant is maintained on his or her side, with the ETT resting on the bed at the same level as the trachea [10].

elevated 30° above the horizontal plane (control group); 14 sheep were intubated with an ETT for CASS; 7 of these 14 sheep were kept prone with the head elevated (CASS-up group), and 7 sheep with the trachea horizontal (CASS-down group). The lower respiratory tract in all sheep kept with the head elevated 30° above horizontal was highly colonized in both of the control and the CASS-up groups. However, in the CASS-down group, the lower respiratory tract was not colonized in 6 of 7 sheep. One sheep showed low levels of bacterial growth.

In yet another study, Bassi et al. [9] investigated the effects of gravitational force on tracheal mucus transport, which is a primary defense mechanisms to prevent lung bacterial colonization. Sixteen intubated sheep were again randomized to be positioned with the orientation of the trachea above (30–45° from horizontal), or below (5°) horizontal (Trendelenburg position). Tracheal mucus velocity was measured via radiographic tracking of tantalum disks. Tracheal mucus flow in sheep in the Trendelenburg position was always towards the ETT cuff with an average speed of 2.1 ± 1.1 mm/min. Mucus flow, constantly moving within the trachea towards the glottis, was mechanically obstructed by inflated ETT cuff and accumulated at the cuff of the ETT, and was either spontaneously drained through the ETT lumen, or was cleared during routine tracheal suction. In sheep in the semirecumbent position, tracheal mucus flow was first towards the glottis in the non-dependent (dorsal) part of the trachea, then mucus accumulated at the inflated ETT cuff and gravitated to the dependent (ventral) part of the trachea, and ultimately revered direction and, by the force of gravity, moved towards the lungs. Six out of 8 sheep in the semirecumbent position developed pneumonia, while no pneumonia was acquired by any of the sheep positioned with the trachea oriented below horizontal. Similar results were reproduced in pigs ventilated for 168 h (fig. 1) to overcome concerns with sheep (ruminants) that may not be a clinically relevant model of infection because of their high colonization of the gastrointestinal tract and abundant production of oropharyngeal secretions [oral commun., unpubl. results].

Table 1. Number (%) of infants and types of microorganisms recovered in tracheal aspirates at days 2 and 5 of mechanical ventilation (χ^2 value = 19.8) [10]

	Supine n = 30	Lateral n = 30	p value
Microbiological results on day 2	20 (67)	14 (47)	0.12
Gram-negative rods	13 (43)	11(37)	
Klebsiella	9 (30)	8 (27)	
Pseudomonus	3 (10)	2 (7)	
Enterobacter	1 (3)	1 (3)	
Gram-positive cocci			
Staphylococcus	1(3)	0 (0)	
Mixed organisms	6(20)	3 (10)	
Microbiological results on day 5	26 (87)	9 (30)	<0.01
Gram-negative rods	18 (60)	6 (20)	
Klebsiella	10 (33)	4 (13)	
Pseudomonus	6 (20)	2 (7)	
Enterobacter	2 (7)	0 (0)	
Gram-positive cocci	0 (0)	2 (7)	
Staphylococcus	0 (0)	1 (3)	
Streptococcus	0 (0)	1 (3)	
Candida	2 (7)	0 (0)	
Mixed	6 (20)	1 (3)	

Clinical Studies

The first clinical trial on the relationship between gravity and bacterial colonization in the lower respiratory system was published in 2008. In that prospective, controlled trial, Aly et al. [10] randomly assigned 60 intubated infants to either supine position (n = 30), or to lateral position (n = 30), to keep the orientation of the neck/trachea at, or below horizontal (fig. 2). After 5 days of mechanical ventilation, tracheal cultures were positive in 26 infants (87%) in the supine position group, and in 9 infants (30%) in the lateral group ($p < 0.05$). Gram-negative bacteria were the main bacteria isolated from the trachea (table 1). In addition to decreased colonization, the lateral position group had a significant decrease in the incidence of self-extubation. It was concluded that when patients were in the lateral position it was more stable to keep the ETT and the breathing circuit resting horizontally on the bed as opposed to suspended in the air for supine patients.

A pilot study [11] was recently conducted to test the feasibility of maintaining ventilated patients in the lateral position in an adult ICU. Ten patients were put in a lateral position and a similar number of patients remained in the semirecumbent position. They examined the incidence of aspiration by detecting pepsin in the tracheal aspirate. The incidence of aspiration did not differ much between groups; 3 patients in the lateral position and 5 patients in the semirecumbent position had aspiration. Of note, patients in the lateral position had a better progression of arterial oxygenation and a significantly shorter duration of mechanical ventilation compared to the semirecumbent position Therefore, this pilot study showed that lateral-horizontal orientation of the body and of the ETT is feasible and safe in intubated adult patients.

Conclusion

From this review, we conclude that gravity is a key component in bacterial colonization of the lower respiratory tract. Keeping ventilated patients in the lateral position is feasible and possibly advantageous. However, large clinical trials are still needed to test the long-term clinical outcomes related to positioning of ventilated patients. Until then it is important to understand that supine and/or semirecumbent positioning is not optimal and such practice is unfounded.

References

1 Chastre J, Fagon JY: Ventilator-associated pneumonia. Am J Respir Crit Care Med 2002;165:867-903.
2 Young PJ, Pakeerathan S, Blunt MC, Subramanya S: A low-volume, low-pressure tracheal tube cuff reduces pulmonary aspiration. Crit Care Med 2006;34:632–639.
3 Rello J, Sonora R, Jubert P, Artigas A, Rue M, Valles J: Pneumonia in intubated patients: role of respiratory airway care. Am J Respir Crit Care Med 1996;154:111–115.
4 Inglis TJ, Millar MR, Jones JG, Robinson DA: Tracheal tube biofilm as a source of bacterial colonization of the lung. J Clin Microbiol. 1989;27:2014–2018.
5 Recommendations of the CDC and the Healthcare Infection Control Practices Advisory Committee: Guidelines for preventing health-care-associated pneumonia, 2003. Respir Care 2004;49:926–939.
6 Drakulovic MB, Torres A, Bauer TT, Nicolas JM, Nogue S, Ferrer M: Supine body position as a risk factor for nosocomial pneumonia in mechanically ventilated patients: a randomised trial. Lancet 1999;354:1851–1858.
7 Panigada M, Berra L, Kolobow T: Bacterial colonization of the respiratory tract under artificial ventilation: trachea and tracheal tube orientation. Crit Care Med 2003;31:2715.
8 Berra L, De Marchi L, Panigada M, Yu ZX, Baccarelli A, Kolobow T: Evaluation of continuous aspiration of subglottic secretion in an in vivo study. Crit Care Med 2004;32:2071–2078.
9 Bassi GL, Zanella A, Cressoni M, Stylianou M, Kolobow T: Following tracheal intubation, mucus flow is reversed in the semirecumbent position: possible role in the pathogenesis of ventilator-associated pneumonia. Crit Care Med. 2008;36:518–525.
10 Aly H, Badawy M, El-Kholy A, Nabil R, Mohamed A: Randomized, controlled trial on tracheal colonization of ventilated infants: can gravity prevent ventilator-associated pneumonia. Pediatrics 2008;122:770–774.
11 Mauri T, Berra L, Kumwilaisak K, Pivi S, Ufberg J, Kueppers F, Pesenti A, Bigatello L: Lateral-horizontal patient position and horizontal orientation of the endotracheal tube to prevent aspiration in adult surgical intensive care unit patients: a feasibility study Respir Care 2010;55:294–302.

Hany Aly, MD
Division of Newborn Services, The George Washington University
900 23rd Street, NW, Suite G-2092, Room G-132
Washington, DC 20037 (USA)
Tel. +1 202 715 5236, Fax +1 202 715 5354, E-mail haly@mfa.gwu.edu

Esquinas AM (ed): Applied Technologies in Pulmonary Medicine. Basel, Karger, 2011, pp 156–162

Use of Gram Stain or Preliminary Bronchoalveolar Lavage Culture Results to Guide Discontinuation of Empiric Antibiotics in Ventilator-Associated Pneumonia

Joseph M. Swanson[a,b,c] · G. Christopher Wood[a]

[a]Departments of Clinical Pharmacy, [b]Pharmaceutical Sciences, and [c]Pharmacology, College of Pharmacy and Medicine, University of Tennessee Health Science Center, Memphis, Tenn., USA

Abbreviations

BAL Bronchoalveolar lavage
HFCC Hold for colony count
NG No growth
pBAL Preliminary BAL cultures
PSB Protected specimen brushing
PTC Protected telescoping catheter
VAP Ventilator-associate pneumonia

VAP remains a significant infectious complication in the ICU, occurring in up to 27% of mechanically ventilated patients, increasing hospital stay by up to 9 days, hospital costs by USD 40,000, and attributable mortality by 33–50%. The profound affect of VAP necessitates the use of a rapid and accurate diagnostic method. Unfortunately, the diagnosis of VAP is problematic. The lack of a 'gold standard' for diagnosis poses a significant problem when comparing different approaches [1]. As a result, practicing clinicians use methods ranging from clinical parameters alone (chest radiograph, temperature, white blood cell count, characterization of sputum, oxygenation, etc.) to invasive diagnostic procedures (BAL, PSB, PTC). Additionally, the lack of a standard diagnostic method has prompted research efforts toward improving the sensitivity and specificity of diagnostic tools for VAP.

Additional important considerations related to therapy of VAP include (1) ensuring appropriate empirical antibiotic therapy and (2) avoiding overexposure to antibiotics. Appropriate empirical therapy is essential because inappropriate empirical antibiotic therapy is associated with increased mortality. Unfortunately, inappropriate empirical antibiotic therapy generally requires broad-spectrum antibiotics and final culture results are generally not available until 72–96 h following culture obtainment [2, 3]. Since only approximately 40% of patients with clinically suspected VAP are actually diagnosed with VAP, many may receive unneeded antibiotics. Increased exposure to antibiotics can increase bacterial resistance, leaving the clinician with a delicate balance to maintain [4]. A potential way to decrease antibiotic use would be to rapidly identify patients without VAP so that empiric antibiotics could be discontinued before the final culture results are reported. This review will focus on the use of preliminary BAL culture results and Gram stain results to adjust empirical antibiotic therapy.

Gram Stain and Preliminary Culture Results

Gram Stain

Logic dictates that the presence or absence of bacteria in pulmonary cultures alludes to the diagnosis of VAP. Gram stain can be used to immediately identify bacteria in pulmonary cultures. Studies have investigated the ability of the Gram stain to enhance the diagnosis of VAP.

In 1994, Marquette et al. [5] were the first to report the ability of Gram stain to identify VAP prior to final culture results. Definitions for VAP or absence thereof were complex, including postmortem examination, PSB (threshold of 10^3 cfu/ml), and chest radiograph 'rapid cavitation'. This report was followed by other studies evaluating Gram stain as a diagnostic tool for VAP. All of the studies used clinical criteria as an indicator of VAP and confirmed the diagnosis using various procedures including BAL, PSB, and PTC. Microbiologic thresholds used to confirm the diagnosis of VAP were the same for PSB and PTC (10^3), whereas thresholds for BAL ranged from 10^3 to 10^5. The use of Gram stain for diagnosis of VAP produced sensitivities ranging from 67 to 90%, specificities ranging from 49 to 100%, positive predictive values from 45 to 100%, and negative predictive values from 42 to 96% (table 1) [5–14]. Several studies addressed the important factor of correlating Gram stain with all pathogens identified on final culture results. This correlation is described differently based on the study. For example, Duflo et al. [10] described partial correlation as meaning some of the Gram stain morphotypes grew on final culture, while Goldberg et al. [14] provided a more detailed description '(e.g. Gram stain G+, culture with G– alone or G+ and G– together) and did not use the terms 'complete correlation' or 'partial correlation. Not all studies evaluated correlation when the Gram stain was negative, but Croce et al. [6] described the best correlation when patients did not have VAP (88%). When a correlation between Gram stain and organism causing VAP were reported, results varied. Goldberg et al. [14] demonstrated the best correlation of Gram stain with VAP organisms at 71%, while others ranged from 46 to 60% [8, 11, 13]. Two studies reported statistical scores for correlation; Raghavendran et al. [15] reported a fair correlation with a κ score of 0.314 and Croce et al. [6] reported φ coefficients ranging from –0.297 to 0.484 depending on the comparison. Overall, these results were disappointing and led most investigators to suggest against the use of Gram stain to guide empirical therapy. This resulted in research into other methods to predict final culture results earlier.

Preliminary Results

Based on published data, use of Gram stain has been abandoned by many clinicians. Without Gram stain, many wait for final culture results to adjust or discontinue empirical antibiotic therapy for VAP. Mueller et al. [2] first investigated the ability of pBAL cultures to predict the final cultures. This study was a retrospective analysis using a pharmacist-maintained microbiologic culture database. Due to the nature of the database, data were only saved in 24-hour increments. Thus, preliminary results >24 h following sample procurement were evaluated. Bronchoscopic BALs were performed in all patients with suspected VAP using techniques previously described [6, 16, 17]. Preliminary results were categorized as no growth (NG), insignificant (1–99,999 cfu/ml), or significant (≥100,000 cfu/ml). Diagnosis of VAP was ruled out if final cultures yielded <100,000 cfu/ml or VAP was confirmed if ≥100,000 cfu/ml. Preliminary culture results demonstrated an overall sensitivity of 90% and specificity >99% for

Table 1. Studies evaluating Gram stain for VAP diagnosis

Reference (first author)	Sample size	Gold standard	Sensitivity %	Specificity %	Positive predictive value, %	Negative predictive value, %
Marquette 1994 [5]	75	PSB, 10^3	85	94	88	92
Croce 1998 [6]	232	BAL, 10^5	57	60	47	69
Prekates 1998 [7]	75	BAL, 10^5	77	87	71	90
Allaouchiche 1999 [8]	118	BAL, PSB	90.2	73.7	64.8	93.3
Mimoz 2000 [9]	186	PSB/ PTC, 10^3	74, 81	94, 100	91,100	82, 88
Duflo 2001 [10]	116	BAL, 10^3	76	100	100	75
Davis 2005 [11]	155	BAL, 10^5	GN 73 GP 87	GN 49 GP 59	GN 78 GP 68	GN 42 GP 83
Veinstein 2006 [12]	76	PTC, 10^3	83	74	79	79
Kopelman 2006 [13]	227	BAL, 10^4	GN 67 GP 80	GN 74 GP 66	GN 69 GP 48	GN 71 GP 70
Goldberg 2008 [14]	309	BAL, 10^5	90	67	45	96

GN = Gram-negative; GP = Gram-positive.

the presence of VAP. Preliminary results accurately predicted the presence or absence of VAP in 96.5% of cases. Interestingly, pBAL results demonstrating NG had a higher false negative rate when compared to those demonstrating insignificant growth (7.9 vs. 2.4%, $p < 0.001$). These results were counterintuitive and a clear explanation was not identified. These data suggested the use of insignificant pBAL culture results could potentially reduce empirical antibiotic duration by 2–3 days. Considering that only ~40% of patients with clinical signs are actually diagnosed with VAP, this could potentially reduce antibiotic exposure in a significant number of patients.

This study prompted changes to the original Presley Memorial Trauma Center VAP clinical guideline (fig. 1). The modified guideline included the use of pBAL results to determine empirical antibiotic duration (fig. 2).

Subsequently, a prospective validation of the retrospective study was conducted with the additional goal of evaluating duration of empirical antibiotics in cases where VAP is ultimately ruled out by using pBAL results [3]. Prospective data

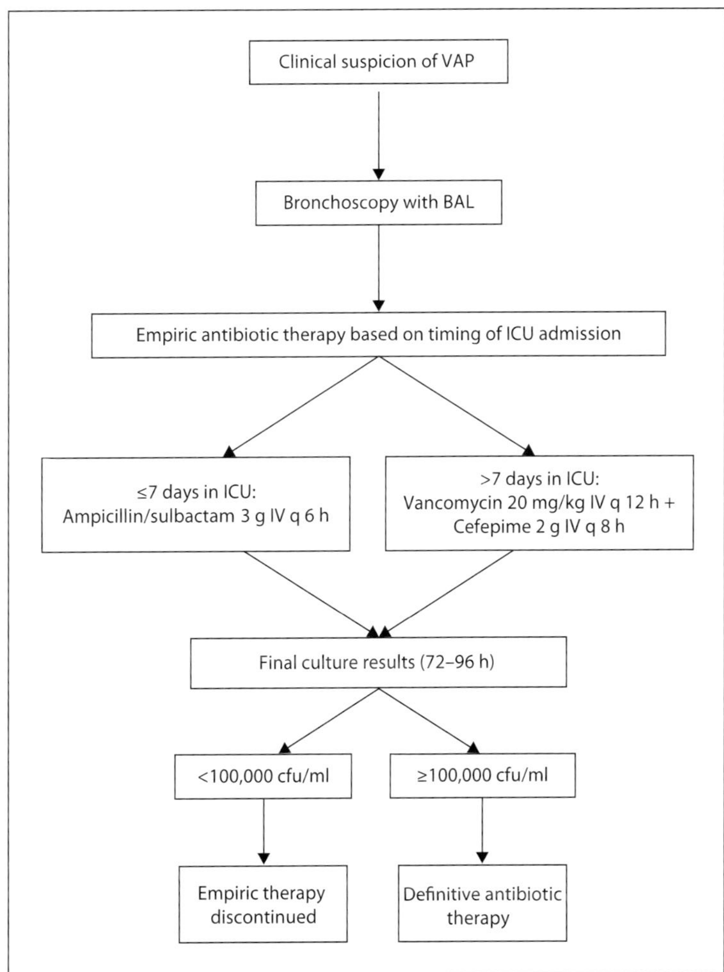

Fig. 1. Original Presley Memorial Trauma Center VAP clinical guideline using final BAL culture results.

collection revealed that the retrospective database had combined two different preliminary culture results into the category of NG. In fact, preliminary BAL culture results could be reported as NG, HFCC, insignificant growth (1–99,999 cfu/ml), or significant growth (≥100,000 cfu/ml). Using these new classifications of preliminary culture results, 474 BALs from 176 patients were analyzed. The positive predictive value of significant preliminary culture results was 100%. The negative predictive values of insignificant and NG preliminary culture results were 95 and 99% respectively. Interestingly, the presence of antibiotics did not alter these results. Unfortunately, not all preliminary results were helpful in determining the final diagnosis. The preliminary culture result HFCC was indeterminate for the final results, yielding final results significant for VAP in only 40% of cases. Additionally, significant preliminary results always yielded significant final results, but in 22% of cases significant growth of an additional pathogen was identified between the first preliminary result and final results. Use of insignificant preliminary culture results resulted in

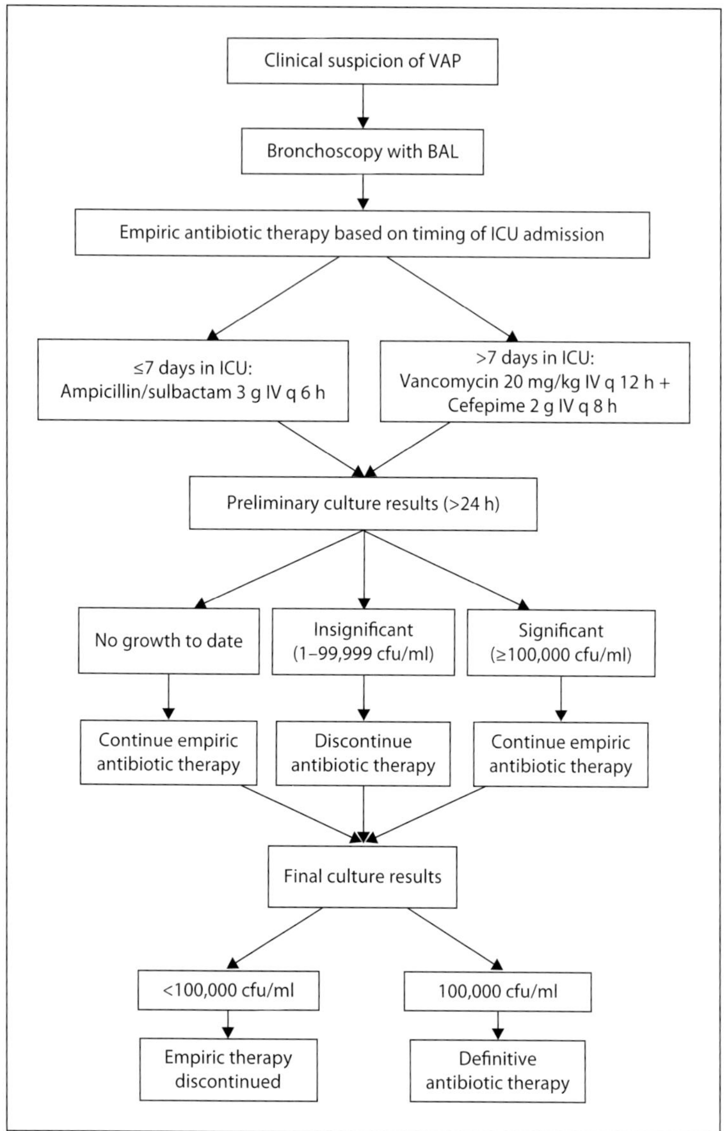

Fig. 2. Updated Presley Memorial Trauma Center VAP clinical guideline using preliminary BAL culture results.

significantly shorter durations of empirical antibiotics when compared to the use of final results [median 1.5 (1.25, 2) vs. 3 (3, 4) days, $p < 0.001$]. These data resulted in an additional change to the Presley Memorial Trauma Center VAP clinical guideline.

Discussion

The intent of using Gram stain or pBAL culture results was to provide a more rapid diagnosis of VAP, with the ultimate goal being the guidance of empirical antibiotic therapy. The ability of Gram stain to predict VAP is debatable. Several studies demonstrated acceptable sensitivities, specificities, positive predictive and negative predictive values [5, 9]. However, others reported less favorable results. More importantly, Gram stain was not shown to be effective in identifying final VAP pathogen morphotypes. This renders Gram stain less helpful in guiding empirical antibiotic therapy, including discontinuing or narrowing of broad-spectrum antibiotics. Current guidelines recommend using quantitative culture results for VAP diagnosis when possible rather than Gram stain.

Preliminary culture results provide more information than Gram stain, mostly related to the quantity of pathogens identified. This additional information is provided at the cost of time. The two studies addressing preliminary cultures investigated results reported ≥24 h post-BAL, whereas Gram stain is available in a few hours. Preliminary results demonstrated excellent positive and negative predictive values in both studies. Finally, insignificant preliminary culture results were used to significantly reduce antibiotic exposure in patients where VAP is ultimately ruled out. This is an important result because it is the first to demonstrate a reduction of unnecessary empirical antibiotic therapy. The prospective study evaluating preliminary results demonstrated NG results had a >99% negative predictive value. This suggests that combining insignificant and NG preliminary culture results could further reduce empirical antibiotic exposure in patients that ultimately have VAP ruled out. Indeed, the most important finding of the prospective study was a significant reduction in the duration of empiric antibiotic therapy when pBAL was used to guide empiric therapy. The decrease of 1.5 days seen in this study may not seem immediately impressive, but there will be a large cumulative reduction in antibiotic use with this method because of the large number of patients who receive empiric antibiotics for a VAP work-up. Also, the use of pBAL to guide discontinuation of antibiotics compares very favorably to another recent study that waited until final culture results were known (1.5 [3] vs. 6 [18] days). Thus, using pBAL to discontinue antibiotics is another tool to potentially reduce the development of resistant bacteria.

However, pBAL culture results are not infallible. In fact, preliminary results yielding HFCC or significant quantities do not provide enough information to completely determine final culture results. This causes the potential misinterpretation of final results and thus requires empirical antibiotics to remain broad until final results are available. Additionally, the validity of preliminary culture results has not been studied outside of one institution. Variations in diagnostic techniques, quantitative thresholds, and laboratory practices may alter the ability of preliminary culture results to accurately predict final results. Overall, the use of preliminary culture results to predict final results and alter empirical therapy are promising.

Recommendations

- The ability of Gram stain to predict VAP and organisms causing VAP is questionable.
- Preliminary culture results demonstrating NG and insignificant growth predict final culture results.
- Preliminary culture results demonstrating insignificant growth have been used to reduce antibiotic exposure in patients suspected of having VAP.

References

1 American Thoracic Society; Infectious Diseases Society of America: Guidelines for the management of adults with hospital-acquired, ventilator-associated, and healthcare-associated pneumonia. Am J Respir Crit Care Med 2005;171:388–416.

2 Mueller EW, Wood GC, Kelley MS, et al: The predictive value of preliminary bacterial colony counts from bronchoalveolar lavage in critically ill trauma patients. Am Surg 2003;69:749–755.

3 Swanson JM, Wood GC, Croce MA, et al: Utility of preliminary bronchoalveolar lavage results in suspected ventilator-associated pneumonia. J Trauma 2008; 65:1271–1277.

4 Trouillet JL, Chastre J, Vuagnat A, et al: Ventilator-associated pneumonia caused by potentially drug-resistant bacteria. Am J Respir Crit Care Med 1998;157: 531–539.

5 Marquette CH, Wallet F, Neviere R, et al: Diagnostic value of direct examination of the protected specimen brush in ventilator-associated pneumonia. Eur Respir J 1994;7:105–113.

6 Croce MA, Fabian TC, Waddle-Smith L, et al: Utility of Gram's stain and efficacy of quantitative cultures for posttraumatic pneumonia: a prospective study. Ann Surg 1998;227:743–751.

7 Prekates A, Nanas S, Argyropoulou A, et al: The diagnostic value of Gram stain of bronchoalveolar lavage samples in patients with suspected ventilator-associated pneumonia. Scand J Infect Dis 1998;30:43–47.

8 Allaouchiche B, Jaumain H, Chassard D, et al: Gram stain of bronchoalveolar lavage fluid in the early diagnosis of ventilator-associated pneumonia. Br J Anaesth 1999;83:845–849.

9 Mimoz O, Karim A, Mazoit JX, et al: Gram staining of protected pulmonary specimens in the early diagnosis of ventilator-associated pneumonia. Br J Anaesth 2000;85:735–739.

10 Duflo F, Allaouchiche B, Debon R, et al: An evaluation of the Gram stain in protected bronchoalveolar lavage fluid for the early diagnosis of ventilator-associated pneumonia. Anesth Analg 2001;92: 442–447.

11 Davis KA, Eckert MJ, Reed RL 2nd, et al: Ventilator-associated pneumonia in injured patients: do you trust your Gram's stain? J Trauma 2005;58:462–466.

12 Veinstein A, Brun-Buisson C, Derrode N, et al: Validation of an algorithm based on direct examination of specimens in suspected ventilator-associated pneumonia. Intensive Care Med 2006;32:676–683.

13 Kopelman TR: Can empiric broad-spectrum antibiotics for ventilator-associated pneumonia be narrowed based on Gram's stain results of bronchoalveolar lavage fluid. Am J Surg 2006;192:812–816.

14 Goldberg AE, Malhotra AK, Riaz OJ, et al: Predictive value of bronchoalveolar lavage fluid Gram's stain in the diagnosis of ventilator-associated pneumonia: a prospective study. J Trauma 2008;65: 871–876.

15 Raghavendran K, Wang J, Belber C, et al: Predictive value of sputum gram stain for the determination of appropriate antibiotic therapy in ventilator-associated pneumonia. J Trauma 2007;62:1377–1382.

16 Mueller EW, Croce MA, Boucher BA, et al: Repeat bronchoalveolar lavage to guide antibiotic duration for ventilator-associated pneumonia. J Trauma 2007;63:1329–1337.

17 Croce MA, Fabian TC, Schurr MJ, et al: Using bronchoalveolar lavage to distinguish nosocomial pneumonia from systemic inflammatory response syndrome: a prospective analysis. J Trauma 1995;39: 1134–1139.

18 Micek ST, Ward S, Fraser VJ, et al: A randomized controlled trial of an antibiotic discontinuation policy for clinically suspected ventilator-associated pneumonia. Chest 2004;125:1791–1799.

Joseph M. Swanson, PharmD
Department of Clinical Pharmacy, College of Pharmacy and Medicine
University of Tennessee Health Science Center
901 Madison Ave., Suite 308, Memphis, TN 38163 (USA)
Tel. +1 901 448 1418, Fax +1 901 448 1221, E-Mail jswanson@uthsc.edu

Esquinas AM (ed): Applied Technologies in Pulmonary Medicine. Basel, Karger, 2011, pp 163–167

Patterns of Resolution in Ventilator-Associated Pneumonia

Pavlos M. Myrianthefs · Penelope Evagelopoulou · George J. Baltopoulos

Intensive Care Unit, KAT Hospital, Athens University School of Nursing, Athens, Greece

Abbreviations

ARDS Acute respiratory distress syndrome
cfu Colony-forming units
CPIS Clinical pulmonary infection score
CRP C-reactive protein
MRSA Methicillin-resistant *Staphylococcus aureus*
ODIN Organ dysfunctions and/or infection
PCT Procalcitonin
SOFA Sepsis-related organ failure assessment
VAP Ventilator-associated pneumonia
WBC White blood cells

VAP is the most frequent ICU-acquired infection among patients receiving mechanical ventilation. VAP prolongs the length of ICU stay and increases the costs and the risk of death in critically ill patients. It has been associated with an attributable mortality of approximately 30% depending on the pathogen isolated, especially when initial antibiotic treatment is inappropriate.

The American Thoracic Society [1] suggests a combination of clinical and microbiological criteria for VAP diagnosis. These include the emergence of a new or progressive radiographic infiltrate, the presence of fever >38.3°C, the presence of increased purulent tracheal aspirates, leukocytosis or leukopenia (>12,000 or <4,000 cells/mm^3) and the deterioration of gas exchange (decreased PaO_2/FiO_2 ratio, increased needs in oxygen or increased need for positive end-expiratory pressure).

The clinical criteria of VAP diagnosis could also be used as patterns of VAP resolution. Beyond their diagnostic role, they could also contribute for the monitoring of VAP evolution and to the evaluation of the efficacy of the appropriate antibiotic therapy and recognition of patients with clinical deterioration or antibiotic failure. The application of the optimum duration of antibiotic therapy decreases relapse rates and prevents reinfection and other complications. As literature is focused on the optimal duration of antibiotic treatment, the study of the natural history of the response to appropriate therapy may help to better justify short-term antibiotic therapy for VAP.

Main Topics

The Infectious Diseases Society of America guidelines suggest 72 h of therapy as the time to record 'failure to improve' in patients with community-acquired pneumonia. Sensitivity information from microbiological cultures is usually available in most patients with pneumonia after

48 h of therapy; at this timepoint the patient is usually reassessed and de-escalation is discussed. Resolution of infectious variables after follow-up of 27 patients with VAP was first evaluated in 1997. These authors reported that resolution occurred in a median of 6 days after diagnosis.

The patterns that have been studied for VAP resolution include the temperature, the WBC count, the PaO_2/FiO_2 ratio and the CPIS. CPIS includes parameters such as oxygenation, radiographic findings and their evolution, temperature, WBC count, tracheal aspirates and microbiological culture results with a maximum score of 12. Values of 6 or higher are considered diagnostic for VAP. Chest radiographs are generally considered to be of limited value for defining clinical improvement in patients with pneumonia, since comorbidities (chronic obstructive pulmonary disease, chronic heart failure) exist in many of them. Although radiologic findings do not reflect VAP severity, deteriorating abnormalities (progressive infiltrates and evolution of abscess) are suggestive of progressive or recurrent episodes of VAP. CRP and PCT have also been evaluated in some studies as markers for VAP monitoring.

Discussion

Hypoxemia and fever are clinical variables that can be easily followed at the bedside of the patient simply by physical examination to monitor clinical response to antibiotic therapy. Most studies report that the oxygenation index (PaO_2/FiO_2 ratio) is the earliest parameter to be improved. PaO_2/FiO_2 ratio improves from the first day of the initiation of appropriate antibiotic therapy and its improvement goes on until 7 days later, so identifying patients with a good prognosis.

Montravers et al. [2] observed a significant decrease in temperature and increase in PaO_2/FiO_2 ratio within 3 days of antibiotic treatment, which was accompanied by eradication of bacteria from distal airways in the majority of patients, as demonstrated by repeated protective specimen brushes. The authors found that microbial growth of $\leq 10^3$ cfu/ml after several days of the initiation of antimicrobial therapy is accompanied by clinical failure in <7% of the patients and that microbial growth of $>10^3$ cfu/ml is related with clinical failure in 55.8% of the patients.

Dennesen et al. [3] demonstrated that among patients treated with initial appropriate antibiotic therapy, significant improvements were observed for all clinical parameters (temperature, PaO_2/FiO_2, leukocyte counts) starting from day 1, most apparently and rapidly for the PaO_2/FiO_2 ratio within the first 6 days. Little further improvement in fever, WBC count or the PaO_2/FiO_2 ratio occurred beyond 7 days of antibiotic treatment. The microbiologic monitoring with bronchoalveolar lavage was also correlated with VAP resolution, as a gradual fall in the mean number of cfu in endotracheal aspirates was observed. Appropriate antimicrobial therapy rapidly eradicates endotracheal colonization with *Streptococcus pneumoniae*, *Haemophilus influenzae* and *Staphylococcus aureus,* but fails to eradicate colonization with *Enterobacteriaceae* and *Pseudomonas aeruginosa*, indicating that follow-up of this parameter is an unreliable parameter for therapy success when these pathogens are involved. These findings, which are completely different from those reported by Montravers et al. [2] emphasize that endotracheal colonization is not equivalent to infection of distal airways and that bacterial eradication from endotracheal aspirates is a poor marker for determination of clinical response of VAP, especially when caused by Gram-negative bacteria. Only when VAP is caused by *H. influenzae* or *S. pneumoniae* may follow-up of endotracheal aspirates be useful.

Luna et al. [4] found that patients who survived VAP due to different pathogens had a clinical improvement by days 3–5 reflected by increased PaO_2/FiO_2 ratio which was the first parameter achieving 'normal' values by day 3 and best correlated to outcome. They also reported that $PaO_2/$

FiO_2 improvement within the first 3 days distinguished survivors from non-survivors.

Shorr et al. [5] in a large randomized trial confirmed that the PaO_2/FiO_2 ratio may be the most valuable tool in assessing response to therapy in VAP. Failure of the PaO_2/FiO_2 ratio to improve by day 3 or the temperature to fall identifies patients with clinical failure and at increased risk for poor outcomes. By day 3, failure of improvement should be considered as a sign for revaluation of the patient. Therefore, intensivists should not focus on the precise value for the PaO_2/FiO_2 but should track it over time.

Core temperature as a clinical variable of VAP resolution is useful mainly in patients with VAP and ARDS, although the feverish period is longer in these patients. Vidaur et al. [6] observed that fever and hypoxemia were the best indicators of resolution in patients with VAP and absence of ARDS within 48 h of therapy. In patients with ARDS, monitoring core temperature is the most useful indicator although fever takes twice as long to resolve, while the oxygenation index should be ignored. The evolution of hypoxemia is the main differential factor in the resolution of VAP between patients with and without ARDS.

Garrard et al. [7] investigated the clinical response to antimicrobial therapy in 83 patients with VAP due to different pathogens using CPIS. In this study, CPIS which was evaluated daily, increased progressively over the 2 days prior to the clinical diagnosis of pneumonia (CPIS $\geq$6) and gradually fell after the commencement of antibiotic therapy over the next 9 days. The authors concluded that CPIS may be useful in identifying pneumonia and evaluating response to therapy. In another study, Luna et al. [4] confirmed the same findings in 63 patients with VAP diagnosis. They found that serial measurements of the CPIS could be used to identify survivors who differed from non-survivors as early as day 3 of therapy. In addition, the evolution of CPIS correlated with mortality rate making it an important variable to monitor during VAP therapy. The authors attributed the good correlation between CPIS and outcome to one component of it, the index of PaO_2/FiO_2 with its value improving rapidly in patients on adequate therapy. They found that improvement in the PaO_2/FiO_2 ratio was best correlated to clinical response, whereas changes in the radiographic infiltrate, secretions, fever and leukocytes were not helpful.

Combes et al. [8], using data from a large prospective multicenter randomized trial, the PNEUMA trial, studied the predictors for infection recurrence and death in VAP patients. They concluded that persistent fever on day 8 after VAP onset was strongly associated with infection recurrence whereas persistently elevated WBC count was not. In contrast, leukocyte count increased for patients who ultimately died, whereas temperature did not discriminate between survivors and non-survivors. WBCs which are persistently increased after 2 weeks of therapy may indicate infection relapse. Also, failure of temperature improvement by day 8 or weak improvement in oxygenation after 2 weeks may indicate reinfection or relapse. In that study [8] it was also patients without infection recurrence who had a rapid improvement of SOFA, ODIN and radiologic scores. The type of bacteria responsible for VAP, non-fermenting Gram-negative bacteria and MRSA, affected outcomes independently despite appropriate antibiotic therapy.

In terms of outcome, it was found [8] that progressive WBCs increase despite antibiotic administration which is a bad prognostic factor as well as oxygenation decline after 2 weeks of treatment. Temperature was not found as an accurate prognostic factor. On the other hand, rapid improvement in SOFA and ODIN as well as chest x-ray scores are predictors of good outcome. A bad prognostic factor is the failure of improvement of chest x-ray infiltrates which further deteriorate within 2 weeks of antibiotic administration.

In another recent prospective observational study trial by Vidaur et al. [9] it was reported that the rate of VAP resolution depends on the pathogen isolated and its susceptibility to treatment. This study which included 60 VAP episodes showed that the clinical variables of VAP resolution (fever, PaO_2/FiO_2, WBC count) were improved during the first 3 days in >70% of patients on appropriate antibiotic therapy when VAP was due to methicillin-sensitive *S. aureus*, *H. Influ*enzae and susceptible *P. aeruginosa*. However, the resolution of the same clinical variables was significantly delayed (8–10 days) in the group of patients with VAP due to MRSA while receiving appropriate antibiotic therapy and due to *P. aeruginosa* with inappropriate antibiotic therapy. Independently of the disease severity, MRSA VAP was significantly associated with poor clinical resolution and a longer duration of mechanical ventilation.

Several studies have shown that CRP is useful in the diagnosis of sepsis in different clinical situations. Póvoa et al. [10] evaluated the CRP levels in the clinical resolution of VAP. In a cohort of 47 VAP patients, CRP levels were monitored daily. The authors observed that on day 4 of the antibiotic therapy, the CRP level of survivors was 0.62 times the initial value, whereas in non-survivors it was 0.98. By day 4, a CRP >0.6 times the initial level or a CRP that relapses or has biphasic kinetics was a marker of poor outcome and was associated with the diagnosis of non-resolving VAP.

PCT, the precursor molecule of calcitonin, is another biomarker that could be used as a tool for VAP prognosis. PCT is a 116-amino-acid peptide that is devoid of known hormonal activity. Serum levels of PCT are very low in healthy individuals. PCT levels rise during bacterial infections. The role of PCT kinetics as a prognostic marker during VAP has been recently investigated by Luyt et al. [11]. The authors observed that higher PCT values during VAP therapy identified patients at higher risk for death or clinical failure. Serum PCT levels decreased during the clinical course of VAP but were significantly higher from day 1 to day 7 in patients with unfavorable outcome. Therefore, failure of PaO_2/FiO_2 to improve by day 3 may be the clinical manifestation of the same inflammatory process as indicated by the persistently elevated PCT.

The value of daily measurements of PCT and CRP and other biological markers as well as soluble triggering receptor expressed on myeloid cells as reliable and useful markers in VAP resolution must be elucidated in further studies. In conclusion, monitoring of VAP evolution can be easily applied by the same parameters used for the diagnosis including oxygenation index (PaO_2/FiO_2), temperature, WBCs and CPIS. The most useful parameter to assess VAP resolution seems to be the oxygenation improvement which is obvious from the first days and continuous for at least 7 days. CPIS seems to be the second most useful parameter which should be improved by day 3. Failure of oxygenation and CPIS to improve by day 3 are signs for patients' re-evaluation and possibly clinical failure. Temperature may be useful only in ARDS patients. Persistently increased WBCs and temperature as well as failure of oxygenation to improve after 2 weeks may be indicators of relapse or reinfection.

Recommendations

- The optimum duration of antibiotic therapy in VAP imposes the monitoring of clinical variables for the definition of VAP resolution. The best indicator of VAP resolution is the oxygenation index (PaO_2/FiO_2) which improves from the first day of antibiotic therapy and reaches 'normal' values within the first 3 days.
- In patients with VAP and ARDS, monitoring core temperature is the most useful indicator although the feverish period is much longer in these patients, while the oxygenation ratio must be ignored.
- Serial measurements of CPIS can define the clinical course of VAP resolution, identifying those with good outcome as early as day 3 and could possibly be of help to define strategies to shorten the duration of therapy.

- Daily CRP measurements after onset of antibiotic therapy are useful in the identification as early as day 4 of VAP patients with poor outcome. Retained PCT serum levels on day 7 of antibiotic therapy are strong predictors of unfavorable outcome. Their role in everyday clinical use must be elucidated.
- Clinical resolution of VAP is associated with the implemented pathogen. MRSA VAP resolution is slower than in episodes due to other pathogens when receiving appropriate antibiotic therapy. The progression of radiologic infiltrates, the persistence of increased WBCs and a non-improved ratio of PaO_2/FiO_2 after 2 weeks of treatment are predictors of poor outcome.

References

1 American Thoracic Society, Infectious Diseases Society of America: Guidelines for the management of adults with hospital-acquired, ventilator-associated, and healthcare-associated pneumonia. Am J Respir Crit Care Med 2005;171:388–416.

2 Montravers P, Fagon JY, Chastre J, et al: Follow-up protected specimen brushes to assess treatment in nosocomial pneumonia. Am Rev Respir Dis 1993;147:38–44.

3 Dennesen PJ, Van der Ven AJ, Kessels AG, et al: Resolution of infectious parameters after antimicrobial therapy in patients with ventilator-associated pneumonia. Am J Respir Crit Care Med 2001;163:1371–1375.

4 Luna CM, Blanzaco D, Niederman MS, et al: Resolution of ventilator-associated pneumonia: prospective evaluation of the clinical pulmonary infection score as an early clinical predictor of outcome. Crit Care Med 2003;31:676–682.

5 Shorr AF, Cook D, Jiang X, et al, for the Canadian Critical Care Trials Group: Correlates of clinical failure in ventilator-associated pneumonia: insights from a large, randomized trial. J Crit Care 2008;23:64–73.

6 Vidaur L, Gualis B, Rodriguez A, et al: Clinical resolution in patients with suspicion of ventilator associated pneumonia: A cohort study comparing patients with and without acute respiratory distress syndrome. Crit Care Med 2005;33:1248–1253.

7 Garrard CS, A'Court CD: The diagnosis of pneumonia in the critically ill. Chest 1995;108(suppl 2):17S–25S.

8 Combes A, Luyt CE, Fagon JY, et al: Early predictors for infection recurrence and death in patients with ventilator-associated pneumonia. Crit Care Med 2007;35:146–154.

9 Vidaur L, Planas K, Sierra R, et al: Ventilator-associated pneumonia impact of organisms on clinical resolution and medical resources utilization. Chest 2008;133:625–632.

10 Póvoa P, Coelho L, Almeida E, et al: C-reactive protein as a marker of ventilator-associated pneumonia resolution: a pilot study. Eur Respir J 2005;25:804–812.

11 Luyt CE, Guerin V, Combes A, et al: Procalcitonin kinetics as a prognostic marker of ventilator-associated pneumonia. Am J Respir Crit Care Med 2005;171:48–53.

Pavlos M. Myrianthefs, MD, PhD
Intensive Care Unit, KAT Hospital, Athens University School of Nursing
Sokratous 4A'
GR–14561 Kifissia, Athens (Greece)
Tel. +30 210 623 4434, Fax +30 210 623 1949
E-Mail pmiriant@nurs.uoa.gr

Esquinas AM (ed): Applied Technologies in Pulmonary Medicine. Basel, Karger, 2011, pp 168–171

Viral Infections in the Intensive Care Unit

C.E. Luyt

Service de Réanimation Médicale, Institut de Cardiologie, Groupe Hospitalier Pitié-Salpêtrière, Paris, France

Abbreviations

ARDS Acute respiratory distress syndrome
CAP Community-acquired pneumonia
CMV Cytomegalovirus
HSV Herpes simplex virus
PCR Polymerase chain reaction
RSV Respiratory syncytial virus

The incidence of viral infection has been long underestimated because of the scarcity of diagnostic tests. Modern diagnosis methods, such as PCR, that can detect small amounts of viral nucleic acid, have markedly improved the identification of viral infections. Viral diseases are in fashion, and the recent A(H1N1) influenza pandemic will not attenuate it. However, it is important to bear in mind that viral detection does not necessarily mean viral infection: actually, viral detection can correspond to asymptomatic carriage, or viral replication without organ involvement, and true viral infection. In the ICU, viral disease can be roughly divided in two categories: community-acquired viral disease, with respiratory viruses at the head [1], and/or nosocomial viral infection, represented by infection due to *Herpesviridae*, namely HSV and CMV [2]. We will not discuss viral infections in specific populations, namely HIV-related infections and those occurring in bone-marrow or solid-organ transplants.

Analysis

Community-Acquired Viral Infections

Community-acquired viral infections are common diseases that can lead to ICU admission. HSV encephalitis is rare, but it should be promptly recognized because of the availability of a curative treatment. Infection of the respiratory tract is more frequent: either infection of the upper respiratory tract, which can lead to ICU admission by triggering exacerbation of chronic obstructive pulmonary disease or heart failure decompensation [3], or infection of the lower respiratory tract, corresponding to a true pneumonia [1]. Respiratory viruses can trigger up to 40% of acute exacerbation of chronic obstructive pulmonary disease requiring ICU [4], and can be involved in cardiopulmonary failure of elderly [3].

Viruses were found to cause CAP in roughly 10% of cases, with some studies reaching up to 40% [1]. In those studies, influenza and rhinovirus were the most frequent viruses detected, followed by other respiratory viruses, like parainfluenza, adenovirus, RSV, coronaviruses and, more recently, human metapneumovirus [2]. These viruses can cause severe pneumonia with ARDS requiring mechanical ventilation, but the frequency of this complication is not known.

Nosocomial Viral Infections
Nosocomial viral infections are due to latent viruses that are reactivated in critically ill individuals. Actually, after the initial phase of the disease (in which the inflammatory response predominates), the anti-inflammatory response becomes predominant, leading to 'immunoparalysis', nosocomial infections and viral reactivation [5]. The viruses responsible for these episodes are mostly *Herpesviridae*.

HSV reactivation in the throat occurs in 22–54% of ICU patients [2, 6, 7]. In a recent study on 201 non-immunocompromised patients ventilated for at least 5 days, HSV reactivation in the throat was diagnosed in 109 patients (54%), asymptomatically in 56% of them, whereas it was associated with herpetic ulceration of the lip or gingivostomatitis in 48 (44%) [6]. HSV can be detected in the lower respiratory tract of 5–64% of ICU patients, depending on the population and the diagnostic method used. In most cases, HSV recovery from lower respiratory tract samples of non-immunocompromised ventilated patients corresponds to viral contamination of the lower respiratory tract from mouth and/or throat, but for some patients, a real HSV bronchopneumonitis (corresponding to HSV infection of the lung parenchyma) can develop. In 201 non-immunocompromised patients with prolonged mechanical ventilation, HSV bronchopneumonitis was diagnosed in 42 (21%) [6]. Although HSV reactivation in the throat can occur early in ICU patients [6, 7], HSV bronchopneumonitis occurs generally later, after a mean of 14 days of mechanical ventilation [6].

CMV reactivation seems also frequent in ICU patients. A recent large multicenter study of critically ill non-immunocompromised patients found that up to 33% of them experienced CMV viremia at any level during their ICU stay, and that 20% had a CMV viremia >1,000 copies/ml [8]. These data confirmed other previously published studies that underlined the role of CMV in unexplained fever, pneumonia or ARDS [9–11]. In ICU patients, CMV can be detected in the blood after a median of ICU stay of 12 days, the highest viremia being detected after a median of 26 days of ICU stay. For patients with CMV lung disease, the infection occurs after prolonged mechanical ventilation, roughly after a mean of 3 weeks of mechanical ventilation [8, 11].

The role of respiratory viruses as a cause of nosocomial pneumonia is probably limited. Daubin et al. [12], in a prospective study on 139 mechanically ventilated patients, showed that only 2 out of the 39 patients suspected of having developed VAP had a respiratory sample (tracheal aspirate) positive for respiratory viruses (1 enterovirus and 1 influenza). Notably, in that study, 12 (31%) patients had a sample positive for HSV and 1 for CMV [12]. Another study found that among 185 patients whose BAL fluid was tested for several respiratory viruses (influenza A and B, rhinovirus, RSV, adenovirus, human metapneumovirus), 21 (11%) [6] were positive: 1 BAL sample was positive for influenza A, 1 for RSV, 5 for rhinovirus and 4 for adenovirus; none were positive for human metapneumovirus [13].

Recently, *Acanthamoeba polyphaga mimivirus* has been considered a possible cause of pneumonia, but its responsibility as pathogen responsible for real cases of pneumonia has never been categorically demonstrated [14]. Because of conflicting data, no definite conclusion can be drawn concerning a possible role of *A. p. mimivirus* in CAP or nosocomial viral pneumonia at present [2, 15].

Discussion

Community-Acquired Viral Infections
Although encephalitis (with HSV encephalitis at the head) are not common, every patient suspected should be promptly treated with acyclovir until

the result of cerebrospinal fluid testing for HSV is obtained.

Viral CAP is common, but as discussed above, it is important to bear in mind that viral detection does not necessarily mean viral infection. The identification of viral infection is mostly done by PCR. However, the reliability of PCR-positive samples could be doubtful. Like other diagnostic tests, there are false positive results, caused by contamination of PCR reactions with amplification products from previous tests or by carryover of homologous genomic DNA. Alternatively, false positive results may arise from non-specific binding of primers to irrelevant sequences. On the other side, the relevance of viral detection in diagnostic samples may be also doubtful. Viral excretion does not mean viral infection; some patients can have asymptomatic carriage, or a viral excretion without organ involvement. Thus, the results of a positive viral sample must be confronted with the clinical status of the patient.

Another issue is the relevance of performing extensive investigations to diagnose viral infection, whereas except for influenza, no specific antiviral drug is available. It is probably relevant to perform rapid tests for influenza in specific conditions, during seasonal influenza, or during epidemic or pandemic. Influenza can be treated by neuraminidase inhibitors, oseltamivir and zanamivir. Oseltamivir is the first-choice drug, although its efficacy is probably limited, even when given in the first 48 h of symptom onset. It should be given only in patients with proven influenza, or in special situations (epidemic or pandemic influenza). Vaccine is probably the best way to fight against seasonal influenza, especially in selected populations (elderly, care workers, immunocompromised), by decreasing the number of severe cases, including viral pneumonia requiring ICU admission, and by reducing the mortality rate.

Nosocomial Viral Infections

Although *Herpesviridae* infections are frequent in ICU patients, screening every patient is probably not meaningful. It is justified to look for HSV reactivation and/or infection in patients with suspected pneumonia, either immunocompromised, non-immunocompromised with clinical reactivation of HSV (herpes labialis or gingivostomatitis), or those with unexplained acute respiratory distress syndrome (ARDS) [6]. The diagnosis of HSV reactivation in the throat can be done by virus isolation in cell culture. For lower respiratory tract infection, HSV can be isolated in tracheal aspirate, BAL or mini-BAL samples by cell culture or PCR. Recently, the virus load, performed by real-time PCR, has been highlighted, and might, in the future, become a way to diagnose HVS lung involvement [6].

For CMV reactivation in the blood, the exact timing and frequency of tests remain to be determined for non-immunocompromised patients, whereas a weekly assay is sufficient in immunocompromised patients [8]. DNA can be detected in the blood by PCR, and quantified by real-time PCR [8]. For CMV pneumonia in non-immunocompromised patients, BAL fluid should be tested for CMV in case of unexplained ARDS or pneumonia symptoms without a pathogen being identified. CMV can be isolated in the BAL fluid by cell culture or PCR [9–11].

However, virus isolation in BAL fluid does not necessarily mean viral infection or viral disease. For example, HSV recovery in the lower respiratory tract might be a local virus excretion or a contamination from the mouth and/or throat. For suspected viral pneumonia, cytologic examination of the cells collected during bronchoscopic BAL is the cornerstone for HSV bronchopneumonitis and CMV pneumonia diagnosis [2, 6]. Actually, *Herpesviridae* lung infections can be confirmed by a histological involvement, i.e. a HSV- or CMV-specific cytopathic effect on cells collected during bronchoscopic BAL [2, 6]. The cytopathic effect seen depends on the *Herpesviridae* considered: nuclear inclusions are specific of HSV infection whereas cytoplasmic inclusions are specific of CMV infection.

Recommendations

- In patients suspected of having developed viral CAP, testing for influenza should be during an epidemic or pandemic.
- In ICU patients suspected of having developed ventilator-associated pneumonia, testing for HSV reactivation should be performed in immunocompromised patients, non-immunocompromised patients with clinical reactivation of HSV (herpes labialis or gingivostomatis), patients with no bacteria but clinical signs of pneumonia, and those with unexplained ARDS.
- CMV reactivation and/or pneumonia should be considered also in ICU patients with unexplained pneumonia, ARDS.

References

1 Jennings LC, Anderson TP, Beynon KA, et al: Incidence and characteristics of viral community-acquired pneumonia in adults. Thorax 2008;63:42–48.
2 Luyt CE, Combes A, Nieszkowska A, et al: Viral infections in the ICU. Curr Opin Crit Care 2008;14:605–608.
3 Carrat F, Leruez-Ville M, Tonnellier M, et al: A virologic survey of patients admitted to a critical care unit for acute cardiorespiratory failure. Intensive Care Med 2006;32:156–159.
4 Cameron RJ, de Wit D, Welsh TN, et al: Virus infection in exacerbations of chronic obstructive pulmonary disease requiring ventilation. Intensive Care Med 2006;32:1022–1029.
5 Hotchkiss RS, Coopersmith CM, McDunn JE, et al: The sepsis seesaw: tilting toward immunosuppression. Nat Med 2009;15:496–497.
6 Luyt CE, Combes A, Deback C, et al: Herpes simplex virus lung infection in patients undergoing prolonged mechanical ventilation. Am J Respir Crit Care Med 2007;175:935–942.
7 Bruynseels P, Jorens PG, Demey HE, et al: Herpes simplex virus in the respiratory tract of critical care patients: a prospective study. Lancet 2003;362:1536–1541.
8 Limaye AP, Kirby KA, Rubenfeld GD, et al: Cytomegalovirus reactivation in critically ill immunocompetent patients. JAMA 2008;300:413–422.
9 Papazian L, Fraisse A, Garbe L, et al: Cytomegalovirus. An unexpected cause of ventilator-associated pneumonia. Anesthesiology 1996;84:280–287.
10 Papazian L, Doddoli C, Chetaille B, et al: A contributive result of open-lung biopsy improves survival in acute respiratory distress syndrome patients. Crit Care Med 2007;35:755–762.
11 Chiche L, Forel JM, Roch A, et al: Active cytomegalovirus infection is common in mechanically ventilated medical intensive care unit patients. Crit Care Med 2009;37:1850–1857.
12 Daubin C, Parienti JJ, Vincent S, et al: Epidemiology and clinical outcome of virus-positive respiratory samples in ventilated patients: a prospective cohort study. Crit Care 2006;10:R142.
13 Luyt CE, Le Goff J, Deback C, et al: Atteintes respiratoires virales nosocomiales autres qu'à *Herpesviridae* (abstract). XXXVI Conference of the Société de Réanimation de Langue Française, Paris, 2008, suppl 58.
14 Vincent A, La Scola B, Forel JM, et al: Clinical significance of a positive serology for mimivirus in patients presenting a suspicion of ventilator-associated pneumonia. Crit Care Med 2009;37:111–118.
15 Dare RK, Chittaganpitch M, Erdman DD: Screening pneumonia patients for mimivirus. Emerg Infect Dis 2008;14:465–467.

C.E. Luyt, MD, PhD
Service de Réanimation Médicale, Institut de Cardiologie
Groupe Hospitalier Pitié-Salpêtrière
FR–75651 Paris Cedex 13 (France)
Tel. +33 42 16 38 16, Fax +33 42 16 38 17, E-Mail charles-edouard.luyt@psl.aphp.fr

Esquinas AM (ed): Applied Technologies in Pulmonary Medicine. Basel, Karger, 2011, pp 172–177

Healthcare-Associated Pneumonia among Hospitalized Patients

Yuichiro Shindo · Yoshinori Hasegawa

Department of Respiratory Medicine, Nagoya University Graduate School of Medicine, Nagoya, Japan

Abbreviations

CAP Community-acquired pneumonia
HAP Hospital-acquired pneumonia
HCAP Healthcare-associated pneumonia
MDR Multidrug-resistant
MRSA Methicillin-resistant *Staphylococcus aureus*
PDR Potentially drug-resistant

HCAP is a relatively new designation [1]. A substantial number of HCAP patients were previously defined as having CAP. However, recent reports suggest that HCAP should be recognized as a distinct entity because of differences in epidemiological patterns of HCAP and CAP patients [2–6]. Patients with HCAP have greater risks of infection with PDR or MDR pathogens (e.g., *Pseudomonas aeruginosa* and MRSA). These patients also have a higher mortality rate than patients with CAP. HCAP is a heterogeneous disease; its epidemiological findings are different among countries and institutions (fig. 1) [2–5]. In this chapter we consider the current issues that need to be discussed and clinical implications regarding HCAP, based on our results and other recent reports [2–6].

Analysis of Main HCAP-Related Topics

Definition of HCAP

Details of the definition of HCAP differ among recent studies [2–6]. The following are current consensus-derived criteria for HCAP: (1) prior hospitalization for ≥2 days in the preceding 90 days; (2) residence in a nursing home or extended care facility; (3) recent receipt of intravenous antibiotic therapy, chemotherapy, or wound care in the preceding 30 days, or (4) attending a hospital or dialysis clinic [7]. These criteria were developed mainly in North America. However, there are several differences in epidemiological factors associated with HCAP (e.g., age distribution and frequency of occurrence of PDR pathogens) among countries and institutions, probably as a result of differences in healthcare systems. When discussing the definition of HCAP, it should be noted that physicians are required to immediately identify patients with risks of PDR pathogen infection in order to approach the optimal decision on the initial appropriate antibiotic treatment. Therefore, considering the epidemiological differences among countries, minor modifications of the criteria of HCAP should be allowed,

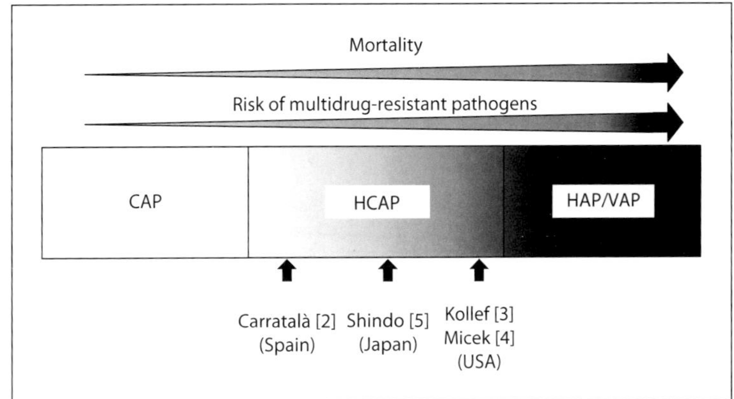

Fig. 1. Position of HCAP in all pneumonias. HCAP is a heterogeneous disease. There are epidemiological differences in the position of HCAP in each country. VAP = Ventilator-associated pneumonia.

keeping in mind their different healthcare systems. Further validation studies are needed.

Baseline Characteristics of Patients with HCAP

Common findings of HCAP patients in recent papers were that they had the following characteristics more often than CAP patients: elderly, severe pneumonia, central nervous system disorder, chronic renal disease, confusion, respiratory failure, aspiration, and previous use of antibiotics [2, 3, 5]. Furthermore, we found that the following findings were more often detected in patients with HCAP than those with CAP: high level of blood urea nitrogen, acidemia, hyponatremia, and anemia [5]. Therefore, we suggest that patients with HCAP require more active intervention for systemic management and appropriate treatment of their underlying diseases in addition to early initiation of appropriate and adequate antibiotic therapy.

Pathogen Distribution

In our study, PDR pathogens (MRSA, *Pseudomonas* species, *Acinetobacter* species, and extended-spectrum β-lactamase-producing *Enterobacteriaceae*) occurred more frequently among HCAP patients than CAP patients [5], as shown in other studies [3, 4]. However, pathogen distribution differed among reports (table 1). In general, *S. pneumoniae* and *H. influenzae* tend to occur among CAP patients, whereas *S. aureus*, *P. aeruginosa*, and MRSA occur among HAP patients. Comparing the frequencies of *S. pneumoniae*, *H. influenzae*, *S. aureus*, *P. aeruginosa*, and MRSA in four studies, we found differences in the position of HCAP among countries or institutions, i.e. whether HCAP was closer to CAP or HAP, as shown in figure 1. This is one of the reasons why HCAP differs among countries and institutions in its epidemiological pattern.

Clinical Outcomes

Table 2 shows a comparison of clinical outcomes among patients with HCAP in five studies [2–6]. In most of these studies, the proportion of 30-day or in-hospital mortality and that of inappropriate initial antibiotic treatment were significantly higher in HCAP patients compared to CAP patients. Furthermore, we reported that in-hospital mortality among HCAP patients with and without initial treatment failure was 62.9% (22/35) and 7.5% (8/106), respectively ($p < 0.001$), and that among CAP patients with and without initial treatment failure was 32.5% (13/40) and 2.5% (4/163), respectively ($p < 0.001$) [5]. Our findings suggest that in-hospital mortality among HCAP patients with initial treatment failure was more

Table 1. Etiology of culture-positive HCAP in four studies*

Microbes	Carratalà et al. [2] (n = 85†) Spain single-center prospective	Shindo et al. [5] (n = 77†) Japan single-center retrospective	Kollef et al. [3] (n = 988) USA multicenter retrospective	Micek et al. [4] (n = 431) USA single-center retrospective
Gram-negative pathogens				
Pseudomonas species	2.6	10.4	25.3	25.5
Acinetobacter species	–	2.1	2.6	–
ESBL‡-producing Gram-negative bacteria	0	1.3	–	–
Klebsiella species	0	13.0	7.6	6.5
Escherichia coli	3.5	6.5	5.2	4.2
Haemophilus influenzae	17.6	5.2	5.8	4.2
Other Gram-negative bacteria	–	10.4	13.0	19.0
Gram-positive pathogens				
Streptococcus pneumoniae	41.2	24.7	5.5	10.4
Staphylococcus aureus	3.5	18.2	46.7	44.5
MRSA§	1.2	6.5	26.5	30.6
Streptococci other than *S. pneumoniae*	–	7.1	7.8	–
Other Gram-positive bacteria	–	2.8	7.7	–

* Data are presented as percentages.
† Cases without identified pathogens were excluded.
‡ Extended-spectrum β-lactamase.
§ Methicillin-resistant *Staphylococcus aureus.*

Table 2. Clinical outcomes among HCAP patients in five studies*

Outcomes	Carratalà et al. [2] (n = 126) Spain single-center prospective	Venditti et al. [6] (n = 90) Italy multicenter prospective	Shindo et al. [5] (n = 141) Japan single-center retrospective	Kollef et al. [3] (n = 988†) USA multicenter retrospective	Micek et al. [4] (n = 431†) USA single-center retrospective
30-Day mortality	10.3	–	15.6	–	–
In-hospital mortality	–	17.8	21.3	19.8	24.6
Inappropriate antibiotic treatment	5.6	18.9	20.8	–	28.3

* Data are presented as percentages.
† Culture-positive pneumonia.

serious than that among CAP patients and indicate that physicians should pay careful attention to the initial treatment of HCAP. Occurrence of PDR pathogens was associated with initial treatment failure and inappropriate initial antibiotic treatment [5]. In particular, HCAP patients with PDR pathogens were 4.2 and 14.0 times as likely to have initial treatment failure and inappropriate initial antibiotic treatment, respectively, than those without PDR pathogens [5]. Therefore, we suggest that physicians should strongly consider PDR pathogens while determining the initial empirical antibiotic treatment of HCAP patients in order to improve their management.

Risk Factors for PDR Pathogens

Which population should be targeted for combination therapy with broad-spectrum antibiotics? First, in our study, the proportion of occurrence of PDR pathogens among HCAP patients was 22.1% [5]. Therefore, it is not necessary that all HCAP patients receive combination therapy with broad-spectrum antibiotics. Furthermore, the frequency of PDR pathogens was not dependent on the severity of pneumonia in HCAP patients, as indicated in our study [5]. Thus, identifying risk factors for PDR pathogens is important in selecting initial empirical antibiotic agents. In our analysis of risk factors for PDR pathogen occurrence, use of broad-spectrum antibiotics on more than 2 days within the previous 90 days and tube feeding were found to be significant, the risk ratios being 3.1 and 2.5, respectively [5].

Discussion

As the first step in clinical management of HCAP, the most important process for physicians is to identify HCAP patients during diagnosis of pneumonia. Pneumonia in hospitalized patients was previously divided into two categories: CAP and HAP. Most patients admitted to hospital with a diagnosis of pneumonia were simply categorized as patients with CAP. However, recent reports revealed that a substantial number of patients with risk of PDR pathogen infection and high mortality, similar to those with HAP, were included among patients with traditionally defined CAP. Such patients are essential to the concept of HCAP. Both patients with newly defined HCAP and CAP present from the community. However, the fact that HCAP was more life-threatening than CAP to patients with initial treatment failure suggests the importance of identifying HCAP patients during diagnosis of pneumonia, especially in the emergency department, to improve their outcome. Therefore, physicians need to understand that HCAP should be identified as a distinct entity.

After identifying HCAP patients, how should we select the initial empirical antibiotic agents? The initial empirical antibiotic strategy for HCAP is currently under discussion because of differences in the etiology of HCAP in each country or institute. The current priorities that need to be discussed are encapsulated in the following questions: (1) What are the acceptable risk factors for infection with PDR or MDR pathogens? (2) Should we stratify those risk factors? and (3) Should we consider the severity of illness in selection of initial empirical antibiotic agents? Additional epidemiological studies are needed to answer the above questions, and interventional studies should be performed to assess the antibiotic treatment strategy. Until such studies are performed, physicians should consider the local risk factors for infection with PDR pathogens, such as use of broad-spectrum antibiotics on more than 2 days within the previous 90 days and tube feeding, as shown in our study.

Figure 2 shows a schematic for identifying patients with HCAP and the potential implications for initial antibiotic treatment. This algorithm is a proposal and needs validation, particularly with regard to selection of initial empirical antibiotic agents after identification of HCAP patients.

Recently, some authors have stated that the concept of HCAP is not needed, because it potentially leads to overtreatment [8]. In considering

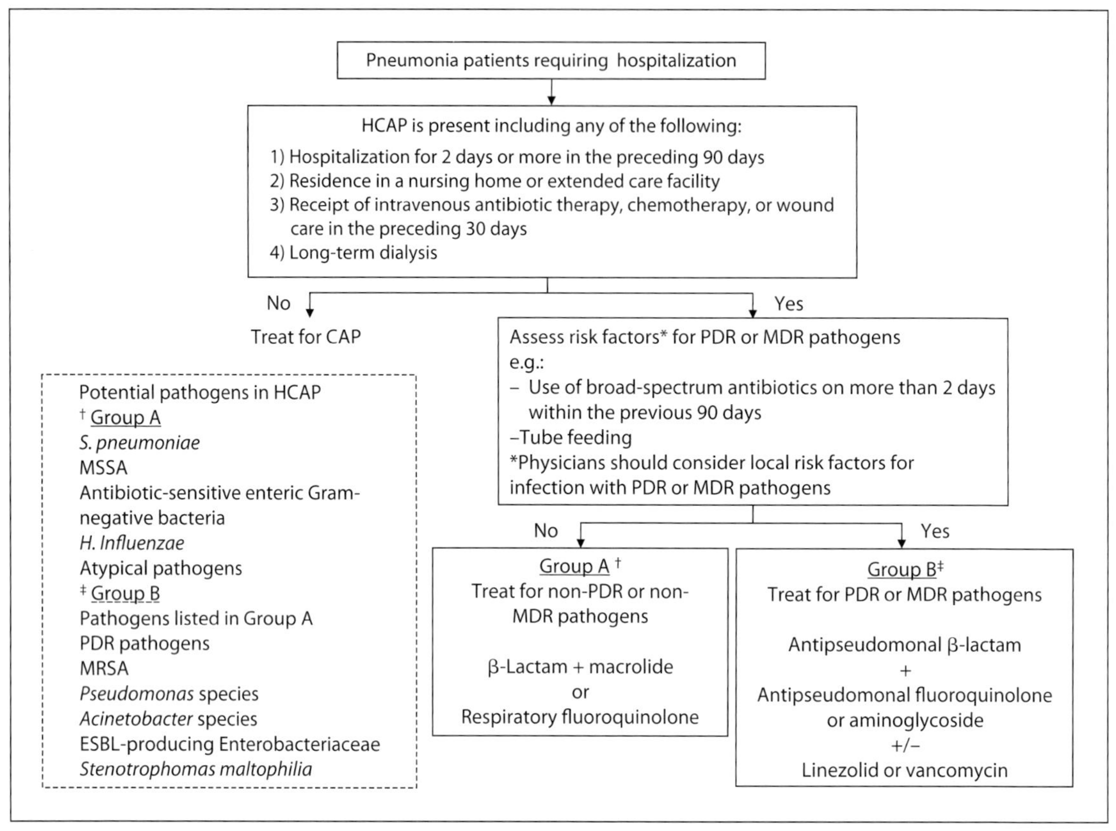

Fig. 2. Schema for evaluation of pneumonia patients requiring hospitalization. This proposed algorithm needs to be validated. The following issues need to be discussed with regard to selection of initial empirical antibiotic agents: (1) What are the acceptable risk factors for infection with PDR or MDR pathogens? (2) Should we stratify those risk factors? and (3) Should we consider the severity of illness? Although use of broad-spectrum antibiotics on more than 2 days within the previous 90 days and tube feeding were found to be significant risk factors for PDR pathogens in our recent study, other factors such as immune suppression may also be possible risk factors.

categories of pneumonia, the most important key perspective is to provide the appropriate initial assessment and empirical treatment for patients with pneumonia. Therefore, identifying HCAP patients is one of the most important approaches to assure appropriate treatment for patients with pneumonia. In order to provide the appropriate treatment or to avoid overtreatment, we consider that it is important to answer three questions, as described above, regarding the selection of initial empirical antibiotic agents in HCAP patients.

In conclusion, many countries are facing the problem of an aging society, and the number of elderly people in close contact with healthcare services will increase in the near future. Therefore, the number of patients with HCAP is also expected to increase, and it is therefore becoming an important challenge for physicians to improve the quality of management for patients with HCAP.

Recommendations

- To recognize that patients with HCAP have greater risks of infection with PDR or MDR pathogens and higher mortality than patients with CAP.
- To identify patients with HCAP during diagnosis of pneumonia, especially in the emergency department.
- To assess risk factors for infection with PDR or MDR pathogens in selecting initial empirical antibiotic agents after identifying HCAP patients.

References

1 American Thoracic Society, Infectious Diseases Society of America: Guidelines for the management of adults with hospital-acquired, ventilator-associated, and healthcare-associated pneumonia. Am J Respir Crit Care Med 2005;171:388–416.

2 Carratalà J, Mykietiuk A, Fernandez-Sabe N, et al: Healthcare-associated pneumonia requiring hospital admission: epidemiology, antibiotic therapy, and clinical outcomes. Arch Intern Med 2007;167:1393–1399.

3 Kollef MH, Shorr A, Tabak YP, et al: Epidemiology and outcomes of healthcare-associated pneumonia: results from a large US database of culture-positive pneumonia. Chest 2005;128:3854–3862.

4 Micek ST, Kollef KE, Reichley RM, et al: Healthcare-associated pneumonia and community-acquired pneumonia: a single-center experience. Antimicrob Agents Chemother 2007;51:3568–3573.

5 Shindo Y, Sato S, Maruyama E, et al: Healthcare-associated pneumonia among hospitalized patients in a Japanese community hospital. Chest 2009;135:633–640.

6 Venditti M, Falcone M, Corrao S, et al: Outcomes of patients hospitalized with community-acquired, healthcare-associated, and hospital-acquired pneumonia. Ann Intern Med 2009;150:19–26.

7 Kollef MH, Morrow LE, Baughman RP, et al: Healthcare-associated pneumonia: a critical appraisal to improve identification, management, and outcomes. Proceedings of the HCAP Summit. Clin Infect Dis 2008;46(suppl 4):S296–S334.

8 Ewig S, Welte T, Chastre J, et al: Rethinking the concepts of community-acquired and health-care-associated pneumonia. Lancet Infect Dis 2010;10:279–287.

Yuichiro Shindo, MD
Department of Respiratory Medicine
Nagoya University Graduate School of Medicine
65 Tsurumai-cho, Showa-ku, Nagoya 466-8550 (Japan)
Tel. +81 52 744 2167, Fax +81 52 744 2176, E-Mail yshindo@med.nagoya-u.ac.jp

Esquinas AM (ed): Applied Technologies in Pulmonary Medicine. Basel, Karger, 2011, pp 178–184

Critical Care Outcome of Lung Cancer Patients

Abdulgadir K. Adam[a] · Ayman O. Soubani[b]

[a]Division of Pulmonary, Critical Care and Sleep Medicine, Wayne State University School of Medicine, and [b]Section of Pulmonary and Critical Care Medicine, Karmanos Cancer Center, Wayne State University School of Medicine, Detroit, Mich., USA

Lung cancer is the third most common malignancy, but remains the leading cause of cancer mortality in both men and women in the USA and throughout the world. An estimated 159,390 deaths, accounting for about 28% of all cancer deaths, are expected to occur in 2009 in the USA. Since 1987, more women have died each year from lung cancer than from breast cancer. Death rates among men decreased by 2.0% per year from 1994 to 2005. Female lung cancer death rates have been stable since 2003 after continuously increasing for several decades. The 1-year relative survival for lung cancer has increased from 35% in 1975–1979 to 41% in 2001–2004, largely due to improvement in surgical techniques and combined therapies. However, the 5-year survival rate for all stages combined is only 15% [1–5]. Patients with lung cancer, regardless of type or stage, commonly require ICU care for a variety of acute illnesses related to the underlying malignancy, treatment, or co-morbid illnesses. Lung cancer is the third most common cancer in critically ill patients, and accounts for 16% of all cancer-related admissions to the ICU [6, 7]. There is an ongoing controversy about the value of ICU care to this patient population given the poor overall prognosis associated with lung cancer. This chapter reviews the indications for medical ICU care for the lung cancer patients, and discusses the recent data on the outcome and predictors of outcome of this care. The discussion is not directed towards patients who are admitted to the ICU postoperatively after resection of lung cancer rather to those patients who develop critical illness associated with their underlying malignancy.

Indications for Medical ICU Admission

In general, lung cancer patients are admitted to the medical ICU for diagnoses that are similar to other patient populations. These include acute respiratory failure, sepsis, cardiovascular problems, neurologic impairments, renal or metabolic abnormalities, or bleeding disorders. In a study of critically ill lung cancer patients by Adam and Soubani [8], the main causes for admission to the medical ICU were acute respiratory failure (49%), cardiovascular problems (25%), sepsis (8%), and neurological impairment (5%). The indications for admission to the medical ICU for lung cancer patients may be classified to cancer-related complications, treatment-related complications, and co-morbid illnesses. These indications are summarized in table 1.

Table 1. Main indications for medical ICU admission

Cancer-related complications
Superior vena cava obstruction
Airways obstruction or infiltrations
Hemoptysis
Pleural effusion
Pulmonary embolism
Electrolyte abnormalities
Neurologic complications
Treatment-related complications
Radiation pneumonitis
Chemotherapy-induced pulmonary toxicity
Bronchoscopic or other pulmonary procedure complications
Postoperative complications for cancer resection
Infections
Directly related to the cancer, e.g. obstructive pneumonia
Immunosuppression secondary to chemotherapy
Underlying co-morbid illnesses
Cardiovascular diseases
Pulmonary diseases
Others

Cancer-Related Complications

Lung cancer can cause obstruction of the superior vena cava causing superior vena cava syndrome, which may be a life-threatening emergency. Tumors may cause airways infiltration and obstruction, resulting in respiratory failure and postobstructive pneumonia. Hemoptysis due to bleeding tumors in the airways or vascular invasion can be life-threatening. Cancer-related or malignant pleural effusion can lead to respiratory decompensation. Pulmonary embolism secondary to a hypercoagulable state due to malignancy is another cause of severe respiratory distress. Electrolyte abnormalities such as hypercalcemia, hyponatremia and hypokalemic alkalosis, are not uncommon in these patients and may be the reasons for admission to the medical ICU. A variety of neurological complications might develop secondary to metastasis to the central nervous system leading to altered mental status, seizures, and spinal cord compression with paraplegia or quadriplegia.

Treatment-Related Complications

Radiation pneumonitis is not an uncommon complication, especially when used with concurrent chemotherapy. The severity of this complication is variable, however may progress rapidly to acute respiratory failure in spite of institution of corticosteroid therapy. Diffuse lung injury consistent with acute respiratory distress syndrome has been described in some patients following radiation therapy for lung cancer [9]. Several chemotherapeutic agents used in the treatment of lung cancer are associated with pulmonary toxicity and acute respiratory failure. These agents include gemcitabine, gefitinib, etoposide, paclitaxel, docetaxel, and bevacizumab. Furthermore, chemotherapy may lead to immunosuppression with increased risk of severe infections, including respiratory infections. The differentiation between infectious and treatment-related pulmonary complications may be challenging.

Also, some patients might develop complications following diagnostic or therapeutic surgical or bronchoscopic procedures that may require admission to the medical ICU. For example, patients may develop acute respiratory distress syndrome following pneumonectomy [10]. In addition, patients may develop acute respiratory failure or significant bleeding following bronchoscopy, biopsies, or palliative endobronchial procedures.

Co-Morbid Illnesses

Lung cancer patients are generally at increased risk for a variety of respiratory and cardiovascular problems that are related to their age and cigarette smoking. These patients may need medical ICU care for acute exacerbation of chronic obstructive pulmonary disease, cardiogenic pulmonary edema, acute coronary syndrome or other illnesses

Table 2. Mortality of lung cancer patients admitted to the medical ICU and literature review

Reference (first author)	Patients n	Mechanical ventilation, n	ICU mortality %	Hospital mortality, %	Long-term mortality, %[1]
Ewer, 1986 [28]	46	46	85	91	98
Boussat, 2000 [29]	57	52	67	75	NR
Jennens, 2002 [32]	20	9	NR	NR	85
Lin, 2003 [30]	81	81	72.8	85	NR
Reichner, 2006 [31]	47	23	43	60	NR
Soares, 2007 [33]	143	100	42	59	67
Adam, 2008 [8]	139	68	22	40	48

NR = Not reported.
[1] Long-term survival signifies survival >6 months after medical ICU admission.

such as acute renal failure. Finally, the indication for medical ICU may be due to a combination of the above conditions.

Critical Care Outcome of Lung Cancer Patients

Studies have shown that the ICU outcome of cancer patients in general is poor [11–27]. There are few studies that specifically evaluated lung cancer patients and they suggested that the medical ICU outcome of these patients is also guarded [8, 28–34] (table 2). Ewer et al. [28] in 1986 reported that the ICU mortality among lung cancer patients requiring mechanical ventilation was 85%. Boussat et al. [29] in 2000 reported an overall ICU mortality of 66%, and 71% for those requiring mechanical ventilation. Lin et al. [30] in 2003 reported an ICU mortality of 73% in those patients requiring mechanical ventilation. However, recent literature suggests that the outcome of lung cancer patients admitted to the medical ICU has been steadily improving. Reichner et al. [31] in 2006 reported an overall ICU mortality of 43%, and 74% for those requiring mechanical ventilation. Another study by Soares et al. [33] in 2007 reported ICU mortality of 42%, and 69% for those receiving mechanical ventilation. More recently, Adam and Soubani [8] reported the outcome of 139 lung cancer patients, including 68 mechanically ventilated patients who were admitted to the medical ICU. The overall ICU mortality was 22%, and 38% for those who were on mechanical ventilation. The hospital mortality for the whole group was 40%, and 52% were still alive more than 6 months after medical ICU admission. These data show that there is a clear trend towards improved overall survival of lung cancer patients admitted to the medical ICU, and while those who are mechanically ventilated had a higher mortality; nevertheless, the survival rate for this subgroup has also improved. The other observation is that the ICU outcome of lung cancer patients generally approaches that of other patient populations admitted to the medical ICU.

It is difficult to establish the specific reasons for the improved ICU outcome of lung cancer patients, however factors that have been shown to improve ICU outcome in other patient populations, probably apply to these patients as well. These factors may be related to improved mechanical ventilation strategies that minimize further lung injury and increased utilization of non-

Table 3. Predictors of critical care outcome

Predictors	Reference(s)
Mechanical ventilation	8, 28, 30, 31
Severity of co-morbidities	33
Number of organ system failures	8, 33
Cancer recurrence or progression	31, 33
High sepsis-related or sequential organ failure assessment score	31
Performance status	29
Hemodynamic instability requiring vasopressors	8

invasive ventilation. A few studies have reported that the early use of this strategy has resulted in improved gas exchange, decreased dyspnea, less mechanical ventilation, and lower overall mortality rates [24, 35]. In addition, better management of sepsis and implementation of patient safety bundles of care (such as the ventilator bundle and sepsis bundle) may play a role in better ICU outcome. The improvement in the different therapeutic options for lung cancer and the increased knowledge and experience that developed in those units that routinely deal with cancer patients may contribute to improved outcome of these patients. Furthermore, the multidisciplinary approach to the management of these patients with the involvement of intensivists, oncologists, and other specialists probably contributes to the better management of critically ill lung cancer patients.

Predictors of Critical Care Outcome of Lung Cancer Patients

Despite the improved ICU and hospital outcome of lung cancer patients reported in the recent literature, not all patients benefit from this aggressive care. For many of the patients with lung cancer, ICU care is futile and will not prolong their lives. Such therapy may be associated with a huge emotional and physical toll on these patients and their families. In addition, such care is very expensive and will consume scarce resources. It would be useful to be able to predict, prior to admission to the ICU, whether the patient is going to benefit from this aggressive and expensive therapy.

Several retrospective studies have tried to identify the clinical variables that are associated with poor ICU outcome (table 3). In a study by Soares et al. [33], the predictors of poor ICU outcome were severity of co-morbidities, number of organ system failures, cancer recurrence or progression, and airway infiltration or obstruction by cancer. Some of the predictors that were reported in the study by Reichner et al. [31] were the need for mechanical ventilation, advanced lung cancer stage, and a higher sepsis-related or sequential organ failure assessment score. The death predictive factors in the study by Boussat et al. [29] were acute pulmonary disease and Karnofsky performance status <70. In the study by Adam and Soubani [8], several predictors correlated with poor ICU outcome. These include high admission Acute Physiology and Chronic Health Evaluation (APACHE) III score, the need for mechanical ventilation, the use of vasopressors, positive blood cultures, high serum lactate, the presence of two or more multi-organ system failure, and the need for advanced cardiac life support protocol for cardiopulmonary arrest. On multi-regression analysis only the use of vasopressors and the presence of two or more organ system failures predicted poor ICU outcome, with an odds ratio 8.7 and 40.8 respectively. The stage of lung cancer or the presence of metastasis did not correlate with poor medical ICU outcome. This was similar to the findings in the study by Boussat et al. [29], but in contrast to the findings of Soares et al. [33] and Reichner et al. [31]. Regarding the type of lung cancer the studies have shown variable results. The latest study observed that patients with non-small cell lung cancer had a favorable ICU outcome [8], which is contrary to the findings of other studies [29, 31].

Age was not found to be a predictor of outcome in most of these studies, and should not be a criterion by itself against ICU care. Performance status, on the other hand, appears to be more a significant factor. A recent study by Christodoulou et al. [36], of critically ill cancer patients, including lung cancer, reported that only performance status (3–4) was a predictor of short-term negative ICU outcome.

It is clear from the available studies that there are no absolute predictors of ICU outcome of lung cancer patients. It appears the outcome of these patients is dependent on clinical variables that are similar to other patient populations and include the performance status, the severity of the acute illness and the number of organ system failures.

Given the difficulty in determining the futility of ICU care for patients with lung cancer upon initial evaluation of their critical illness, it is reasonable to offer this care to all critically ill lung cancer patients except those who have advanced malignancy unresponsive to therapy, or have made a decision against aggressive therapy. Treatment of these patients who are admitted to the medical ICU should include appropriate diagnostic studies, ventilatory support (either by non-invasive positive pressure ventilation or mechanical ventilation), hemodynamic support and, when necessary, renal replacement therapy. These patients should be re-evaluated in a few (3–5) days to assess their response to therapy [19–21]. If they are not responding to therapy, continue to require mechanical ventilation, or develop multiorgan system failure, then the patients and/or their family should be approached regarding limiting aggressive therapy and considering palliative care. While aggressive therapy is appropriate in patients with lung cancer, it appears that performing advanced cardiac life support on those with critical illness is futile. Few studies have shown that it is unusual for those patients to survive their hospitalization [8, 33]. This observation may be conveyed to patients and their family members to avoid subjecting the patients to this measure if their conditions deteriorate.

An important aspect in the care of the lung cancer patient should be an early discussion about the extent of treatment the patient wishes and end-of-life issues. It has been our experience, and documented in the literature, that the majority of the lung cancer patients admitted to the medical ICU did not have discussions with their oncologists about the extent of treatment they wish, nor have they addressed their code status. This adds an extra burden, and sometimes confusion, among physicians and family members about the patient's wishes. Critically ill lung cancer patients may not be able to make informed decisions and their family may not know the patients' wishes. Thoughtful decisions about end-of-life issues are difficult under these stressful situations. In a study by Reichner et al. [31], only 26% of lung cancer patients admitted to the medical ICU had 'do-not-resuscitate' orders, and 64% of patients with stage IV non-small cell lung cancer were full code. Of those patients who were full code on admission to the medical ICU, there was no record of end-of-life discussions documented in any of the available outpatient records. The code status was subsequently changed to do-not-resuscitate in 49% of the patients a mean of 7 days after admission to the medical ICU. The pulmonary and critical care physician was solely responsible for the change in the code status in 65% of the cases. Another study by Lamont and Christakis [37] showed that physicians provide a frank estimate of prognosis in only one third of cases, and in the rest provide no estimate or consciously over- or underestimate survival time. It may be understandable for the oncologists not to discuss end-of-life care as they are starting treatment for these patients, however they are in the best position to have frank discussions with their patients and family members, in the outpatient setting, after they had a good rapport with them and had a time to assess the patients' health and response to therapy. An important resource to physicians caring for lung cancer patients is consultation with palliative care services that support the patient, family and physicians as they are going through treatment and in making end-of-life decisions. Recent observations have shown that such services are underutilized, especially in critically ill patients. Furthermore, making use of the palliative care services has been associated with lowered cost for care of cancer patients [38]. The recent American College of Chest Physicians guidelines for the diagnosis and management of lung cancer recommend that palliative care, including a consultation with a palliative care team, be integrated into the treatment of patients with advanced lung cancer, even those pursuing curative or life-prolonging therapies [39].

Recommendations

Lung cancer patients are increasingly being admitted to the medical ICU for conditions related to their malignancy, side effects of treatment, or co-morbid illnesses. The outcome of these patients has been progressively improving, and is approximating that of the general critically ill population. There are no absolute predictors of critical care outcome of these patients. The severity and the acuity of illness and the number of organ system failures appear to be more important than the characteristics of the underlying malignancy. Full ICU care should be considered for all lung cancer patients who wish to have it, or those whose wishes are not known, except those who clearly have an advanced refractory disease. A multidisciplinary team approach including an intensivist, medical oncologist, and palliative care service is important for the appropriate management of these patients. It is reasonable to reassess the clinical status of these patients after 3–5 days of their care in the ICU to decide on further management. Every effort should be made to discuss the patient's end-of-life wishes and code status by their oncologist in the outpatient setting.

References

1 American Cancer Society: Cancer Facts and Figures 2009. Atlanta, American Cancer Society, 2009 (www.cancer.org).
2 Jemal A, Siegel R, Ward E, et al: Cancer statistics, 2009. CA Cancer J Clin 2009; 59:225–249.
3 Jemal A, Chu KC, Tarone RE: Recent trends in lung cancer mortality in the United States. Cancer surveillance series. J Natl Cancer Inst 2001;93:277–283.
4 Jemal A, Travis WD, Tarone RE, et al: Lung cancer rates convergence in young men and women in the United States: analysis by birth cohort and histologic type. Int J Cancer 2003;105:101–107.
5 Thun MJ, Henley SJ, Burns D, et al: Lung cancer death in lifelong nonsmoker. J Natl Cancer Inst 2006;98:691–699.
6 Griffin JP, Nelson JE, Koch KA, et al: End-of-life care in patients with lung cancer. Chest 2003;123:312S–31S.
7 Kress JP, Christenson J, Pohlman AS, et al: Outcomes of critically ill cancer patients in a university hospital setting. Am J Respir Crit Care Med 1999;160: 1957–1961.
8 Adam AK, Soubani AO: Outcome and prognostic factors of lung cancer patients admitted to the medical intensive care unit. Eur Respir J 2008;31: 47–53.
9 Byhardt RW, Abrams R, Almagro U: The association of adult respiratory distress syndrome with thoracic irradiation. Int J Radiat Oncol Biol Phys 1988;15:1441–1446.
10 Tang SS, Redmond K, Griffiths M, et al: The mortality from acute respiratory distress syndrome after pulmonary resection is reducing: a 10-year single institutional experience. Eur J Cardiothorac Surg 2008;34:898–902.
11 Groeger JS, White P, Nierman DM, et al: Outcome for cancer patients requiring mechanical ventilation. J Clin Oncol 1999;17:991–997.

12 Staudinger T, Stoiser B, Mullner M, et al: Outcome and prognostic factors in critically ill cancer patients admitted to the intensive care unit. Crit Care Med 2000;28:1322–1328.

13 Thiery G, Azoulay E, Darmon M, et al: Outcome of cancer patients considered for intensive care unit admission: a hospital-wide prospective study. J Clin Oncol 2005;23:4406–4413.

14 Groeger JS, Lemeshow S, Price K, et al: Multicenter outcome study of cancer patients admitted to the intensive care unit: a probability of mortality model. J Clin Oncol 1998;16:761–770.

15 Azoulay E, Moreau D, Alberti C, et al: Predictors of short-term mortality in critically ill patients with solid malignancies. Intensive Care Med 2000;26: 1817–1823.

16 Ghosen M, Kanso C, Kattan J, et al: Outcome of cancer patients admitted to the intensive care unit. J Med Liban 2002;50: 132–136.

17 Groeger JS, Glassman J, Nierman DM, et al: Probability of mortality of critically ill cancer patients at 72 h of intensive care unit management. Support Care Cancer 2003;11:686–695.

18 Hauser MJ, Tabak J Baier H: Survival of patients with cancer in a medical critical care unit. Arch Intern Med 1982;142: 527–529.

19 Schapira DV, Studnicki J, Bradham DD, et al: Intensive care, survival and expense of treating critically ill cancer patients. JAMA 1993;269:783–786.

20 Maschmeyer G, Bertschat FL, Moesta KT, et al: Outcome analysis of 189 consecutive cancer patients referred to the intensive care unit as emergencies during a 2-year period. Eur J Cancer 2003; 39:783–792.

21 Kongsgaard UE, Meidell NK: Mechanical ventilation in critically ill cancer patients: outcome and utilization of resources. Support Care Cancer 1999;7: 95–99.

22 Benoit DD, Vandewoude KH, Decruyenaere JM, et al: Outcome and early prognostic indicators in patients with a hematologic malignancy admitted to the intensive care unit for a life-threatening complication. Crit Care Med 2003;31: 104–112.

23 Soubani AO, Kseibi E, Bander JJ, et al: Outcome and prognostic factors of hematopoietic stem cell transplantation recipients admitted to a medical ICU. Chest 2004;126:1604–1611.

24 Azoulay E, Alberti C, Bornstain C, et al: Improved survival in cancer patients requiring mechanical ventilatory support: impact of noninvasive mechanical ventilatory support. Crit Care Med 2001; 29:519–525.

25 Azoulay E, Thiery G, Chevret S, et al: The prognosis of acute respiratory failure in critically ill cancer patients. Medicine (Baltimore) 2004;83:360–370.

26 Mendoza V, Lee A, Marik PE: The hospital – survival and prognostic factors of patients with solid tumors admitted to an ICU. Am J Hosp Palliat Care 2008;25:240–243.

27 Taccone FS, Artigas AA, Sprung CL, et al: Characteristics and outcomes of cancer patients in European ICUs. Crit Care 2009;13:R15.

28 Ewer MS, Ali MK, Atta MS, et al: Outcome of lung cancer patients requiring mechanical ventilation for pulmonary failure. JAMA 1986;256:3364–3366.

29 Boussat S, El'rini T, Dubiez A, et al: Predictive factors of death in primary lung cancer patients on admission to the intensive care unit. Intensive Care Med 2000;26:1811–1816.

30 Lin YC, Tsai YH, Huang CC, et al: Outcome of lung cancer patients with acute respiratory failure requiring mechanical ventilation. Respir Med 2004;98:43–51.

31 Reichner CA, Thompson JA, O'Brien S, et al: Outcome and code status of lung cancer patients admitted to the medical ICU. Chest 2006;130:719–723.

32 Jennens RR, Rosenthal MA, Mitchell P, Presneill JJ: Outcome of patients admitted to the intensive care unit with newly diagnosed small cell lung cancer. Lung Cancer 2002;38:291–296.

33 Soares M, Darmon M, Salluh JI, et al: Prognosis of lung cancer patients with life-threatening complications. Chest 2007;13:840–846.

34 Sharma G, Freeman J, Zhang D, Goodwin JS: Trends in end-of-life ICU use among older adults with advanced lung cancer. Chest 2008;133:72–78.

35 Cuomo A, Delmastro M, Ceriana P, et al: Noninvasive mechanical ventilation as a palliative treatment of acute respiratory failure in patients with end-stage solid cancer. Palliat Med 2004;18:602–610.

36 Christodoulou C, Rizos M, Galani E, et al: Performance status: a simple predictor of short-term outcome of cancer patients with solid tumors admitted to the intensive care unit. Anticancer Res 2007;27:2945–2948.

37 Lamont EB, Christakis NA: Prognostic disclosure to patients with cancer near the end of life. Ann Intern Med 2001;134:1096–105.

38 Fadul N, Elsayem A, Palmer JL, et al: Predictors of access to palliative care services among patients who died at a comprehensive cancer center. J Palliat Med 2007;10:1146–52.

39 Griffin JP, Koch KA, Nelson JE, Cooley ME: Palliative care consultation, quality-of-life measurements, and bereavement for end-of-life care in patients with lung cancer: ACCP evidence-based clinical practice guidelines, ed 2. Chest 2007;132:404S–422S.

Ayman O. Soubani, MD
Division of Pulmonary, Critical Care and Sleep Medicine
Wayne State University School of Medicine
3990 John R Street, 3 Hudson, Detroit, MI 48201 (USA)
Tel. +1 313 745 8471, Fax +1 313 993 0562, E-Mail asoubani@med.wayne.edu

Esquinas AM (ed): Applied Technologies in Pulmonary Medicine. Basel, Karger, 2011, pp 185–191

Readmission to the Intensive Care Unit for Patients with Lung Edema or Atelectasis

Yoshinori Matsuoka · Akinoro Zaitsu · Makoto Hashizume

Department of Emergency and Critical Care Center, School of Medicine, Kyushu University Japan, Fukuoka, Japan

Abbreviations

PaO_2	Partial pressure of arterial oxygen
P/F ratio	PaO_2/FiO_2 ratio
FiO_2	Function of inspired O_2 concentration
PEEP	Positive-pressure respiration

Of 1,835 patients who entered the ICU during the 36 months from January 2003 to December 2005, 141 were readmitted within 1 month of their initial discharge. Acute respiratory failure by lung edema or atelectasis was present in 21 of these patients (14.9% of the readmitted patients, and 1.1% of all ICU patients). For these 21 patients, the body weight on the last day of the first ICU stay was markedly higher than that on the first day. In addition, most of the patients had normalized respiratory states at the time of initial ICU discharge, but aggravation of the respiratory state occurred immediately after discharge, with lung consolidation. Patients requiring a longer period of artificial respiration and those with a shorter ICU stay after extubation had a shorter time to ICU readmission. After readmission, their respiratory state was improved by decreasing the body weight based on strict water management.

It is generally thought that weight reduction by muscle contraction of 0–0.5 kg/day occurs during bed rest [1–3] and body weight gain due to improved nourishment occurs about 4 weeks later [4–6]; therefore, we thought that the body weight gain may have occurred due to internal surplus water. In turn, this might cause lung edema or atelectasis and worsening of the respiratory state. This suggests that surplus lung water that was not removed during the first ICU stay may be associated with subsequent development of lung edema or atelectasis and early readmission to the ICU. Therefore, we performed a retrospective investigation of patient management during the first ICU stay for patients readmitted to the ICU with lung edema or atelectasis.

Analysis Main Topics Related with Your Title

During the 36-month period from January 1, 2003 to December 31, 2005, 1,835 patients were admitted into our ICU. Of these patients, 141 (7.6% of the total number of admissions) were readmission cases, and 21 of the 141 patients were suffering from acute respiratory failure due to lung edema or atelectasis. Thus, patients with lung edema or atelectasis comprised 14.9% of readmitted

Table 1. Clinical data during the first ICU admission period for the 21 readmitted acute respiratory failure patients (1)

	Initial body weight, kg	Final body weight, kg	Body weight gain, %	Time to ICU readmission, days
1	56.1	62.7	12	1
2	60.3	71.1	11.8	2
3	49.9	55.3	11	2
4	53.2	58.9	10.8	2
5	55.9	61.7	10.3	2
6	64.1	70.6	10.2	2
7	67.3	74	10	3
8	66	71.9	9	4
9	49.2	53.1	8	4
10	55	59.4	8	4
11	67	71.7	7	8
12	60.3	63.9	6	10
13	61.5	64.6	5	10
14	54	56.6	4.8	10
15	46.7	48.6	4	11
16	58.3	60.5	3.7	11
17	62.2	64.1	3	15
18	63	64.3	2.1	16
19	50.3	51.3	1.9	16
20	52.6	53.2	1.2	17
21	54.1	54.6	1	18

Body weight gain (%) = Final body weight (kg) ÷ Initial body weight (kg).

patients and 1.1% of the total number of ICU patients. We investigated the patients who had lung consolidation and were diagnosed with acute respiratory failure due to lung edema or atelectasis. Patients with a diagnosis of a disease due to a specific bacterial cause, such as pneumonia, were excluded from the study. Since almost all patients readmitted to the ICU more than 1 month after their initial ICU stay did not have a condition that was connected directly with the disease that caused the first ICU admission, we only investigated patients who were readmitted to the ICU within 1 month of their initial ICU stay.

Acute respiratory failure was defined as PaO_2 <60 Torr for indoor inspiration or a respiratory disorder equivalent to PaO_2 <60 Torr [7]. This threshold is the definition of respiratory failure in Japan. Respiratory function was evaluated using the P/F ratio [8]. The initial and final body weight during the first ICU period, body weight gain at the time of ICU discharge (weight upon discharge from the ICU ÷ weight when entering the ICU), the time to ICU readmission, the P/F ratio on the last day of the first ICU stay and on the first day of the second admission, the period using the respirator, the length of the initial ICU stay after

Table 2. Clinical data during the first ICU admission period for the 21 readmitted acute respiratory failure patients (2)

	P/F ratio 1	P/F ratio 2	R value	E value	R/E ratio
1	388	120	18	1	18
2	368	132	17	2	8.5
3	378	123	16	2	8
4	400	149	16	2	8
5	410	161	13	2	6.5
6	441	176	15	2	7.5
7	399	155	12	2	6
8	387	166	10	2	5
9	412	185	8	2	4
10	433	199	12	2	6
11	412	195	11	2	5.5
12	450	200	10	3	3.33
13	399	211	8	3	2.66
14	421	253	8	3	2.66
15	419	258	7	4	1.75
16	367	345	5	4	1.25
17	421	309	9	4	2.25
18	403	321	9	4	2.25
19	367	339	12	5	2.4
20	410	297	11	6	1.83
21	400	344	10	6	1.66

P/F ratio 1 = P/F ratio on the last day of the first ICU stay (mm Hg); P/F ratio 2 = P/F ratio on the first day of ICU readmission (mm Hg); R value = the period using a respirator (days); E value = length of ICU stay after extubation (days); R/E ratio = R value ÷ E value.

extubation, and the R/E ratio (the period using a respirator (R) ÷ the length of the ICU stay after extubation (E)) were measured retrospectively. Correlations were investigated between body weight gain at the time of ICU discharge and the time to ICU readmission, between body weight gain and the P/F ratio at ICU readmission, between the R/E ratio and the time to ICU readmission, between the R/E ratio and body weight gain, and between body weight gain until extubation and the time to extubation.

Clinical data during the first ICU admission period for the 21 readmitted acute respiratory failure patients are shown in tables 1 and 2. A negative linear relationship was found between body weight gain at the time of initial ICU discharge and the time to ICU readmission (fig. 1). A weight increase of more than 10% at the time of ICU discharge was likely to cause readmission to the ICU within 3 days. A negative linear relationship was also found between body weight gain at the time of ICU discharge and the P/F ratio at ICU readmission (fig. 2). A weight increase of more than 10% at ICU discharge and a P/F ratio <150 were likely to result in readmission to the ICU due to severe respiratory failure.

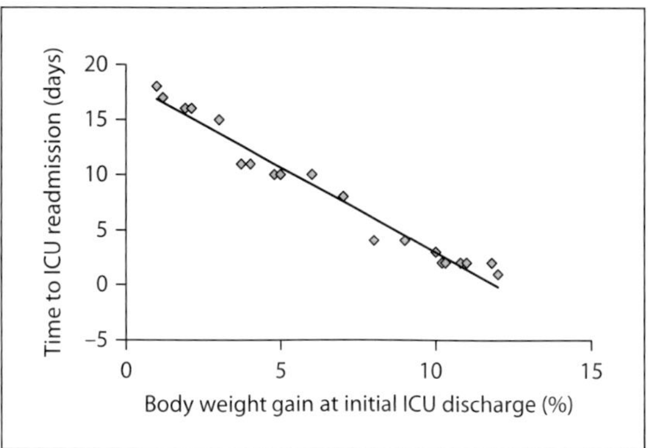

Fig. 1. A negative linear relationship (R = –0.98) was found between body weight gain at the initial ICU discharge and the time to ICU readmission. A weight increase of more than 10% at the time of ICU discharge suggested readmission to the ICU within 3 days was likely.

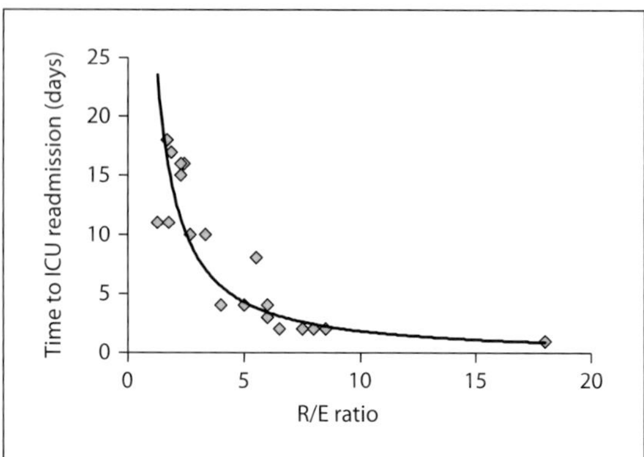

Fig. 3. An inverse proportional relationship (R = –0.74) was found between the R/E ratio and the time to ICU readmission. A large R/E ratio correlated with a short time to ICU readmission.

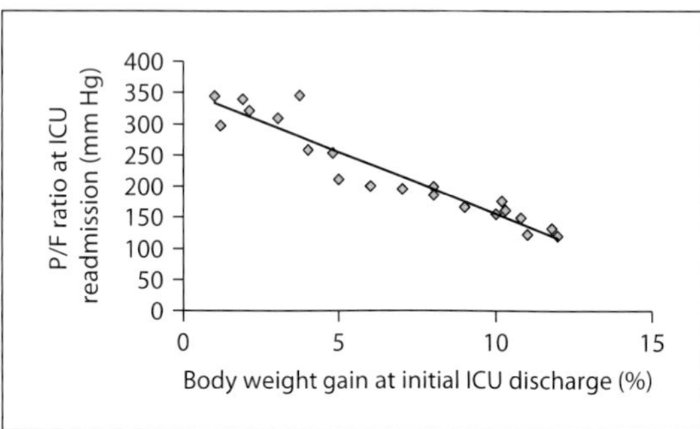

Fig. 2. A negative linear relationship (R = –0.96) was found between body weight gain at the initial ICU discharge and the P/F ratio at ICU readmission. A weight increase of more than 10% at ICU discharge or a P/F ratio below 150 indicated probable readmission to the ICU with severe respiratory failure.

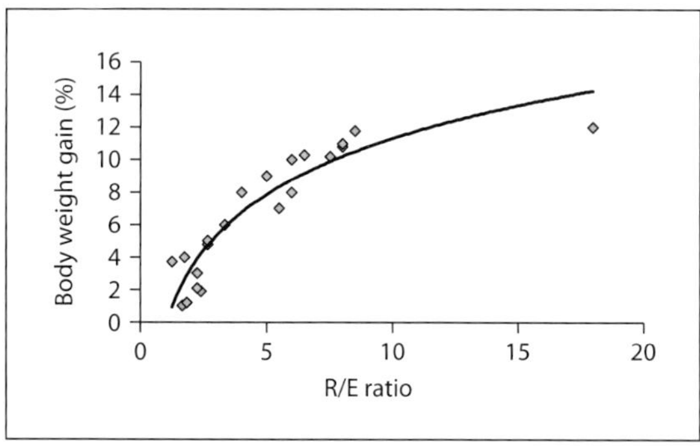

Fig. 4. A proportional relationship (R = 0.81) was found between the R/E ratio and body weight gain. A large R/E ratio correlated with a large body weight gain at the time of initial ICU discharge.

An inverse relationship was found between the R/E ratio and the time to ICU readmission (fig. 3). A large R/E ratio indicates that the patient left the ICU soon after long-term respirator management, and this was associated with a short period before ICU readmission. An R/E ratio of over 5 indicated that a patient was likely to return to the ICU within 5 days. Conversely, a patient with an R/E ratio of around 1 had a very low possibility of readmission to the ICU. A direct relationship was found between the R/E ratio and body weight gain (fig. 4); hence, a large R/E ratio correlated with high body weight gain at the time of ICU discharge. As shown in figure 1 or 2, a large body weight gain at ICU discharge or a poor P/F ratio were associated with readmission to the ICU due to severe respiratory failure. A positive linear relationship was found between

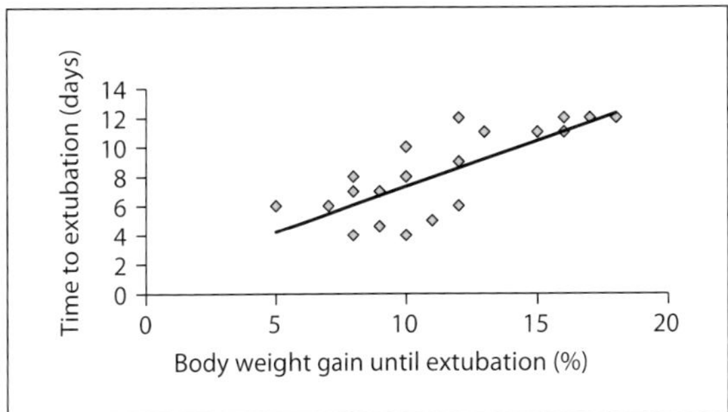

Fig. 5. A positive linear relationship (R = 0.75) was found between body weight gain until extubation and the time to extubation. As the weight increased during respirator use, the time to extubation was prolonged.

body weight gain until extubation and the time to extubation (fig. 5); as weight increased during the period of respiratory support, the time to extubation lengthened.

Discussion

Cytokine release is stimulated by inflammation, and these cytokines stimulate adherence of leukocytes and monocytes to endothelial cells of blood vessels. Elastase and oxygen radicals released by leukocytes may then cause damage to the endothelial cells [9–11], causing circulation failure and increased blood-vessel permeability [12–15]. Transfusion can be performed to compensate for the insufficient amount of plasma due to increased blood-vessel permeability and this may stabilize the circulation dynamics.

The lungs are especially prone to leukocyte-induced damage. Once the blood-vessel endothelial cells are damaged by activated leukocytes in the acute phase, increased blood-vessel permeability in the lungs allows plasma to move into the alveolar space from outside the lung blood vessels [16–18]. Transfusion can be performed to stabilize the circulation, but plasma may leak outside of the lung blood vessels due to the increased permeability. The relative increase in the amount of fluid outside the lung blood vessels causes alveolar collapse, a fall in lung compliance, lung edema, and atelectasis, and this leads to pre-lung failure. This kind of lung failure reflects a state in which alveolar regions with poor ventilation are formed locally. Even if breathing movement is satisfactory and alveolar ventilation is maintained, full inspiration of oxygen cannot occur because a blood-flow shunt has arisen in the lungs [19–22].

Once the lung blood-vessel endothelium is restored, the permeability is reduced and the circulation is stabilized, the transfusion procedure should enter the refilling stage [23]. At this stage, since extracellular fluid has returned to the lung blood vessels, diuresis is used to normalize the amount of fluid outside the blood vessels. This requires immediate reduction of transfusion, performance of diuresis and prompt discharge of the extracellular fluid from the body. Improvement of oxygenation is also important for recovery from pre-lung failure. However, judgment of the timing of this procedure is not easy in practice, and often there is a failure to normalize the extracellular fluid due to continuation of superfluous transfusion and inadequate diuresis. Consolidation of the lungs may therefore arise, and this kind of lung failure might be viewed as iatrogenic respiratory failure. Many cases of lung edema in the ICU may not also be due to bacteria [24, 25].

The development of respirators has allowed maintenance of oxygenation, even in patients with severe lung failure, by providing the correct amount of ventilation. PEEP is particularly effective for atelectasis caused by lung edema, because it increases the lung expiration capacity, widens the peripheral respiratory tract, and re-expands the collapsed alveolar space. As a result, oxygenation appears to improve, but if PEEP is stopped the respiratory state worsens; hence, this procedure does not address the fundamental causes of lung failure. The basic treatment for lung failure is simply to normalize surplus extracellular fluid outside the lung blood vessels. Extubation by

PEEP before the extracellular fluid is normalized does allow oxygenation to be maintained at a high concentration of oxygen, but the alveolar space opened by PEEP collapses in a short time and this may cause lung consolidation in this region.

In the current work, a negative linear relationship was found between body weight gain at the time of ICU discharge and the time to ICU readmission (fig. 1) and between body weight gain at the time of ICU discharge and the P/F ratio at the time of ICU readmission (fig. 2). A weight increase of more than 10% at ICU discharge or a P/F ratio of below 150 was associated with readmission to the ICU within 3 days. Body weight should decrease steadily from entering the ICU by about 0.5 kg/day due to muscle wasting by bed rest, as mentioned above; therefore, the actual body weight gain at ICU discharge is larger than the measured value, since some weight loss should have occurred in the ICU.

A large R/E ratio, which indicates that a patient left the ICU soon after long-term respirator management, was associated with a large body weight gain at the time of ICU discharge (fig. 4). Since a large body weight gain tends to lead to ICU readmission (fig. 1 or 2), it is desirable to have a small R/E ratio. From figure 3, readmission to the ICU is extremely unlikely when the R/E ratio is around 1, suggesting that it is preferable to keep patients in the ICU after extubation for the same period for which a respirator was used. However, in practice this is difficult due to medical costs and the desire to limit the number of hospitalization days. Reduction of the R value (the period of respiratory support) would also have a favorable effect on the R/E ratio.

From figure 5, losing weight during the period of respiratory support is likely to lead to early extubation, since the time to extubation was related to body weight gain. In other words, losing body weight at the refilling stage prevents ICU readmission and may decrease the length of the ICU stay. Fluid management failure during the first ICU stay may result in ICU readmission due to lung edema or atelectasis. A key for prevention of ICU readmission is to obtain complete reversal of lung failure before ICU discharge, using strict water management based on weight measurements and with care not to assume that an apparent improvement in the respiratory state will be sustained, since this improvement may be due to respiratory support.

Recommendations

- Prevention of ICU readmission requires complete recovery from lung failure before initial ICU discharge.
- Strict water management based on body weight measurement is essential at the refilling stage.
- A decrease in body weight at this stage prevents ICU readmission and may decrease the length of the initial ICU stay.

References

1 Forbes GB: Weight loss during fasting: implications for the obese. Am J Clin Nutr 1970;23:1212–1219.

2 Benedict FG: A Study of Prolonged Fasting. Washington, Carnegie Institute of Washington, 1915, pp 69–87.

3 Drenick EJ, Swendseid ME, Blahd WH, Tuttle SG: Prolonged starvation as treatment for severe obesity. JAMA 1964;187: 100–105.

4 Spady DW, Payne PR, Picou D, Waterlow JC: Energy balance during recovery from malnutrition. Am J Clin Nutr 1976;29: 1073–1088.

5 Long CL: Energy balance and carbohydrate metabolism in infection and sepsis. Am J Clin Nutr 1977;30:1301–1310.

6 Long CL, Kinney JM, Geiger JW: Nonsuppressability of gluconeogenesis by glucose in septic patients. Metabolism 1976;25:193–201.

7 Zaitsu A: The latest trends in the treatment of acute respiratory failure. Fukuoka Igaku Zasshi 1990;81:391–295.
8 Covelli HD, Nessan VJ, Tuttle WK: Oxygen derived variables in acute respiratory failure. Crit Care Med 1983;11:646–649.
9 Nakae H, Endo S, Inada K, Kasai T, Yoshida M: Significance of α-tocopherol and interleukin-8 in septic adult respiratory distress syndrome. Res Commun Chem Pathol Pharmacol 1994;84:197–202.
10 Endo S, Inada K, Inoue Y, Kuwata Y, Suzuki M, Yamashita H, Hoshi S, Yoshida M: Two types of septic shock classified by the plasma levels of cytokines and endotoxin. Circ Shock 1992;38:264–274.
11 Endo S, Inada K, Yamada Y, Kasai T, Takakuwa T, Nakae H, Kikuchi M, Hoshi S, Suzuki M, Yamashita H, et al: Plasma tumour necrosis factor-α levels in patients with burns. Burns 1993;19:124–127.
12 Endo S, Inada K, Yamashita H, Takakuwa T, Nakae H, Kasai T, Kikuchi M, Ogawa M, Uchida K, Yoshida M: Platelet-activating factor acetylhydrolase activity, type II phospholipase A_2, and cytokine levels in patients with sepsis. Res Commun Chem Pathol Pharmacol 1994;83:289–295.
13 Endo S, Inada K, Ceska M, Takakuwa T, Yamada Y, Nakae H, Kasai T, Yamashita H, Taki K, Yoshida M: Plasma interleukin-8 and polymorphonuclear leukocyte elastase concentrations in patients with septic shock. J Inflamm 1995;45:136–142.
14 Petty TL: Protease mechanisms in the pathogenesis of acute lung injury. Ann NY Acad Sci 1991;624:267–277.
15 Edens HA, Parkos CA: Neutrophil transendothelial migration and alteration in vascular permeability: focus on neutrophil-derived azurocidin. Curr Opin Hematol 2003;10:25–30.
16 Su X, Camerer E, Hamilton JR, Coughlin SR, Matthay MA: Protease-activated receptor-2 activation induces acute lung inflammation by neuropeptide-dependent mechanisms. J Immunol 2005;175:2598–2605.
17 Guo M, Wu MH, Granger HJ, Yuan SY: Focal adhesion kinase in neutrophil-induced microvascular hyperpermeability. Microcirculation 2005;12:223–232.
18 Brigham KL, Meyrick B: Endotoxin and lung injury. Am Rev Respir Dis 1986;133:913–927.
19 Dantzger DR: Pulmonary gas exchange; in Dantzger DR (ed): Cardiopulmonary Critical Care, ed 2. Philadelphia, Saunders, 1991, pp 25–43.
20 Lanken PN: Ventilation-perfusion relationships; in Grippi MA (ed): Pulmonary Pathophysiology. Philadelphia, Lippincott, 1995, pp 195–210.
21 Buohuys A: Respiratory dead space; in Fenn WO, Rahn H (eds): Handbook of Physiology: Respiration. Bethesda, American Physiological Society, 1964, pp 699–714.
22 D'Alonzo GE, Dantzker DR: Mechanisms of abnormal gas exchange. Med Clin North Am 1983;67:557–571.
23 Matsui M, Kudo T, Kudo M, Ishihara H, Matsuki A: The endocrine response after burns. Agressologie 1991;32:233–235.
24 Meduri GU, Mauldin GL, Wunderink RG, et al: Causes of fever and pulmonary densities in patients with clinical manifestations of ventilator-associated pneumonia. Chest 1994;106:221–235.
25 Bates JH, Campbell GD, Barron AL, et al: Microbial etiology of acute pneumonia in hospitalized patients. Chest 1992;101:1005–1012.

Yoshinori Matsuoka, MD
Department of Emergency and Critical Care Center
School of Medicine, Kyushu University Japan
3-1-1 Maidashi Higashiku, Fukuokashi, Fukuoka 812-8582 (Japan)
Tel. +81 92 642 5871, Fax +81 92 642 5874, E-Mail yoshinori216@h2.dion.ne.jp

Esquinas AM (ed): Applied Technologies in Pulmonary Medicine. Basel, Karger, 2011, pp 192–196

Early Mobilization in the Intensive Care Unit: Safety, Feasibility, and Benefits

Radha Korupolu[a] · Jeneen M. Gifford[b] · Jennifer M. Zanni[c] · Alex Truong[a] · Gangadhar Vajrala[a] · Scott Lepre[d] · Dale M. Needham[a,d]

[a]Division of Pulmonary and Critical Care Medicine, Johns Hopkins University, [b]Department of Internal Medicine, Johns Hopkins Bayview Medical Center, [c]Department of Physical Medicine and Rehabilitation, Johns Hopkins Hospital, and [d]Department of Physical Medicine and Rehabilitation, Johns Hopkins University, Baltimore, Md., USA

Deconditioning and weakness are problems commonly experienced by ICU patients [1–4]. Bed rest and immobility contribute to the development of these neuromuscular complications, which can be severe and long lasting in ICU survivors [1–3]. The benefits of physical medicine and rehabilitation in patients with prolonged mechanical ventilation have been well recognized [5–8], and recently there has been growing interest in evaluating early initiation of mobilization activities in the acute ICU setting [4, 9, 10]. Existing studies have demonstrated that early mobilization is safe, feasible, and associated with short-term benefits in critically ill patients.

In this chapter, we will briefly review the relevant epidemiology and pathophysiology of immobility and bed rest. Thereafter, we will discuss early mobilization of critically ill patients specifically addressing its safety, feasibility and potential benefits.

Epidemiology

Routine use of physical medicine and rehabilitation therapy in the ICU is relatively rare. In one study, physical therapy was given to only 8 of 135 (6%) patients receiving 'usual care' in the ICU [11]. In another study of 150 acute lung injury patients in the ICU, only 27% received physical therapy which occurred on only 6% of all ICU days [12]. Likewise, in a smaller study of 20 physiologically stable ICU patients, physical activity was observed over two separate 4-hour periods that were variably scheduled throughout the day. During a total of 156 h of observation, only two instances of sitting and one instance of standing were recorded. No patient ambulated, and all other activities consisted solely of a passive range of motion and turning the patient in bed [13].

One systematic review included 24 studies which evaluated neuromuscular abnormalities in 1,421 adult ICU patients with sepsis, multiorgan dysfunction, or prolonged mechanical ventilation [14]. In this review, 46% of subjects had critical illness neuromuscular abnormalities diagnosed using electrophysiological testing, with or without associated physical examination. A separate study used physical examination to diagnose neuromuscular weakness in awake patients who required >7 days of mechanical ventilation. In this cohort, ICU-acquired weakness was clinically diagnosed in 25% of 95 patients [1]. Neuromuscular weakness acquired in the ICU can persist for months or years after hospital discharge, causing impairments in physical function and quality of life [2, 3, 15].

Pathophysiology of Bed Rest and Immobility

Immobility has deleterious effects on muscle that may contribute to the development of ICU-acquired weakness. Experimental studies in animals have demonstrated that immobility activates multiple molecular pathways which result in an overall imbalance between protein degradation and protein synthesis, resulting in a net loss of muscle fibers [16–18]. Studies in healthy individuals have demonstrated that long-term bed rest (i.e. >30 days) leads to a state of systemic inflammation, with increased reactive oxide species [19] and inflammatory cytokines [20], as well as a transient decrease in protective antioxidants [21]. Together, these changes create an inflammatory environment that is toxic to muscles through inhibition of anabolic pathways, activation of catabolic pathways, and direct interaction with muscle fibers to interrupt contractile force. Insulin resistance and increased sensitivity to the catabolic effects of cortisol are other mechanisms that have been implicated in muscle atrophy associated with bed rest [22–24].

Bed rest also results in important cardiovascular changes that can decrease exercise tolerance. Underlying physiological mechanisms include abnormal baroreceptor response contributing to postural hypotension and tachycardia, and decreased stroke volume, cardiac output, and peak oxygen uptake [25, 26]. In addition, patients exposed to prolonged periods of bed rest often experience changes in mood which may also contribute to one's decreased physical function [27].

Early Mobilization in the ICU

The goals of early mobilization in the ICU are to mitigate the effects of decreased physical activity, preserve patients' physical function, and expedite recovery. The term 'early' is used to emphasize the important difference in timing between this strategy and current ICU practice where mechanically ventilated patients frequently are heavily sedated and unable to actively participate in mobilization activities until after extubation or ICU discharge. By contrast, with early mobilization, heavy sedation is avoided, with a goal of balancing patient alertness and comfort. In this setting, physical activity may commence immediately after major physiological derangements have been stabilized, often within 24–72 h of ICU admission [28]. Mobilization of patients may occur despite their ongoing requirements for moderate levels of support from mechanical ventilation, vasopressor infusions, and other ICU therapies.

Safety

The safety of early physical medicine and rehabilitation activities is of particular concern in patients who are critically ill. Three published studies have specifically analyzed this issue. In one study conducted in a respiratory ICU, 103 mechanically ventilated patients with acute respiratory failure performed a total of 1,449 activity events, including sitting on the edge of the bed, sitting in a chair, and ambulation. Safety-related issues occurred in less than 1% of all activity events, and all were corrected promptly without any negative sequelae attributable to the issue. Of all activities, 41% were conducted in intubated patients without any extubations occurring during therapy [28]. Similarly, a controlled trial in a medical ICU analyzed the effect of an early mobility protocol, initiated within 48 h of mechanical ventilation. None of the 106 patients in the early mobility protocol arm experienced accidental dislodgement of any medical device or any life-threatening situation [11]. Finally, in a third study conducted in a medical ICU, 69 mobilization activity events were performed on 31 patients. Only three adverse events were reported: all were desaturation episodes which only required a temporary increase in oxygen requirement [29].

Based on these studies, we have proposed an algorithm for selecting ICU patients who are appropriate for early mobilization [10]. Patients are assessed daily for the ability to actively participate. Early mobilization is deferred in patients who are deeply sedated or comatose. Criteria for cardiac and pulmonary stability include (1) $FiO_2 \leq 0.6$, (2) PEEP ≤ 10 cm H_2O, (3) no increase in vasopressor dose in the past 2 h, (4) no continuous infusion of a vasodilator medication, (5) no new anti-arrhythmic agent, and (6) no new cardiac ischemia. Clinical judgment from all clinicians participating in patient care is necessary to determine other contraindications and to identify patients who may benefit from a trial of therapy despite failing to meet these specific criteria.

Feasibility

Common mobilization activities that are feasible for mechanically ventilated patients in the ICU setting include transferring from the supine position to an unsupported sitting position at the edge of the bed, standing, transferring into a chair, and ambulation [11, 28–30]. Ambulation in the typical mechanically ventilated patient requires the combined efforts of a physical therapist, nurse, respiratory therapist and technician to safely manage the patient and the associated lines, tubes and life support equipment [11, 28]. In addition to mobilization activities, patients may benefit from resistance training and range of motion activities to promote muscle strengthening and joint mobility. As previously outlined, these activities are feasible and safe, even in ICU patients requiring mechanical ventilation via an endotracheal tube [28, 31]. Additionally, this therapy can be accomplished without any increase in cost [28, 31].

Promoting early mobilization in the ICU requires a multidisciplinary team approach to patient care with the goal of minimizing barriers to rehabilitation and promoting safety and efficiency. Challenging long-standing assumptions about the need for heavy sedation and bed rest in critically ill patients is important in instituting 'culture change' in the ICU. Successful culture change involves interdisciplinary training, support from all levels of leadership, and a commitment from the ICU clinical staff and administration to make mobilization a priority in patient care. If successful, such changes can improve teamwork, safety and consistency of ICU care, as well as minimize ICU-acquired weakness and impairments in physical function [10, 30, 31].

Potential Benefits of Early Mobilization

Mobilization of patients in the ICU can prevent the negative sequelae of immobility and enhance physical function in the hospital. In patients with chronic pulmonary disease or requirement for long-term mechanical ventilation, physical medicine and rehabilitation therapy improves mobility, increases overall strength, improves weaning from mechanical ventilation, increases independence with activities of daily living, and reduces ICU length of stay [5–8]. There is growing evidence that these benefits may also occur with physical medicine and rehabilitation therapy in ICU patients who have a greater acuity of illness. Recent studies of early mobility in the ICU have demonstrated improved physical function [11, 28, 30], shortened length of stay in ICU and hospital [11, 31], and improved weaning from mechanical ventilation [31].

One study of an early mobility program involving 103 mechanically ventilated patients demonstrated that 69% of patients walked more than 100 ft by ICU discharge. A subsequent study at the same medical center used a different cohort of 104 mechanically ventilated patients and demonstrated that 91 patients (88%) walked a median (interquartile range) distance of 200 (0–800) ft by ICU discharge [31]. During a 6-year period in which the early mobility program was ongoing at this hospital, ICU and hospital length of stay steadily decreased, the proportion of patients receiving tracheotomy decreased from 29 to 5%, and the proportion of patients with weaning failure decreased from 12 to 3% [31]. Collectively, these reports demonstrate mobilization in the ICU can be beneficial for patient outcomes and hospital resource utilization. Beneficial results were observed at another hospital where a controlled trial demonstrated that an early mobility protocol was associated with a shorter time from ICU admission to getting out of bed (5.0 days in the mobility group vs. 11.3 days in the 'usual care' control group, $p < 0.001$), a shorter risk-adjusted ICU length of stay (5.5 vs. 6.9 days, $p = 0.025$), and a decreased risk-adjusted hospital length of stay (11.2 vs. 14.5 days, $p = 0.006$) [11]. This controlled trial again demonstrates that early mobilization in the ICU is associated with improved physical function and decreased resource utilization.

Conclusion

Neuromuscular complications in survivors of critical illness are common and may cause long-lasting impairments in physical function and quality of life. Prolonged bed rest and immobility are important factors in the development of these complications. Early mobilization may diminish the detrimental effects of bed rest. Recent studies have demonstrated that early mobilization is safe, feasible, and beneficial for mechanically ventilated ICU patients. Large multicenter randomized trials will enhance the validity and generalizability of these existing studies. Future research should address the effects of early mobility on ICU patients' long-term outcomes, including muscle strength, physical function, quality of life, and resource utilization after hospital discharge.

References

1 De Jonghe B, Sharshar T, Lefaucheur JP, et al: Paresis acquired in the intensive care unit: a prospective multicenter study. JAMA 2002;288:2859–2867.

2 Fletcher SN, Kennedy DD, Ghosh IR, et al: Persistent neuromuscular and neurophysiologic abnormalities in long-term survivors of prolonged critical illness. Crit Care Med 2003;31:1012–1016.

3 Herridge MS, Cheung AM, Tansey CM, et al: One-year outcomes in survivors of the acute respiratory distress syndrome. N Engl J Med 2003;348:683–693.

4 Needham DM: Mobilizing patients in the intensive care unit: improving neuromuscular weakness and physical function. JAMA 2008;300:1685–1690.

5 Nava S: Rehabilitation of patients admitted to a respiratory intensive care unit. Arch Phys Med Rehabil 1998;79:849–854.

6 Martin UJ, Hincapie L, Nimchuk M, Gaughan J, Criner GJ: Impact of whole-body rehabilitation in patients receiving chronic mechanical ventilation. Crit Care Med 2005;33:2259–2265.

7 Make B, Gilmartin M, Brody JS, Snider GL: Rehabilitation of ventilator-dependent subjects with lung diseases. The concept and initial experience. Chest 1984;86:358–365.

8 Chiang LL, Wang LY, Wu CP, Wu HD, Wu YT: Effects of physical training on functional status in patients with prolonged mechanical ventilation. Phys Ther 2006;86:1271–1281.

9 Herridge MS: Mobile, awake and critically ill. CMAJ 2008;178:725–726.

10 Korupolu R, Gifford JM, Needham DM: Early mobilization of critically ill patients: reducing neuromuscular complications after intensive care. Contemp Crit Care 2009;6:1–12.

11 Morris PE, Goad A, Thompson C, et al: Early intensive care unit mobility therapy in the treatment of acute respiratory failure. Crit Care Med 2008;36:2238–2243.

12 Needham DM, Wang W, Desai SV, et al: Intensive care unit exposures for long-term outcomes research: development and description of exposures for 150 patients with acute lung injury. J Crit Care 2007;22:275–284.

13 Winkelman C, Higgins PA, Chen YJ: Activity in the chronically critically ill. Dimens Crit Care Nurs 2005;24:281–290.

14 Stevens RD, Dowdy DW, Michaels RK, Mendez-Tellez PA, Pronovost PJ, Needham DM: Neuromuscular dysfunction acquired in critical illness: a systematic review. Intensive Care Med 2007;33:1876–1891.

15 Dowdy DW, Eid MP, Dennison CR, et al: Quality of life after acute respiratory distress syndrome: a meta-analysis. Intensive Care Med 2006;32:1115–1124.

16 Paddon-Jones D, Sheffield-Moore M, Cree MG, et al: Atrophy and impaired muscle protein synthesis during prolonged inactivity and stress. J Clin Endocrinol Metab 2006;91:4836–4841.

17 Taillandier D, Aurousseau E, Meynial-Denis D, et al: Coordinate activation of lysosomal, Ca^{2+}-activated and ATP-ubiquitin-dependent proteinases in the unweighted rat soleus muscle. Biochem J 1996;316:65–72.
18 Tidball JG, Spencer MJ: Calpains and muscular dystrophies. Int J Biochem Cell Biol 2000;32:1–5.
19 Pawlak W, Kedziora J, Zolynski K, Kedziora-Kornatowska K, Blaszczyk J, Witkowski P: Free radicals generation by granulocytes from men during bed rest. J Gravit Physiol 1998;5:131–132.
20 Schmitt DA, Schwarzenberg M, Tkaczuk J, et al: Head-down tilt bed rest and immune responses. Pflugers Arch 2000;441(suppl):R79–R84.
21 Pawlak W, Kedziora J, Zolynski K, et al: Effect of long-term bed rest in men on enzymatic antioxidative defence and lipid peroxidation in erythrocytes. J Gravit Physiol 1998;5:163–164.
22 Ferrando AA, Lane HW, Stuart CA, Davis-Street J, Wolfe RR: Prolonged bed rest decreases skeletal muscle and whole-body protein synthesis. Am J Physiol 1996;270:E627–E633.
23 Hamburg NM, McMackin CJ, Huang AL, et al: Physical inactivity rapidly induces insulin resistance and microvascular dysfunction in healthy volunteers. Arterioscler Thromb Vasc Biol 2007;27:2650–2656.
24 Wang X, Hu Z, Du J, Mitch WE: Insulin resistance accelerates muscle protein degradation: activation of the ubiquitin-proteasome pathway by defects in muscle cell signaling. Endocrinology 2006;147:4160–4168.
25 Convertino VA, Bloomfield SA, Greenleaf JE: An overview of the issues: physiological effects of bed rest and restricted physical activity. Med Sci Sports Exerc 1997;29:187–190.
26 Fortney SM, Schneider VS, Greenleaf JE: The physiology of bed rest; in Fregly MJ, Blatteis CM (eds): Handbook of Physiology. New York, Oxford University Press, 1996, pp 889–939.
27 Hough CL, Needham DM: The role of future longitudinal studies in ICU survivors: understanding determinants and pathophysiology of weakness and neuromuscular dysfunction. Curr Opin Crit Care 2007;13:489–496.
28 Bailey P, Thomsen GE, Spuhler VJ, et al: Early activity is feasible and safe in respiratory failure patients. Crit Care Med 2007;35:139–145.
29 Stiller K, Phillips A, Lambert P: The safety of mobilisation and its effects on haemodynamics and respiratory status of intensive care patients. Physiother Theory Pract 2004;20:175–185.
30 Thomsen GE, Snow GL, Rodriguez L, Hopkins RO: Patients with respiratory failure increase ambulation after transfer to an intensive care unit where early activity is a priority. Crit Care Med 2008;36:1119–1124.
31 Hopkins RO, Spuhler VJ, Thomsen GE: Transforming ICU culture to facilitate early mobility. Crit Care Clin 2007;23:81–96.

Dale M. Needham, MD, PhD
Division of Pulmonary and Critical Care Medicine, Johns Hopkins University
1830 E. Monument St, 5th Floor, Baltimore, MD 21205 (USA)
Tel. +1 410 955 3467, Fax +1 410 955 0036
E-Mail dale.needham@jhmi.edu

Esquinas AM (ed): Applied Technologies in Pulmonary Medicine. Basel, Karger, 2011, pp 197–201

Evidence-Based Guidelines in Pulmonary Rehabilitation

Andrew L. Ries

School of Medicine, University of California, San Diego, Calif., USA

Abbreviations

AACVPR	American Association of Cardiovascular and Pulmonary Rehabilitation
ACCP	American College of Chest Physicians
ATS	American Thoracic Society
COPD	Chronic obstructive pulmonary disease
ERS	European Respiratory Society

Pulmonary rehabilitation has emerged as a recommended standard of care for patients with chronic lung disease based on a growing body of scientific evidence. Several organizations have taken a lead role in championing pulmonary rehabilitation and developing comprehensive statements, practice guidelines, and evidence-based guidelines. Documenting the scientific evidence underlying clinical practice has been important in overcoming skepticism and convincing health professionals, healthcare institutions, third-party payors, and regulatory agencies to support pulmonary rehabilitation.

The first definition of pulmonary rehabilitation was developed in 1974 by the ACCP, and the first comprehensive statement published by ATS in 1981 [1]. ATS subsequently updated its statement in 1999 [2] and then, in conjunction with ERS, in 2006 [3]. The first systematic review of the scientific basis of pulmonary rehabilitation was published by the AACVPR in 1990 [4] and then, in conjunction with ACCP in 1997, the first evidence-based guidelines [5]. Since that time, the published literature on pulmonary rehabilitation has increased substantially, providing justification for recommending pulmonary rehabilitation as part of standards of care for the management of patients with COPD and other chronic lung diseases [3, 6, 7]. Therefore, ACCP and AACVPR decided to update the 1997 guidelines with a systematic, evidence-based review of the literature that was published recently [8].

Main Topics

The ATS and ERS recently adopted the following definition of pulmonary rehabilitation [3]:

Pulmonary rehabilitation is an evidence-based, multidisciplinary, and comprehensive intervention for patients with chronic respiratory diseases who are symptomatic and often have decreased daily life activities. Integrated into the individualized treatment of the patient, pulmonary rehabilitation is designed to reduce symptoms, optimize functional status, increase participation, and reduce health-care costs through stabilizing or reversing systemic manifestations of the disease.

This definition focuses on three important features of successful rehabilitation: (1) a multidisciplinary approach; (2) an individualized program

Table 1a. Relationship of strength of the supporting evidence to the balance of benefits to risks and burdens [10]

Strength of evidence	Balance of benefits to risks and burdens			
	benefits outweigh risks/burdens	risks/burdens outweigh benefits	evenly balanced	uncertain
High	1A	1A	2A	
Moderate	1B	1B	2B	
Low or very low	1C	1C	2C	2C

1A: strong recommendation. 2A: weak recommendation.
1B: strong recommendation. 2B: weak recommendation.
1C: strong recommendation. 2C: weak recommendation.

Table 1b. Description of balance of benefits to risks/burdens scale

Benefits clearly outweigh the risks and burdens	Certainty of imbalance
Risks and burdens clearly outweigh the benefits	Certainty of imbalance
Risks/burdens and benefits are closely balanced	Less certainty
Balance of benefits to risks and burdens is uncertain	Uncertainty

tailored to the patients needs, and (3) attention to physical, psychological and social function.

Rehabilitation programs for patients with chronic lung disease are well established as a means of enhancing standard therapy in order to control and alleviate symptoms and optimize functional capacity [3, 5, 7, 9]. The primary goal is to restore the patient to the highest possible level of independent function which is accomplished by helping patients learn more about their disease, treatments, and coping strategies.

Pulmonary rehabilitation is appropriate for any patient with stable chronic lung disease who is disabled by respiratory symptoms. Programs typically include components such as patient assessment, exercise training, education, nutritional intervention, and psychosocial support. These programs have been successfully applied to patients with diseases other than COPD such as interstitial diseases, cystic fibrosis, bronchiectasis, and thoracic cage abnormalities.

In the recently updated evidence-based guidelines, the ACCP/AACVPR Panel focused on studies published since the previous 1997 review, concentrating on published literature in patients with COPD. Because of the many advances and new areas of investigation, the Panel not only updated the areas reviewed and recommendations in the previous guideline [5] but also reviewed additional new topics. Recommendations were developed for several outcomes of comprehensive pulmonary rehabilitation programs including lower extremity exercise training, dyspnea, health-related quality of life, healthcare utilization, survival, psychosocial outcomes, and long-term benefits. Additional topics reviewed include duration of

Table 2. Recommendations and ratings of the evidence-based guidelines

1.	Recommendation: A program of exercise training of the muscles of ambulation is recommended as a mandatory component of pulmonary rehabilitation for patients with COPD. *Grade of Recommendation: 1A*
2.	Recommendation: Pulmonary rehabilitation improves the symptom of dyspnea in patients with COPD. *Grade of Recommendation: 1A*
3.	Recommendation: Pulmonary rehabilitation improves health-related quality of life in patients with COPD. *Grade of Recommendation: 1A*
4.	Recommendation: Pulmonary rehabilitation reduces the number of hospital days and other measures of healthcare utilization in patients with COPD. *Grade of Recommendation: 2B*
5.	Recommendation: Pulmonary rehabilitation is cost-effective in patients with COPD. *Grade of Recommendation: 2C*
6.	Statement: There is insufficient evidence to determine if pulmonary rehabilitation improves survival in patients with COPD. *No recommendation is provided.*
7.	Recommendation: There are psychosocial benefits from comprehensive pulmonary rehabilitation programs in patients with COPD. *Grade of Recommendation: 2B*
8.	Recommendation: 6–12 weeks of pulmonary rehabilitation produces benefits in several outcomes that decline gradually over 12–18 months. *Grade of Recommendation: 1A* Some benefits, such as health-related quality of life, remain above control at 12–18 months. *Grade of Recommendation: 1C*
9.	Recommendation: Longer pulmonary rehabilitation programs (beyond 12 weeks) produce greater sustained benefits than shorter programs. *Grade of Recommendation: 2C*
10.	Recommendation: Maintenance strategies following pulmonary rehabilitation have a modest effect on long-term outcomes. *Grade of Recommendation: 2C*
11.	Recommendation: Lower extremity exercise training at higher exercise intensity produces greater physiologic benefits than lower intensity training in patients with COPD. *Grade of Recommendation: 1B*
12.	Recommendation: Both low- and high-intensity exercise training produce clinical benefits for patients with COPD. *Grade of Recommendation: 1A*
13.	Recommendation: Addition of a strength training component to a program of pulmonary rehabilitation increases muscle strength and muscle mass. *Strength of evidence: 1A*
14.	Recommendation: Current scientific evidence does not support the routine use of anabolic agents in pulmonary rehabilitation for patients with COPD. *Grade of Recommendation: 2C*
15.	Recommendation: Unsupported endurance training of the upper extremities is beneficial in patients with COPD and should be included in pulmonary rehabilitation programs. *Grade of Recommendation: 1A*
16.	Recommendation: The scientific evidence does not support the routine use of inspiratory muscle training as an essential component of pulmonary rehabilitation. *Grade of Recommendation: 1B*
17.	Recommendation: Education should be an integral component of pulmonary rehabilitation. Education should include information on collaborative self-management and prevention and treatment of exacerbations. *Grade of Recommendation: 1B*
18.	Recommendation: There is minimal evidence to support the benefits of psychosocial interventions as a single therapeutic modality. *Grade of Recommendation: 2C*

Table 2. Continued

19.	Statement: Although no recommendation is provided since scientific evidence is lacking, current practice and expert opinion support the inclusion of psychosocial interventions as a component of comprehensive pulmonary rehabilitation programs for patients with COPD.
20.	Recommendation: Supplemental oxygen should be used during rehabilitative exercise training in patients with severe exercise-induced hypoxemia. *Grade of Recommendation: 1C*
21.	Recommendation: Administering supplemental oxygen during high-intensity exercise programs in patients without exercise-induced hypoxemia may improve gains in exercise endurance. *Grade of Recommendation: 2C*
22.	Recommendation: As an adjunct to exercise training in selected patients with severe COPD, noninvasive ventilation produces modest additional improvements in exercise performance. *Grade of Recommendation: 2B*
23.	Statement: There is insufficient evidence to support the routine use of nutritional supplementation in pulmonary rehabilitation of patients with COPD. *No recommendation is provided.*
24.	Recommendations: Pulmonary rehabilitation is beneficial for some patients with chronic respiratory diseases other than COPD. *Grade of Recommendation: 1B*
25.	Statement: Although no recommendation is provided since scientific evidence is lacking, current practice and expert opinion suggest that pulmonary rehabilitation for patients with chronic respiratory diseases other than COPD should be modified to include treatment strategies specific to individual diseases and patients in addition to treatment strategies common to both COPD and non-COPD patients.

pulmonary rehabilitation intervention, post-rehabilitation maintenance strategies, intensity of aerobic exercise training, strength training, anabolic drugs, upper extremity training, inspiratory muscle training, education, psychological and behavioral components, oxygen supplementation, noninvasive ventilation, nutritional supplementation, and rehabilitation for patients with disorders other than COPD. The new document also makes recommendations for future research in pulmonary rehabilitation.

Through a thorough and systematic review of the published literature from 1996 to 2004, the Panel developed recommendations on rehabilitation for patients with chronic lung disease. Based on the published evidence systematically evaluated, ratings of the recommendations followed guidelines developed by ACCP and are indicated in table 1 [10]. These ratings evaluate both the strength of the evidence (A – high; B – moderate; C – low or very low) as well as the balance of benefits to risks and burdens (grade 1, strong recommendation – certainty that benefits do, or do not, outweigh risks and burdens; grade 2, weak recommendation – evenly balanced or uncertainty regarding benefits versus risks and burdens). The recommendations developed by the Panel are presented in table 2, along with the rating for each.

Discussion

Overall, this new guideline provides an excellent summary of the literature published over the past decade. The increasingly solid base of scientific evidence further strengthens the justification for including pulmonary rehabilitation as a standard of care for patients with chronic lung diseases. These new guidelines clearly represent a major step forward in advancing the practice of pulmonary rehabilitation and provide a road map for future research and needed areas for further development in this field.

Recommendations

- Pulmonary rehabilitation should be considered for any patient with symptomatic, disabling chronic lung disease.
- Effective pulmonary rehabilitation can improve symptoms, exercise tolerance, and health-related quality of life and reduce hospitalization and healthcare utilization for patients with chronic lung diseases.
- Pulmonary rehabilitation should be considered for patients with chronic respiratory diseases other than COPD.

References

1 American Thoracic Society: Pulmonary rehabilitation. Am Rev Respir Dis 1981; 124:663–666.

2 American Thoracic Society: Pulmonary rehabilitation – 1999. Am J Respir Crit Care Med 1999;159:1666–1682.

3 American Thoracic Society/European Respiratory Society: ATS/ERS statement on pulmonary rehabilitation. Am J Respir Crit Care Med 2006;173:1390–1413.

4 Ries AL: Scientific basis of pulmonary rehabilitation. J Cardiopulm Rehabil 1990;10:418–441.

5 ACCP-AACVPR Pulmonary Rehabilitation Guidelines Panel: Pulmonary rehabilitation: joint ACCP/AACVPR evidence-based guidelines. Chest 1997; 112:1363–1396.

6 Global Initiative for Chronic Obstructive Lung Disease: Workshop Report: Global Strategy for Diagnosis, Management, and Prevention of COPD – Updated 2008 (http://goldcopd.org).

7 American Thoracic Society-European Respiratory Society Task Force: Standards for the diagnosis and management of patients with COPD (Internet). Version 1.2. (http://www-test.thoracic.org/copd). New York, American Thoracic Society, 2005.

8 Ries AL, Bauldoff GS, Carlin BW, et al: Pulmonary rehabilitation: joint ACCP/AACVPR evidence-based clinical practice guidelines. Chest 2007;131(suppl 5):4S–42S.

9 American Association of Cardiovascular and Pulmonary Rehabilitation: Guidelines for Pulmonary Rehabilitation Programs, ed 3. Champaign/IL, Human Kinetics, 2004.

10 Guyatt G, Gutterman D, Baumann MH, et al: Grading strength of recommendations and quality of evidence in clinical guidelines: report from an American College of Chest Physicians task force. Chest 2006;129:174–181.

Andrew L. Ries, MD, MPH
Professor of Medicine and Family and Preventive Medicine
School of Medicine, University of California, San Diego
9500 Gilman Drive–0602, La Jolla, CA 92093 (USA)
Tel. +1 858 534 4877, Fax +1 858 534 0338
E-Mail aries@ucsd.edu

Esquinas AM (ed): Applied Technologies in Pulmonary Medicine. Basel, Karger, 2011, pp 202–204

Ward Mortality in Patients Discharged from the ICU with Tracheostomy

Rafael Fernandez Fernandez

Hospital Sant Joan de Deu, Fundacio Althaia, Manresa, Spain

Critically ill ventilated patients commonly need tracheostomy as an alternative method for airway management. Whereas some patients need tracheostomy due to anatomical reasons (e.g. upper airway obstruction, ORL surgery) without any choice, in the majority of ICU patients, tracheostomy is an elective method restricted to patients needing long-term mechanical ventilation. Despite the lower invasiveness of the today commonly percutaneous approach, tracheostomy still carries some morbidity. Physicians should therefore balance the expected benefit (greater comfort, lower work of breathing, and better clearance of secretions) against the risks (anesthetics, surgical wound, infection, and hemorrhage).

In this scenario, tracheostomy is very commonly performed in the ICU, ranging from 8 to 35% of ventilated patients depending on the case mix and local practices. Whether tracheostomy has an impact on the patient's outcome remains controversial. Some authors report faster tapering of sedatives with shortening in ICU length of stay, whereas others suggest that such short-term improvements only transfer morbidity and mortality to wards, with null advantages on medium and long-term outcomes.

Main Topics

We recently published our experience in this field [1]. Our hypothesis was that the supposed morbidity of remaining tracheotomized in the ward will differently affect patients depending on their clinical conditions. Accordingly, we review clinical charts of patients admitted in our 16-bed ICU between 2003 and 2006. We excluded patients who received <24 h mechanical ventilation in the postoperative period. Variables recorded on admission included age, sex, diagnosis, APACHE II score, and comorbidities. During the ICU stay, we recorded major procedures and adverse events. At ICU (or step-down unit, when applicable) discharge, the attending physician classified the patient according to the Sabadell score, a subjective tool explained in detail elsewhere [2]. Briefly, it has four levels of expected prognosis: score 0 is for patients with good prognosis, score 1 is for patients with poor prognosis in the medium to long term, score 2 is for patients with poor prognosis in the short term, and score 3 is for patients who are expected to die before discharge from the hospital.

Patients who remained tracheotomized at ICU discharge were placed in dedicated rooms in ordinary wards. The ward team responsible for their care always included dedicated laryngologists and physiotherapists, but was not informed of the Sabadell score. We reviewed the wards' clinical charts to determine the appropriateness of airway care, characteristics of secretions, time to decannulation, technical complications, and cause of death in patients who died.

From 3,065 admissions, 1,502 needed mechanical ventilation for at least 24 h. Only 936 (62%) of these patients survived the ICU and were transferred to the ward; 130 (13.9%) patients had a tracheostomy cannula in place when transferred to the ward. The overall ward mortality was 87/936 (9.3%) and was higher in patients with a tracheostomy cannula in place at ICU discharge than in those without (34/130 (26%) vs. 53/806 (7%), $p < 0.001$). Patients that remained cannulated at discharge were sicker and had more complications (blood transfusion, renal replacement therapy, ICU infection, pneumothorax, acute renal failure, upper gastrointestinal bleeding, and reintubation). A multivariate analysis found three factors associated with ward mortality: age, tracheostomy, and Sabadell score, with a global accuracy of 93.1% for predicting ward mortality. We found that the mortality increase associated with tracheostomy was restricted to patients with intermediate Sabadell scores, whereas minimal or no difference was found between patients with tracheostomy cannulae and those without in the 'good prognosis' and 'expected to die in hospital' groups.

Discussion

Our study offers conclusions that should be carefully framed. First, treatment in the ward in our center was optimal, and our results cannot be extrapolated to any other institution without taking into account this very sensitive aspect. Every hospital should evaluate their outcome for tracheotomized patients in the ward before adopting any new strategy.

Due to the lower rate of death in the ward attributable to airway care problems, we may suggest that the excess in mortality risk should be due to underlying conditions and progressive deterioration. Then, efforts to avoid tracheotomized patients in the ward by extending ICU stay or accelerating decannulation may be futile, or not cost-effective approaches.

The clinical impact of our study will result from a better definition of the population most likely to benefit from outreach team surveillance in the ward or from a prolonged stay in the step-down unit until decannulation, when feasible.

We conclude that lack of tracheostomy decannulation in the ICU appears to be associated with ward mortality, but only in the group with a Sabadell score of 1. Whether discharge without decannulation is a direct risk factor or a marker of sicker patients remains to be elucidated.

Recommendations

- Tracheostomy in the ICU remains common despite recent improvements in weaning techniques and protocols.
- Despite optimal ward treatment, patients with tracheostomy cannula in the ward are at higher risk for death.
- This additional risk is only important in patients with medium and long-term bad prognosis, whereas patients with good prognosis were not affected.
- Whether a longer ICU stay for allowing safer decannulation may improve outcome remains an unanswered question.

References

1 Fernandez R, Bacelar N, Hernandez G, Tubau I, Baigorri F, Gili G, Artigas A: Ward mortality in patients discharged from the ICU with tracheostomy may depend on patient's vulnerability. Intensive Care Med 2008;34:1878–1882.

2 Fernandez R, Baigorri F, Navarro G, Artigas A: A modified McCabe score for stratification of patients after ICU discharge: the Sabadell score. Crit Care 2006;10:R179.

Dr. Rafael Fernandez Fernandez
Hospital Sant Joan de Deu, Fundacio Althaia, Manresa
ES–08243 Manresa (Spain)
Tel. +34 938742112, Fax +34 938736204
E-Mail rfernandezf@althaia.cat

Esquinas AM (ed): Applied Technologies in Pulmonary Medicine. Basel, Karger, 2011, pp 205–209

Exogenous Surfactant in Respiratory Distress Syndrome

Andrea Calkovska[a] · Egbert Herting[b]

[a]Department of Physiology, Jessenius Faculty of Medicine, Comenius University and Martin Faculty Hospital, Martin, Slovakia, and [b]Department of Pediatrics, University of Lübeck, Lübeck, Germany

Abbreviations

ARDS	Acute respiratory distress syndrome
LA	Large surfactant aggregates
RDS	Respiratory distress syndrome
rSP-C	Recombinant SP-C
SA	Small surfactant aggregates
SP	Surfactant protein
SP-A–D	Surfactant proteins A–D

Surfactant replacement therapy is an established part of routine clinical management of neonates with RDS and this treatment may also be effective in other forms of lung diseases including meconium aspiration syndrome, neonatal pneumonia and the 'adult' form of ARDS. In the present chapter we discuss the factors influencing the efficacy of exogenous surfactant therapy in the ARDS.

Pulmonary Surfactant

Pulmonary surfactant is a lipoprotein complex that covers the inner surface of the lungs. It prevents collapse of the alveoli and small airways during expiration by reducing surface tension at the air-liquid interface and allows efficient gas exchange at low transpulmonary pressures. It is synthesized in the type II alveolar epithelial cells and composed of several phospholipids, neutral lipids and surfactant-specific proteins. The largest proportion of phospholipids is phosphatidylcholine, of which dipalmitoylphosphatidylcholine is the major surface-active component. Four native SPs have been identified: hydrophobic SP-B and SP-C are thought to have a role in the surface tension-lowering properties of pulmonary surfactant, and SP-A and SP-D are hydrophilic and play a role in surfactant metabolism and pulmonary host defense [1].

Changes of Pulmonary Surfactant in ARDS

RDS is the most common respiratory disorder of premature babies. Typically, idiopathic RDS affects infants below 35 weeks of gestational age and the key element in the pathophysiology is the structural and functional immaturity of the lung with a primary deficiency of the endogenous surfactant system. In contrast, the 'adult' form of ARDS is characterized by secondary abnormalities of the surfactant system. Several possible mechanisms responsible for surfactant changes in ARDS have been suggested [2]. The most important mechanism in the pathogenesis of ARDS seems to be alveolar flooding by plasma proteins which occurs early in the course of the disease. Plasma proteins such as albumin, fibrinogen and fibrin monomer inhibit surfactant adsorption, prevent the establishment of low alveolar surface tension during surface compression and interfere with the surfactant-related parameters of lung function.

As patients with ARDS exhibit an intense pulmonary inflammatory reaction, a variety of mediators may directly or indirectly interfere with surfactant function. Increased phospholipolytic and proteolytic activities with a consequent decrease in surfactant activity were demonstrated in the alveolar compartment as a result of the inflammatory process.

The change in the ratio between LA and SA is another typical finding. Under physiological conditions, up to 90% of the surfactant material in bronchoalveolar lavage fluid is recovered in the fraction of LA with high surface activity and a relatively high SP-B content. The amount of the functionally inferior SA fraction, which is considered to be a degradation product of surfactant, is increased in bronchoalveolar lavage fluid in patients with ARDS. Alterations in endogenous pulmonary surfactant further include the decrease in total phospholipid content, changes in relative distribution of the phospholipid classes, increased levels and altered neutral lipid profile, decreased levels of surfactant-specific proteins and inactivation of endogenous surfactant by incorporation into hyaline membranes.

Surfactant Replacement Therapy

Taken together, beside neonatal RDS, surfactant replacement therapy can also be helpful in other forms of lung disease, in which endogenous surfactant is inactivated by aspirated material or leakage of plasma proteins into the airspaces. Although the mortality associated with the ARDS in adults has decreased significantly in the past, it is still over 30%. Treatment of these patients is mainly supportive and interventions improving outcome are of great interest. The importance of pulmonary surfactant in maintaining normal lung function and the observation that alterations in the endogenous surfactant system contribute to the pathophysiology of ARDS, provide a rationale for treatment of ARDS patients with exogenous surfactant. The effects of surfactant therapy are however influenced by several factors.

Timing of Surfactant Administration

Both experimental and clinical studies demonstrated the superior physiological and clinical effects of early administration of surfactant ('prophylaxis') in comparison to replacement at later stages of the disease ('rescue'). In contrast to neonatal RDS, in the 'adult' form of ARDS there is no consensus on which patient would benefit most from early surfactant therapy since there is a lack of reliable and sensitive markers of lung injury. Theoretically, administration of surfactant earlier in the course of ARDS may help to modulate pulmonary inflammation before severe lung dysfunction occurs.

Mode of the Surfactant Administration

Commonly, exogenous surfactant is instilled *as a bolus* into the central airways. With this method, large doses of the surface-active material can be given in a relatively short time and a rapid response to the treatment is expected. Disadvantages of this technique include airway obstruction by the liquid bolus and non-uniform distribution. In comparison to the bolus administration, *aerosolization* of exogenous surfactant requires smaller amounts of material and may facilitate a more uniform distribution. However, surfactant will mainly be deposited in ventilated parts of the lungs. On the other hand, the loss of surfactant in the delivery system is high, and the response may need several hours or even days. The promising technique of *lung lavage* may help to remove aspirated material, plasma inhibitors and/or inflammatory mediators from the lungs and at the same time replace inactivated surfactant and stabilize the lungs. Moreover, surfactant applied by lavage technique spreads more homogenously throughout the lungs, and a higher volume of diluted surfactant washes out the airspaces more effectively. Lavage methods of surfactant administration were shown to be effective in some respiratory disorders like meconium aspiration syndrome and may become an alternative in ARDS patients in the future. *Bronchoscopic application* of surfactant with or without lavage in patients with severe ARDS was also recommended as both feasible and safe resulting in an improvement of gas exchange.

Ventilation Patterns

The goal of ventilatory management during the early stages of RDS is to maintain adequate oxygenation and ventilation, while minimizing ventilator-induced lung injury. The mode of ventilation preceding the surfactant administration influences the physiological effects of exogenous surfactant as the surfactant-deficient lungs are very susceptible to epithelial disruption due to e.g. large tidal volumes. In patients with ARDS the ventilation with low tidal volumes and sufficiently high levels of positive end-expiratory pressure after reopening of the collapsed alveoli will both protect the lungs and reduce mortality. Moreover, an appropriate positive end-expiratory pressure is required for optimal function of some synthetic surfactant preparations.

Dosing

The individual dose of the surfactant depends on the disorder being treated, for example on whether the exogenous material is given to compensate for primary surfactant deficiency in premature newborns, or administered to overcome the inhibitory effects of aspirated meconium or plasma proteins leaking into the airspaces in the patients with ARDS [1]. The initial dose, required for clinical response and eventually the need for retreatment, depends on the quality of the surfactant preparation, the severity of the disease and the clearance rate of exogenous surfactant. The initial surfactant dose currently recommended ranges from 50 to 200 mg/kg b.w. In premature babies with RDS this dose should be close to the estimated pool size of alveolar surfactant in a normal full-term newborn, about 100 mg/kg b.w. In adult patients with ARDS the optimal dose is not yet known. However, large quantities of exogenous surfactant are needed to overcome the inhibitory effects of plasma proteins in the airspaces and to optimize surfactant distribution. In individual patients with ARDS, cumulative doses up to 800 mg/kg b.w. have been applied. Based on clinical experience, it seems that more than 2–4 repeated doses of instilled surfactant have no additional benefit.

Type of Surfactant Preparation

The clinical response depends on the quality of the exogenous surfactant preparation. Modified natural surfactants containing the native hydrophobic peptides SP-B and SP-C are more effective than protein-free synthetic surfactants. However, surfactant preparations derived from animal lungs are expensive with a limited supply and they pose a potential danger of viral or prion disease or allergic reactions. Thus, there is a need for synthetic surfactant substitutes, which can be produced in large quantities at (hopefully) reasonable costs [3].

If the alveoli are flooded with protein-rich edema fluid (e.g. in ARDS), the inhibitory effects of plasma proteins can only be counterbalanced by relatively large amounts of surfactant and/or by administration of surfactant preparations resistant to plasma protein inhibition. Therefore, preventing surfactant inactivation is an important new approach that could increase the therapeutic effects of exogenous surfactant in various forms of lung disease. Sensitivity to inactivation varies between different surfactant preparations and is in part related to their protein content. Complete natural surfactant containing all specific proteins is much more resistant to inactivation than the modified natural surfactants isolated from mammalian lungs. The latter contain only lipids and small amounts of the hydrophobic SP-B and SP-C because the hydrophilic SP-A and SP-D are removed by extraction procedures. The resistance of commercially available modified natural surfactants to inactivation by plasma proteins or meconium can be enhanced by enriching the material with SP-A and by addition of polymers such as dextran, polyethylene glycol, hyaluroran, or by polymyxin B.

Current research is focused on the development of a new generation of artificial surfactant substitutes based on synthetic analogues of SP-B and/or SP-C [3]. These SP analogues have been produced by peptide synthesis or recombinant technology to provide a new class of synthetic surfactants that may be a suitable alternative to animal-derived surfactants. Up to this time, two synthetic preparations have been used in clinical trials, rSP-C surfactant (Venticute®) and KL_4 surfactant (Surfaxin®) with the peptide KL_4 designed to mimic the function of SP-B.

Surfactant Metabolism

The effects of therapy also depend on how the exogenous surfactant is metabolized in the treated lungs. The underlying lung injury (uniform vs. non-uniform) which may influence the distribution of exogenous material and the speed of LA to SA conversion belong to the most important factors. If the damage of the alveolar epithelium is not too extensive, an exogenous surfactant may become activated ('recycled') by entering the intra-alveolar metabolism, combining with endogenous surfactant and may be newly secreted into the alveolar space. Thus, the utilization of exogenous surfactant depends on interactions between the material delivered into the lungs and the host alveolar environment.

Perspectives of Surfactant Treatment

Taken together, the treatment of ARDS with exogenous surfactant has a strong rationale, which is firmly founded on experimental data. However, stimulating results obtained in animal experiments were not always reproducible in clinical trials. Firstly, most animal studies have reported on respiratory failure caused by direct injury whereas clinical ARDS is caused more often by indirect injury. Secondly, in animals, surfactant is usually administered in optimal timing whereas in patients this treatment tends to be late. Finally, most of the animal studies are terminated within several hours and thus, they cannot evaluate long-term effects of surfactant therapy in ARDS. Moreover, there are many differences among the various clinical trials. Different types of surfactant and different delivery methods were used that may have resulted in varying concentrations of surfactant reaching the alveoli and altering the effectiveness of therapy. Other differences include different ventilation strategies, the timing of surfactant administration as well as the cause of ARDS (pulmonary vs. extrapulmonary).

In a meta-analysis on surfactant treatment of adults with ARDS published in 2006, the authors identified 251 articles between 1966 and 2005 and five studies met the inclusion criteria [4]. Only studies that were randomized controlled clinical trials, that compared the use of exogenous surfactant to an appropriate control group receiving standard therapy and that evaluated mortality and/or pulmonary physiological parameters were included in the analysis. It was concluded that exogenous surfactant may improve oxygenation but does not reduce mortality, and thus that exogenous pulmonary surfactant cannot currently be considered an effective adjunctive therapy in ARDS patients. The lack of effectiveness of exogenous surfactant is explained firstly by the fact that the patients with ARDS usually die of multiorgan system failure rather than from respiratory failure and thus the treatment of pulmonary disorders may not affect overall mortality. In addition, an optimal regimen for surfactant treatment has not yet been identified [4].

It becomes evident that the success of surfactant replacement therapy in ARDS depends on the appropriate selection of the indication for this treatment. By pooled analysis of five multicenter studies in which patients with ARDS treated with rSP-C surfactant, it was shown that rSP-C surfactant improved oxygenation in patients with ARDS irrespective of the underlying disease. Reduced mortality in association with surfactant treatment was only obtained in patients with direct lung insult such as pneumonia or aspiration [5]. However, a randomized controlled study applying rSP-C surfactant relatively early in the course of ARDS in consequence of pneumonia or aspiration of gastric contents (VALID study) was recently stopped due to lack of effectiveness.

Conclusion

Surfactant replacement therapy is now an established part of routine clinical management of neonatal RDS and the indications are widening to other forms of neonatal diseases (meconium aspiration syndrome, pneumonia). Based on the current knowledge, adults with ARDS are also a possible target group for surfactant replacement. However, large doses of surfactant are necessary to overcome the inhibitory effects of plasma proteins leaking into the airspaces. As a consequence, there is an urgent need to develop a new generation of surfactant preparations that are more resistant to inhibitors and can be produced in large quantities at reasonable costs. At the same time, we need to find out the safe, effective and hopefully non-invasive ways for surfactant administration.

Acknowledgements

This work was supported by the National Scientific Grant Agency (VEGA) (Project No. 1/0061/08), project 'Center of Experimental and Clinical Respirology' co-financed by EC sources and a grant of the German Research Council (DFG He 2072-2/2).

References

The number of references has been limited to five. A complete list is available from the authors on request.

1 Robertson B, Halliday H: Principles of surfactant replacement. Biochim Biophys Acta 1998;1408:346–361.

2 Guenther A, Walmrath D, Grimminger F, et al: Surfactant metabolism and replacement in acute respiratory distress syndrome. Eur Respir Mon 2002;20:119–128.

3 Curstedt T, Johansson J: New synthetic surfactant – how and when? Biol Neonate 2006;89:336–339.

4 Davidson WJ, Dorscheid D, Spragg R, et al: Exogenous pulmonary surfactant for the treatment of adult patients with acute respiratory distress syndrome: results of a meta-analysis. Criti Care 2006;10:R41.

5 Taut FJ, Rippin G, Schenk P, et al: A search for subgroups of patients with ARDS who may benefit from surfactant replacement therapy: a pooled analysis of five studies with recombinant surfactant protein-C surfactant (Venticute®). Chest 2008;134:724–732.

Prof. Andrea Calkovska, MD, PhD
Department of Physiology, Jessenius Faculty of Medicine, Comenius University
Mala Hora 4, SK–037 54 Martin (Slovakia)
Tel./Fax +421 43 4131426
E-Mail calkovska@jfmed.uniba.sk

Esquinas AM (ed): Applied Technologies in Pulmonary Medicine. Basel, Karger, 2011, pp 210–216

Hypercapnia and Hypocapnia in Neonates

Li Tao · Wei Zhou

Department of Neonatology, Guangzhou Children's Hospital, Guangzhou Women and Children's Medical Center, Guangzhou, China

Abbreviations

CBF Cerebral blood flow
IVH Intraventricular hemorrhage
$PaCO_2$ Partial pressure of carbon dioxide
PAH Pulmonary artery hypertension
$PbrO_2$ Brain tissue oxygen tension
PVL Periventricular leukomalacia
VLBW Very low birth weight
VRLI Ventilator-related lung injury

Arterial $PaCO_2$ reflects the balance between CO_2 production and consumption. $PaCO_2$ ranges from 4.7 to 6.0 kPa (35–45 mm Hg) in normal neonates [1]. In newborn infants, hypercapnia caused by elevation of $PaCO_2$ can have an adverse effect on the internal environment and function; hypocapnia (also known as hypocarbia) can increase the incidence of brain injury. In recent years, researchers have focused on the permissive hypercapnia ventilation strategy in neonates with respiratory disease and brain injury. In this article, we review the latest progress in neonatal hypocapnia, hypercapnia and permissive hypercapnia strategy, and discuss their clinical implications.

Influence of Hypocapnia on the Central Nervous System

In the last century it was reported that hypocapnia induced by hyperventilation did not deflate the infarcted area after middle cerebral artery occlusion or increase CBF of the ischemic region, but increased the size of the ischemic area. Subsequent trials demonstrated that hypocapnia could aggravate the decrease in energy-rich phosphate, impair ischemic brain metabolism, and worsen cerebral ischemia [2]. The decrease in CBF reduces oxygen transport, raises nervous excitation, and limits cerebral metabolism, which further limits oxygen transport. The results of Ohyu et al. [3] suggested that hypocapnia under hypotension might cause neuronal cell death in the hippocampus of the neonatal rabbit. Not only ischemia but also metabolic changes induced by hypocapnia might contribute to this apoptotic neuronal cell damage. Alkali poisoning of cerebrospinal fluid is the main adverse effect of hypocapnia on the nervous system. As an important component of the HCO_3^-/H_2CO_3 buffer system of extracellular fluid, CO_2 changes initially alter pH and initiate cerebral vessel contraction and reduce CBF through NO, prostanoid, potassium channels, and intracellular Ca^{2+}. It has been reported [4] that during end-tidal CO_2 changes, $PbrO_2$ is linearly correlated with intracranial blood flow, and $PbrO_2$ is correlated with end-tidal CO_2 ($PbrO_2$ >60 or <20 mm Hg). In addition, it was found that cerebral hypoxic events can be reduced significantly by increasing cerebral perfusion pressure as required [5].

Hypocapnia is a potential risk factor for PVL, cerebral palsy, cognition developmental disorders, and auditory deficits [6, 7]. The studies of Erickson et al. [8] show that the risk of severe IVH/PVL was significantly increased when $PaCO_2$ was <30 mm Hg within 48 h after birth. There was also an association between duration of hypocapnia and the risk of severe IVH/PVL. Fujimoto et al. [9] retrospectively visited 167 survivors of VLBW newborns <35 weeks' gestational age. The results showed that the cystic PVL incidence in infants with and without hypocapnia was 23 and 5%, respectively. Seven years later, Okumura's research gained similar results as Fujimoto et al. [10]. Hypocapnia within the first 2 h after birth increased the risk of brain damage in severely asphyxiated newborns [11]. In an observational cohort study [12] performed in full-term asphyxia neonates with hypoxic ischemic encephalopathy born from 1985 to 1995, mortality and incidence of severe cerebral palsy, blindness, deafness and hypoevolutism were found to be significantly increased in infants with severe hypocapnia. In addition, 34 newborns with severe persistent pulmonary hypertension were treated by hyperventilation or maintenance of $PaCO_2$ >50 mm Hg [13]. The results in a group that received hyperventilation showed that physical development delay and severe neurologic abnormalities were highly correlated with the duration of hyperventilation, especially the incidence of sensorineural hearing loss was the highest. However, none had sensorineural hearing loss in the group treated with maintenance of $PaCO_2$ >50 mm Hg. These data indicated that sensorineural hearing loss is associated with hypocapnia ($PaCO_2$ <25 mm Hg). Collins et al. [14] conducted a prospective cohort study and enrolled 1,105 newborns with a birth weight of 500–2,000 g. 657 two-year-old survivors had both neurodevelopmental assessments and blood-gas data taken the first week after birth. Disabling cerebral palsy was subsequently diagnosed in 2.3% of the 257 unventilated newborns, 9.4% of the 320 ventilated newborns without exposure to unusual levels of hypocapnia, and 27.5% of the 80 ventilated infants with exposure to significant hypocapnia. The researchers recommend that neonatologists avoid arterial PCO_2 levels <35 mm Hg and arterial PO_2 levels >60 mm Hg whenever possible in ventilated LBW infants. There is extensive, albeit retrospective, evidence that hypocapnia in premature infants is associated with poor neurodevelopmental outcome, such as PVL, IVH, and cerebral palsy [14–16], possibly due to cerebral vasoconstriction, decreased CBF and cerebral oxygen delivery. Therefore, prevention of hypocapnia must also be a primary objective in the management of these infants.

Effect of Hypocapnia on the Respiratory System

Neonatal respiratory failure was associated with PAH, right-left shunt, and severe hypoxemia. After hyperventilation to maintain $PaCO_2$ levels at 25–30 mm Hg, the pulmonary arterial pressure of PAH newborns was significantly decreased, and the right-left shunt was reversed, indicating that hyperventilation could lessen PAH and improve circulation oxygenation. Based on the above theory, a hypocapnia strategy is recommended to treat neonatal persistent PAH and congenital diaphragmatic hernia. However, another experimental study suggests that hypocapnia can deteriorate bronchial spasm, airway pressure, microvascular permeability and lung compliance, worsening the acute lung injury following ischemia-reperfusion. Moreover, the degree of lung injury was proportional to the degree of hypocapnic alkalosis [17].

Hypercapnia

The influence of hypercapnia on neonates depends on the degree and speed of $PaCO_2$ elevation, hypoxia or ischemia condition, and intracranial disease or other complications. Generally, the body has good compensation for and tolerance of acute hypercapnia or slowly elevated $PaCO_2$. Many studies have suggested that acute hypercapnia with $PaCO_2$ <10.67 kPa (80 mm Hg) and pH >7.15 can hardly damage the body; when saturation of blood oxygen is normal, $PaCO_2$ slowly elevates to 10.0–14.67 kPa (75–110 mm Hg) and does not cause any noticeable clinical symptoms [2], and even has some benefits, such as increased gangliated nerve excitation, more catecholamine and improved circulation from vasodilation induced by hypercapnia. Mild intracellular acidosis can even protect hypoxic cells [18]. However, $PaCO_2$ >110 mm Hg can lead to organ dysfunction. Hypoxia/ischemia and hypercapnia have an additive effect on body injury. Neonate and preterm cerebral vessels are more sensitive to $PaCO_2$ elevation (vessel expanding) than to $PaCO_2$ decrease (vessel contraction). Rapidly increased $PaCO_2$ to 12.0–14.67 kPa (90–110 mm Hg) can induce central nervous palsy (consciousness alterations, cataphora) and hyperspasmia [19], worsen blood-brain barrier permeability, cerebral interstitial edema, CBF and CBF's autoregulation, and finally cause intracranial hypertension and even intracraninal hemorrhage. If complicated with ischemia, intracellular acidosis from hypercapnia can stimulate cell metabolism and oxygen free radical production, and worsen brain damage, especially in reperfusion injury [18, 20]. Hypercapnia alters neuronal energy metabolism, increases phosphorylation of transcription factors, and increases the expression of apoptotic proteins in the cerebral cortex of newborn piglets; therefore, it may be deleterious to the newborn brain [21]. Hypercapnia in VLBW infants during the first 3 postnatal days is associated with severe IVH [22]. In addition, a retrospective search analyzed blood gas data in the first 4 postnatal days for 849 infants weighing from 401 to 1,250 g and suggested that both extremes of arterial $PaCO_2$ and the magnitude of fluctuations in arterial $PaCO_2$ are associated with severe IVH in preterm infants, so it may be prudent to avoid extreme hypocapnia and hypercapnia during the risk period of IVH [23]. Severe hypercapnia can inhibit the myocardial contractile force, expand vessels leading to blood pressure decrease, and stimulate gangliated nerve excitation, resulting in arrhythmia. Hypercapnia complicates hypoxia and can induce pulmonary vasoconstriction and increase pulmonary circulation resistance, leading to PAH, cardiac ejection fraction reduction, and worsening of cerebral functional lesions [24, 25]. Acute hypercapnia can reduce skeletal muscle contraction, especially diaphragmatic muscle contraction, and exhaust respiratory muscles. By contrast, chronic hypercapnia contributes to an increase in adrenal medulla secretion, adrenocorticotrophic hormone, aldosterone and antidiuretic hormone production.

Permissive Hypercapnia

Traditional ventilation strategies cause adverse effects on newborn infants, such as barotraumas, lung interstitial emphysema, and systemic gas embolism. In our current understanding of the pathology and physiology of the respiratory system, permissive hypercapnia is used in clinic as a novel ventilatory strategy. The term permissive hypercapnia defines a ventilatory strategy for acute respiratory failure, in which the lungs are ventilated with a low inspiratory volume and pressure [26]. The aim of permissive hypercapnia is to minimize lung damage during mechanical ventilation. The small tidal volume ventilation reduces peak inspiratory pressure and mean airway pressure, and minimizes the incidence of air leaks and the effect of mechanical ventilation on returned blood volume and cardiac output.

Permissive Hypercapnia and Disease of the Respiratory System

It was reported by Dariol and Perret [27] in 1984 that controlled mechanical ventilation was performed to maintain $PaCO_2$ at 90 mm Hg to treat severe acute asthma and the effect was favorable. Subsequent studies also suggest that, in the treatment of some respiratory tract diseases, such as acute respiratory distress syndrome, CO_2 elevation to a certain extent can decrease complications and improve survival rate. Some researchers treated newborns with persistent pulmonary hypertension or congenital diaphragmatic hernia by elevating $PaCO_2$ to 60 mm Hg, and found that the newborns were tolerant of the treatment, with no adverse effects [28]. Recent studies have demonstrated that CO_2 elevation can to a certain extent protect lung from ischemia/reperfusion injury [28]. Trials of animals with acute lung injury showed that the lung interstitial edema and cardiac load in the hypercapnic group were significantly relieved compared with a high ventilation group, indicating that hypercapnia could improve acute pulmonary hemorrhage [29]. By the observation of lung mechanical, blood gas and pathological changes, it found that hypercapnia improved the lung mechanics index and dynamic compliance, decreased PIP level and protein content in bronchoalveolar lavage fluid which reflex lung permeability [30]. All of the above-mentioned results suggest that permissive hypercapnia is of help in respiratory disease.

Traditional mechanical ventilation often causes VRLI which prolongs the disease course and is necessary for oxygen. The VRLI's incidence is 13–35% in VLBW and ultra low birth weight infants. Permissive hypercapnia may reduce VRLI and bronchopulmonary dysplasia [31]. However, a meta-analysis from two trials involving 269 newborns shows permissive hypercapnia cannot contribute to reduce the incidence of death or chronic lung disease at 36 weeks, IVH grade 3 or 4, or PVL [32]. At present, the best ventilation strategy and the precision impact of permissive hypercapnia on this strategy is not very clear, however it is important to understand hypercapnia's mechanism which is helpful for determining the safety and therapeutic utility of hypercapnia in protective lung ventilatory strategies [25]. An animal experiment found that the pH and heart rate of neonatal rabbits decreased and mean blood pressure increased progressively as CO_2 was increased [33]. When $PaCO_2$ was increased from 20 to 80 mm Hg, vessel diameter, blood flow velocity, and blood flow rate increased markedly. Cardiac output increased slightly. When CO_2 exceeded 100 mm Hg, all of these variables decreased. When $PaCO_2$ exceeded 150 mm Hg, all variables were significantly lower than the control values. Intravital microscopic visualization of rabbit ear microcirculation showed that 150 mm Hg is the permissive upper limit of acute hypercapnia with respect to maintenance of the peripheral microcirculation.

Permissive Hypercapnia and Central Nervous System Disease

Permissive hypercapnia can protect against ventilation-induced brain injury. Hypoxemia associated with acute hypercapnia ($PaCO_2$ 68 mm Hg) can reduce 30% of cerebral oxygen consumption, and induce synthesis of neuronal nitric oxide synthase-derived nitric oxide which increases the CBF and vasodilation response [34]. At moderate hypercapnia, CBF increases 6% as soon as $PaCO_2$ increases 1 mm Hg [35], and such a response quickly reached a peak within 5–15 min. Monitoring the mean CBF velocity, $PaCO_2$, and mean arterial blood pressure of 43 ventilated VLBW infants during the postnatal first week showed that when $PaCO_2$ was >45 mm Hg, mean CBF velocity increased with increasing $PaCO_2$, suggesting that the progressive loss of cerebral autoregulation and impaired autoregulation during this period may be associated with increased vulnerability to brain injury [20]. Collins et al. [36] carried out a large-scale follow-up survey of 1,105 newborns who weighed 500–2,000 g. 777 of 902 cases received mechanical ventilation with assessment of neurological function for 2 years. The results show the incidence of cerebral palsy was 9.4% in cases treated with a permissive hypercapnia strategy and 27.5% in those treated with traditional ventilation characterized by hypocapnia. These results indicate that permissive hypercapnia in the neonatal period played a protective role in the treatment of brain injury. By targeting mild to moderate hypercapnia during ventilation of premature infants, it has been suggested that permissive hypercapnia may be neuroprotective by avoidance of accidental hypocapnia [37], and it should be noted that the pursuit of permissive hypercapnia should not be at the expense of decreased lung expansion, i.e. an adequate PEEP is essential. Recently, Hagen et al. [38] studied the effect of permissive hypercapnia on brain injury and developmental impairment. There were two groups: permissive hypercapnia in which PCO_2 values fluctuated from 45 to 55 mm Hg, and normocapnia in which PCO_2 values fluctuated from 35 to 45 mm Hg. The analysis shows that Infants who received a permissive hypercapnia strategy were not more likely to have IVH than those with normocapnia. There were no differences in any of the behavioral or functional scores among children according to the respiratory strategy. There was a significant interaction between care strategy and the 1-min Apgar score, indicating that infants with lower Apgar scores may be at higher risk for IVH with permissive hypercapnia. On the other hand, inadvertent hypercapnia may result from this method, and hypercapnia has been associated with IVH [39–41]. In fact, in the initial pilot trial of permissive hypercapnia in premature infants, many infants in the hypercapnic group had maximum $PaCO_2$ >55 mm Hg, perhaps out of the traditional 'safe' range of hypercapnia [42, 43].

Conclusion

Permissive hypercapnia as a novel protective ventilation therapy may to a certain extent improve the survival rate of neonates with brain injury or respiratory tract diseases. However, a large-sample study needs to be conducted to assess its clinical application. During permissive hypercapnia treatment, how to select the appropriate ventilatory index, whether or not permissive hypercapnia can worsen cerebral edema, and the potential risk of intracranial hypertension, still need further exploration and study.

References

1 Brouillette RT, Waxman DH: Evaluation of the newborn's blood gas status. Clin Chem 1997;43:215–221.

2 Laffey JG, Kavanagh BP: Hypocapnia. N Engl J Med 2002;347:43–53.

3 Ohyu J, Endo A, Itoh M, Takashima S: Hypocapnia under hypotension induces apoptotic neuronal cell death in the hippocampus of newborn rabbits. Pediatr Res 2000;48:24–29.

4 Hemphill JC 3rd, Bleck T, Carhuapoma JR, et al: Is neurointensive care really optional for comprehensive stroke care? Stroke 2005;36:2344–2345.

5 Meixensberger J, Jaeger M, Väth A, et al: Brain tissue oxygen-guided treatment supplementing ICP/CPP therapy after traumatic brain injury. J Neurol Neurosurg Psychiatry 2003;74:760–764.

6 Murase M, Ishida A: Early hypocarbia of preterm infants: its relationship to periventricular leukomalacia and cerebral palsy, and its perinatal risk factors. Acta Paediatr 2005;94:85–91.
7 Ambalavanan N, Carlo WA: Hypocapnia and hypercapnia in respiratory management of newborn infants. Clin Perinatol 2001;28:517–531.
8 Erickson SJ, Grauaug A, Gurrin L, et al: Hypocarbia in the ventilated preterm infant and its effect on intraventricular haemorrhage and bronchopulmonary dysplasia. J Paediatr Child Health 2002; 38:560–562.
9 Fujimoto S, Togari H, Yamaguchi N, et al: Hypocarbia and cystic periventricular leukomalacia in preterm infants. Arch Dis Child 1994;71:F107–F110.
10 Okumura A, Hayakawa F, Kato T, et al: Hypocarbia in preterm infants with periventricular leukomalacia: the relation between hypocarbia and mechanical ventilation. Pediatrics 2001;107: 469–475.
11 Klinger G, Beyene J, Shah P, Perlman M: Do hyperoxaemia and hypocapnia add to the risk of brain injury after intrapartum asphyxia? Arch Dis Child Fetal Neonatal Ed 2005;90:F49–F52.
12 Foix-L'helias L, Baud O, Lenclen R, Kaminski M, Lacaze-Masmonteil T: Benefit of antenatal glucocorticoids according to the cause of very premature birth. Arch Dis Child Fetal Neonatal Ed 2005;90:F46–F48.
13 Marron MJ, Crisafi MA, Driscoll JM Jr, Wung JT, Driscoll YT, Fay TH, et al: Hearing and neurodevelopmental outcome in survivors of persistent pulmonary hypertension of the newborn. Pediatrics 1992;90:392–396.
14 Collins MP, Lorenz JM, Jetton JR, Paneth N: Hypocapnia and other ventilation-related risk factors for cerebral palsy in low birth weight infants. Pediatr Res 2001;50:712–719.
15 Greisen G, Munck H, Lou H: Severe hypocarbia in preterm infants and neurodevelopmental deficit. Acta Paediatr Scand 1987;76:401–404.
16 Okumura A, Hayakawa F, Kato T, Itomi K, Maruyama K, Ishihara N, et al: Hypocarbia in preterm infants with periventricular leukomalacia: the relation between hypocarbia and mechanical ventilation. Pediatrics 2001;107: 469–475.
17 Laffey JG, Engelberts D, Kavanagh BP: Injurious effects of hypocapnic alkalosis in the isolated lung. Am J Respir Crit Care Med 2000;162:399–405.
18 Fritz KI, Delivoria-Papadopoulos M: Mechanisms of injury to the newborn brain. Clin Perinatol 2006;33:573–591.
19 Wang X-L: Neonatal respiratory failure; in Zhou X-G, Xiao X, Nong S-H (eds): Therapeutics of Mechanical Ventilation in Neonates (in Chinese). Beijing, People's Medical Publishing House, 2004, pp 75–89.
20 Kaiser JR, Gauss CH, Williams DK: The effects of hypercapnia on cerebral autoregulation in ventilated very low birth weight infants. Pediatr Res 2005;58:931–935
21 Fritz KI, Zubrow A, Mishra OP, Delivoria-Papadopoulos M: Hypercapnia-induced modifications of neuronal function in the cerebral cortex of newborn piglets. Pediatr Res 2005;57:299–304.
22 Kaiser JR, Gauss CH, Pont MM, Williams DK: Hypercapnia during the first 3 days of life is associated with severe intraventricular hemorrhage in very low birth weight infants. J Perinatol 2006;26: 279–285.
23 Fabres J, Carlo WA, Phillips V, Howard G, Ambalavanan N: Both extremes of arterial carbon dioxide pressure and the magnitude of fluctuations in arterial carbon dioxide pressure are associated with severe intraventricular hemorrhage in preterm infants. Pediatrics 2007;119: 299–305.
24 Ni Chonghaile M, Higgins B, Laffey JG: Permissive hypercapnia: role in protective lung ventilatory strategies. Curr Opin Crit Care 2005;11:56–62.
25 Dorrington KL, Talbot NP: Human pulmonary vascular responses to hypoxia and hypercapnia. Pflugers Arch 2004; 449:1–15.
26 Bigatello LM, Patroniti N, Sangalli F: Permissive hypercapnia. Curr Opin Crit Care 2001;7:34–40.
27 Darioli R, Perret C: Mechanical controlled hypoventilation in status asthmaticus. Am Rev Respir Dis 1984;129: 385–387.
28 Feihl F, Eckert P, Brimioulle S, Jacobs O, Schaller MD, Mélot C, et al: Permissive hypercapnia impairs pulmonary gas exchange in the acute respiratory distress syndrome. Am J Respir Crit Care Med 2000;162:209–215.
29 Laffey JG, Tanaka M, Engelberts D, Luo X, Yuan S, Tanswell AK, et al: Therapeutic hypercapnia reduces pulmonary and systemic injury following in vivo lung reperfusion. Am J Respir Crit Care Med 2000;162:2287–2294.
30 Yang LL, Ji XP, Liu Z: Effects of hypercapnia on nuclear factor-κB and tumor necrosis factor-α in acute lung injury models. Chin Med J (Engl) 2004;117: 1859–1861.
31 Ambalavanan N, Carlo WA: Ventilatory strategies in the prevention and management of bronchopulmonary dysplasia. Semin Perinatol 2006;30:192–199.
32 Woodgate PG, Davies MW: Permissive hypercapnia for the prevention of morbidity and mortality in mechanically ventilated newborn. Cochrane Database Syst Rev 2001;CD002061.
33 Komori M, Takada K, Tomizawa Y, et al: Permissive range of hypercapnia for improved peripheral microcirculation and cardiac output in rabbits. Crit Care Med 2007;35:2171–2175.
34 Okamoto H, Hudetz AG, Roman RJ, Bosnjak ZJ, Kampine JP: Neuronal NOS-derived NO plays permissive role in cerebral blood flow response to hypercapnia. Am J Physiol 1997;272: H559–H566.
35 Ito H, Kanno I, Ibaraki M, Hatazawa J, Miura S: Changes in human cerebral blood flow and cerebral blood volume during hypercapnia and hypocapnia measured by positron emission tomography. J Cereb Blood Flow Metab 2003; 23:665–670.
36 Collins MP, Lorenz JM, Jetton JR, et al: Hypocapnia and other ventilation-related risk factors for cerebral palsy in low birth weight infants. Pediatr Res 2001;50:712–719.
37 Thome UH, Carlo WA: Permissive hypercapnia. Semin Neonatol 2002;17: 409–419.
38 Hagen EW, Sadek-Badawi M, Carlton D, et al: Permissive hypercapnia and risk for brain injury and developmental impairment. Pediatrics 2008;122: e583–e589.
39 Levene MI, Fawer CL, Lamont RF: Risk factors in the development of intraventricular haemorrhage in the preterm neonate. Arch Dis Child 1982;57:410–417.

40 Van de Bor M, van Bel F, Lineman R, Ruys JH: Perinatal factors and periventricular-intraventricular hemorrhage in preterm infants. Am J Dis Child 1986;140:1125–1130.
41 Wallin LA, Rosenfeld CR, Laptook AR, Maravilla AM, Strand C, Campbell N, et al: Neonatal intracranial hemorrhage. II. Risk factor analysis in an inborn population. Early Hum Dev 1990;23:129–137.
42 Ambalavanan N, Carlo WA: Hypocapnia and hypercapnia in respiratory management of newborn infants. Clin Perinatol 2001;28:517–531.
43 Mariani G, Cifuentes J, Carlo WA: Randomized trial of permissive hypercapnia in preterm infants. Pediatrics 1999;104:1082–1088.

Prof. Wei Zhou, MD, PhD
Department of Neonatology, Guangzhou Children's Hospital
Guangzhou Women and Children's Medical Center
Guangzhou 510120 (China)
Tel. +86 20 81330578, Fax +86 20 81861650, E-Mail zhouwei_pu002@126.com

Esquinas AM (ed): Applied Technologies in Pulmonary Medicine. Basel, Karger, 2011, pp 217–222

Air Pollution and Health

Regiani Carvalho-Oliveira[a] · Naomi Kondo Nakagawa[a,b] · Paulo Hilário Nascimento Saldiva[a]

[a]Department of Pathology, Laboratory of Experimental Air Pollution, Laboratory of Medical Investigation 05, and [b]Department of Physiotherapy, Communication Science and Disorders and Occupational Therapy, Laboratory of Medical Investigation 34, Faculdade de Medicina da Universidade de São Paulo, Brazil

Abbreviations

CO	Carbon monoxide
COPD	Chronic obstructive pulmonary disease
NO_2	Nitrogen dioxide
NOx	Nitrogen oxide
O_3	Ozone
PM	Particulate matter
SO_2	Sulfur dioxide
UFP	Ultrafine particles
VOCs	Volatile organic compounds

There is strong evidence that ambient air pollution exposure causes adverse health effects. Long- and short-term air pollution exposure have been related to noxious effects on the pulmonary and cardiovascular system in children, elderly, pregnant women and baby birth outcomes, as well as in patients with chronic respiratory diseases such as asthma and COPD. In recent decades, many efforts to understand and to reduce the effects of air pollutants on human health have been employed. Around the world, environmental agencies have developed and set up air pollution indicator standards and criteria which have been widely used to characterize air quality. Table 1 summarizes the health effects of the main air pollutants and points out the populations at greatest risk in the USA [1]. However, the determination of air quality standards for health-balancing risks varies according to several factors, such as technical feasibility, social, political and economical factors (according to the World Health Organization), which in turn depend, among others, on the level of national development and capacity to manage air quality. This heterogeneity and the local characteristics should therefore be carefully considered before adopting a range of pollutant levels as national standards for air quality. Table 2 summarizes typical ranges of major pollutant concentrations found in a selection of regions around the world [2].

Assessment of human health risks due to exposure to air pollution requires the characterization of pollutants, sources and emissions in a specific area (named air quality background). By determination of the concentration of a specific pollutant in the atmosphere, the level of exposure of receptors (humans, other animals, plants and equipment) is indicated as the final process of emission of this specific pollutant in the atmosphere, considering the sources and atmospheric interactions. Conceptually, in this case, the receiver or human exposure occurs along the 'environmental pathway' between the concentration

Table 1. Health effects of air pollutants and populations at great risk

Pollutants	Main source	Groups at risk	Clinical consequences	Comments
CO	Incomplete combustion of carbon-containing fuels	Healthy adults children Patients with ischemic heart disease	Decreased exercise capacity Decreased exercise capacity Angina pectoris (Premature mortality)	Effects increased with anemia or chronic lung disease
NO_2	Fuel and coal combustion Atmospheric chemistry	Healthy adults	Increased airway reactivity	Effects occur at levels found indoors with unvented sources of combustion
SO_2	Combustion of fuels containing sulfur (coal and diesel)	Healthy adults and COPD patients	Increased respiratory symptoms	Highly soluble gas with little penetration to distal airways
O_3	Atmospheric chemistry (from primary NO_x and VOCs)	Healthy adults and children Athletes, outdoor workers Asthmatics (and others with respiratory illnesses)	Decreased lung function Increased airway reactivity Lung inflammation Increased respiratory symptoms Decreased exercise capacity Increased hospitalizations	Effects found at or below current NAAQS; effects increased with exercise Effects seen in combination with acid aerosols
PM_{10}	Fuel and coal combustion Road Traffic Atmospheric chemistry; Soil resuspension	Children Patients with chronic lung/heart disease Asthmatic	Increased respiratory symptoms Increased respiratory illness Decreased lung function Premature mortality Increased asthma exacerbations	Effects seen alone or in combination with SO_2

NAAQS = National ambient air quality standards. The items in parentheses are associations that have been shown in some studies; additional confirmation is suggested.

and dose of pollutants. Air pollution consists of a highly variable and complex mixture of different substances, which may occur in the gas, liquid or solid phase. In the troposphere, several hundred different components have been found and many of them are potentially harmful to human health and to the environment. Air pollution components are generated by human and natural activities (primary air pollutants) and by chemical reactions in the atmosphere (secondary air pollutants). The main source of primary air pollutants is from factory chimneys, vehicle exhaust pipes, suspension of the crust by the action of wind and vehicular traffic, volcanic activity and sea evaporation. Secondary air pollutants are produced by chemical reactions between primary pollutants and natural elements of the composition of the atmosphere. Weather conditions directly affect air pollutant production and concentration. Air quality deteriorates when weather

Table 2. Ranges of annual concentrations of NO_2, SO_2, O_3, PM_{10}, and CO in some regions, standard maximum annual and 24-hour averages

Pollutants	Annual average concentration						Standard average time	
	Africa	Asia	Australia/ New Zeland	Canada / United States	Europe	South America	Annual (Arithmetic mean)	24-hour
NO_2	35–65	20–75	11–28	35–70	18–57	30–82	100 $\mu g{\cdot}m^{-3}$	
SO_2	10–100	6–65	3–17	9–35	8–36	40–70	0.03 ppm	0.14 ppm
O_3	120–300	100–250	120–310	150–180	150–350	200–600	0.12 ppm*	
PM_{10}	40–150	35–220	28–127	20–60	20–70	30–120	150 $\mu g{\cdot}m^{-3}$	50 $\mu g{\cdot}m^{-3}$
CO	–	–	–	–	–	–	10 $\mu g{\cdot}m^{-3}$**	35 $\mu g{\cdot}m^{-3}$*

* One-hour average time.
** Eight-hour average time.

conditions are most unfavorable to pollutant dispersion, which can be observed during the winter periods, that significantly increases CO, PM and SO_2 concentrations in the atmosphere. During spring and summer periods, concentrations of O_3 are increased because the chemical reaction that forms O_3 in the atmosphere depends on the intensity of sunlight. The association of weather conditions and concentration of pollutants allows the development of dispersion models.

For a better understanding of the dynamics of pollutants dispersed in the atmosphere, the geographical location and distribution of sources should be taken into account [2, 3]:

(a) *Local scale:* By source or by having a very short atmospheric lifetime (typically of the order of an hour during daytime), some pollutants such as UFP and volatile pollutants are encountered in elevated concentrations only in areas close to the emission source.

(b) *Urban scale:* Higher concentrations of pollutants from urban sources, such as NOx and CO generated by road traffic, tend to be detected throughout the city. The atmospheric lifetime of these pollutants typically lasts hours (low removal from the atmosphere). CO persists longer and its removal is more difficult.

(c) *Regional scale:* Some gas-phase pollutants and fine particles (<2.5 μm diameter, but not UFP) have atmospheric lifetimes of days or even weeks, which facilitates their spread on a regional scale. For example, O_3, sulfate particles, and black carbon particles (from fossil fuels and biomass burnings) readily travel thousands of kilometers crossing national boundaries in a process known as long-range transport.

(d) *Hemispheric and global scale:* Some pollutants, especially those associated with greenhouse-warming effects (CO_2, nitrous oxide and methane) have atmospheric lifetimes of years and are capable of distribution throughout a hemisphere and ultimately the world. One example of the hemispherical transport of pollutants is the O_3. Because the atmospheric lifetime of O_3 is 1–2 weeks in summer and 1–2 months in winter, O_3 produced in a polluted region of one continent can be transported to another continent all year long [4]. The pollutant concentrations are often marginally higher in locations close to the sources, unless the sources emit very large quantities [1].

The main classical indicators of air pollution in epidemiological studies are PM, measured as particles (an aerodynamic diameter <10 μm, PM_{10}), NO_2, SO_2 and O_3. However, this selection does not imply that other air pollutants do not have significant effects on human health and the adverse effects on the environment. For example, VOCs and polycyclic aromatic hydrocarbons are reported to have deleterious effects on human health. Based on the Assessment System for Population Exposure Nationwide (ASPEN) model, the US Environmental Protect Agency (EPA) [5] showed that almost 50% of the total estimated pollutant-induced cancer cases could be attributed to VOCs, with another 40% of the total estimate to polycyclic aromatic hydrocarbons. The characteristics of pollutants (sources, distribution in the atmosphere) and the effects on human health are briefly discussed below:

(a) PM varies in number, size, shape, surface area, chemical composition, solubility, and origin (dust, fumes and all sorts of solid and liquid materials that remain suspended in the atmosphere). Total suspended particles in the ambient air have trimodal size distribution, including coarse particles, fine particles, and UFP. They also show PM with a diameter of ≤2.5 μm ($PM_{2.5}$), PM_{10}, and UFP fractions, which are typically those measured within the atmosphere for the purposes of epidemiological health effect studies; the first two fractions are also used for compliance monitoring. The main sources of PM emission to the atmosphere are automotive vehicles, industrial processes, biomass burning, and resuspension of dust from the ground, among others. Depending on the compounds and processes involved during its formation, the emission can be classified either as primary or secondary main source with complex composition which may include sulfates, nitrates, and, particularly, polar oxidized organics. The mechanisms by which particles influence human health are only poorly understood. The risk assessment of coarse particles (i.e. the size fraction between 2.5 and 10 μm) is not completely understood. However, it is widely accepted that PM is like a mix container of toxicologically relevant components and others. Thus, local characteristics may influence the toxicological effect of PM, and results from studies carried out in one region may not necessarily be applied somewhere else. The Health Effects Institute has performed an analysis of the quality of past epidemiological studies. Factors such as population socioeconomic status and the slope of the pollutant dose-response relationships from time-series studies needed adjustment due to some problems with statistical analysis programs. Nevertheless, the whole body of knowledge supports that PM plays an important role in pollution-related air disturbances in human health [2, 6, 7].

(b) Gas air pollutants are gases or vapors that are not condensed and discharged into the atmosphere. Gaseous air pollutants are readily taken into the human respiratory system, although if water-soluble they may very quickly be deposited in the upper respiratory tract and not penetrate deeply into the lungs. Currently the most important gaseous pollutants are those from burning fossil fuels such as O_3, SO_2, NOx and VOCs. Both NO_2 and VOCs are the precursors of O_3 in the troposphere. The history of air pollution is directly linked to SO_2 emissions. The first scientific manuscripts reporting air pollution-related problems correlated with episodes of high concentrations of SO_2 and PM. From them, the severe episode of air pollution that occurred at London in 1952, dubbed 'London smog' is one of the most known. Nowadays in developed countries, much of the sulfur element is removed from motor fuels in the refining process and from stack gases prior to emission. However, in developing countries, unabated burning of coal and the use of fuel oils and automotive diesel with higher sulfur content are the major sources of SO_2, which is undoubtedly the main source of SO_2 atmospheric emission and contains expressive amounts of sulfur (typically between 1 and 5%). Another major mechanism of SO_2 production and emission is the sintering process used in metal smelting, which involves roasting metal sulfide [2, 6]. NOx is produced by fuel combustion processes and by chemical atmospheric reactions. From the fuel combustion process, the use of coal is the major nitrogen product source compared with oil or gas combustions (at the same temperature). However, during the high-temperature combustion process, oil and gases produce a great amount of NOx in the atmosphere by the combination of nitrogen and atmospheric oxygen released. For this reason, road traffic and generation of electricity are huge sources of NOx emission nowadays. In NOx products, NO_2 is the most important pollutant that adversely affects human health. Typically, 5% of the total NO_2 is emitted directly into the atmosphere by the combustion process. The majority of NO_2 is a secondary product of an atmospheric chemical reaction (the oxidation of nitrogen monoxide, NO, after dilution in air). The conversion of NO into NO_2 occurs as part of the organic compound oxidation, initiated by reactive species (OH radical). Once this conversion occurs, there are a variety of other chemical reaction pathways that may follow [2, 6]. O_3 is the most important photochemical oxidant in the troposphere, and its production is mostly due to human-related activities (fuel combustion vehicle-related). O_3 is formed by photochemical reactions in the presence of sunlight and other pollutants, such as NOx and VOCs. The complex chemical reaction involving VOCs and NO_x (where NOx = NO + NO_2) leads to the formation of not only O_3, but a variety of additional oxidative species. There is evidence from controlled human and animal exposure studies of the potential for O_3 to cause adverse health effects. In short-term studies that evaluated pulmonary function, lung inflammation and permeability, respiratory symptoms, quantity of medication, morbidity and mortality, O_3 does appear to have an independent effect (especially in the summer periods). However, the role of each independent factor has not been fully determined [2, 6]. The World Health Organization recommends in its air quality guidelines a daily maximum 8-hour mean amount of 100 $\mu g \bullet m^3$ of O_3. However, some health effects may occur below this level. In addition to the health effects, O_3 damages ecosystems, agricultural crops and materials.

Air pollutants can be measured by several instruments that may vary greatly in complexity and costs. To determine the background of air pollution, simple to complex methods can be used to adequately estimate the short- and long-term average pollutant concentrations and trends. One of the simplest methods is the passive samplers of pollutants that are used to screen air quality studies. However, complex, more expensive and advanced monitoring systems are needed to assess air pollution distributions and sources. Currently, mathematics modeling, as well as modeling of receptors, emissions and dispersions, have been used to determine emission sources and the environmental distribution of pollutants. Although studies of mathematical modeling require long-term *a*nd adequate monitoring of pollutants and climatic conditions, these models provide the development of effective control strategies [8, 9].

Conclusion

Despite all efforts to improve air quality, huge problems related to atmospheric contamination are frequently found in urban areas. In addition, developing countries are currently facing other major challenges to control the emission of pollutants with the use of new fuels and their production. According to Ott [10], human exposure can be defined as 'the event that a person comes into contact with a pollutant in a certain concentration during a certain period of time'. Therefore, the accuracy of air quality data and representativeness in area and period are important factors for the assessment of the relative risk of air pollution on human morbidity and mortality.

References

1 Bernard SM, Samet JM, Grambsch A, et al: The potential impacts of climate variability and change on air pollution-related health effects in the United States. Environ Health Perspect 2001; 109:199–209.
2 World Health Organization: Air quality guidelines, Global Update, 2005 (www.who.int/phe/health_topics/outdoorair_agg/en/).
3 Holguin F, Flores S, Ross Z, et al: Traffic-related exposures, airway function, inflammation and respiratory symptoms in children. Am J Respir Crit Care Med 2007;176:1236–1242.
4 Akimoto H: Global air quality and pollution. Science 2003;302:1716–1719.
5 EPA: Handbook for criteria pollutant inventory development: A beginner's guide for point and area sources. Washington, Environmental Protection Agency, 1999.
6 Finlayson-Pitts BJ, Pitts JN Jr: Tropospheric air pollution: ozone, airborne toxics, polycyclic aromatic hydrocarbons, and particles. Science 1997;276: 1045–1050.
7 Englert N: Fine particles and human health: a review of epidemiological studies. Toxicol Lett 2004;149:235–242.
8 Lodge PJ: Methods of Air Sampling and Analysis, ed 3. Washington, Lewis Publishers, 1989, pp 83–214.
9 Krochmal D, Kalina A: A method of nitrogen dioxide and sulphur dioxide determination in ambient air by use of passive samplers and ion chromatography. Atmos Environ 1997;31:3473–3479.
10 Ott WR: Concepts of human exposure to air pollutants. Environ Int 1982;7:179–196.

Regiani Carvalho-Oliveira, PhD
Department of Pathology, Laboratory of Experimental Air Pollution, Laboratory of Medical Investigation 05
Faculdade de Medicina da Universidade de São Paulo
Av. Dr. Arnaldo 455, Rm 1150/1220, São Paulo 01246-903 (Brazil)
Tel. +55 11 3061 8520, Fax +55 11 3068 0072, E-Mail regiani@usp.br

Esquinas AM (ed): Applied Technologies in Pulmonary Medicine. Basel, Karger, 2011, pp 223–230

Air Pollution and Non-Invasive Respiratory Assessments

Naomi Kondo Nakagawa[a,b] · Mayumi Nakao[b] · Danielle Miyuki Goto[a,b] · Beatriz Mangueira Saraiva-Romanholo[c]

[a]Department of Physiotherapy, Communication Science and Disorders and Occupational Therapy, Laboratory of Medical Investigation 34, [b]Department of Pathology, Laboratory of Medical Investigation 05, and [c]Department of Internal Medicine, Laboratory of Medical Investigation 20, Faculdade de Medicina da Universidade de São Paulo, Brazil

Abbreviations

COPD	Chronic obstructive pulmonary disease
EBC	Exhaled breath condensate
FeNO	Nitric oxide in exhaled air
FEV_1	Forced expiratory volume in 1 s
FVC	Forced vital capacity
NL	Nasal lavage
NO	Nitric oxide
STT	Saccharine transit time

The respiratory system represents the route of entry for many environmental and occupational pollutants. Inhalation of toxic particles and noxious gases affects the innate defense mechanisms from the nose to the alveoli by increasing epithelial permeability, reducing mucociliary clearance, activating neutrophils and depressing macrophage function. Documentation of the effects of air pollution on the respiratory tract has been performed in epidemiological studies and established by a variety of methods and techniques that acute episodes of air pollution are associated with an increased risk of adverse pulmonary and cardiovascular events. Non-invasive or relatively non-invasive methods for assessment of the normal biological processes and respiratory inflammation or dysfunction are used in current research. The biomarkers quantitatively or semi-quantitatively measure the extent of lung inflammation and/or damage without any major restriction related to the exposure conditions, age, or health status of the subjects. The analysis of lung function, induced sputum, exhaled air, EBC and STT test are feasible, repeatable and non-invasive assessments to detect early lung damage induced by diseases and external agents. These methods can also be useful to identify new biomarkers of exposure or susceptibility in subjects/patients to enhance the understanding of airways changes due to diseases and noxious exposition to air pollution.

Lung Function Testing

The most important aspects of spirometry are: (a) the FVC, which is the volume delivered during an expiration made as forcefully and completely as possible, which starts from full inspiration, and

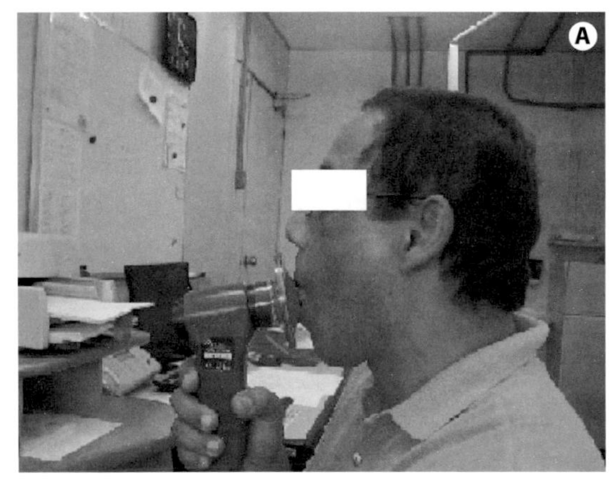

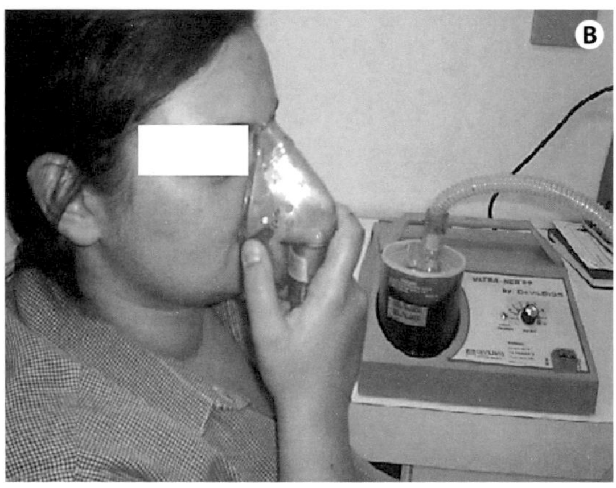

Fig. 1. Lung function testing (**A**) and induced sputum performance with an ultrasonic nebulizer (**B**).

(b) the FEV_1, which is the volume delivered in the first second of an FVC maneuver. FEV_1 is an independent predictor of respiratory and cardiovascular mortality [1]. Other spirometric variables derived from the FVC maneuver are also addressed in epidemiological studies of pollutant effects in children and adult asthmatics, such as peak expiratory flow. Spirometry can be undertaken with many different types of equipment. However, this method requires cooperation of the subject (fig. 1A) and the results obtained will depend on technical as well as personal factors. The interpretation of lung function tests requires the classification of the derived values considering the reference population, and the integration of the results into the diagnosis for an individual patient [2]. It is the gold standard method to measure airflow limitation [3, 4]. However, it does not completely define the extent and severity of the disease. Acute exposition to air pollutants (particulate matter and noxious gases) is associated with respiratory symptoms and a significant decline in lung function in children [5], in young healthy volunteers (FEV_1 and FVC, but not in the FEV_1/FVC ratio parameter) [6, 7], and adult asthmatics [8]. Adverse health effects and worsening of the clinical status have also been reported after chronic air pollution exposition in the general population [9] and adult asthmatics [10].

Sputum Induction

Sputum cells recovered from spontaneous coughing were first examined in stained smears in the 1950s through the 1970s to study lung cancer and respiratory infection. Now, induced sputum is a well-recognized, repeatable, useful and relatively non-invasive sampling method for research and clinical use to diagnose and monitor clinical and subclinical airway and bronchial inflammation, as well as infection and other respiratory and systemic diseases with lung involvement. There is a large body of knowledge on sputum characteristics, particularly in relation to the inflammatory cells content [11–14] and mediators [15, 16], matrix metalloproteinases [17], and physical properties and appearance [18, 19]. Induced sputum tests (fig. 1B) are performed with 3, 3.5, 4, 4.5, 5 or 7% of saline solution that are given

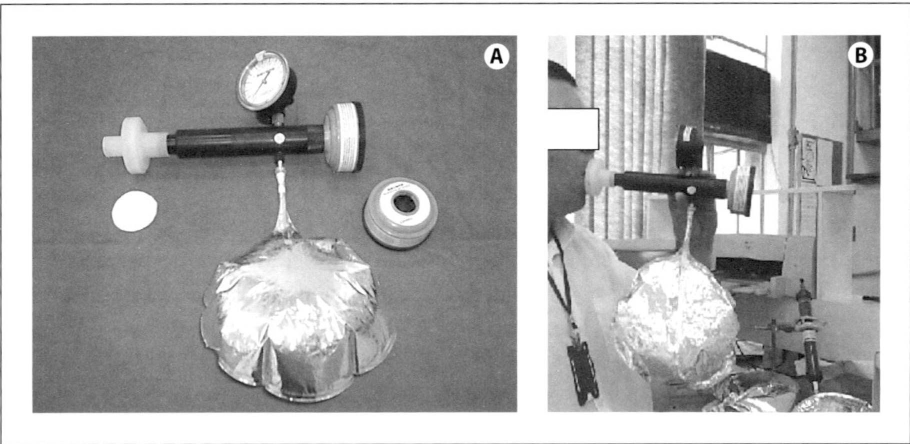

Fig. 2. Equipment and materials for collection of the exhaled breath for NO analysis (**A**); exhaled breath collection for NO analysis (**B**).

sequentially in the amount of 5–7 ml in the form of a spray produced by an ultrasonic nebulizer. Following each dose of inhaled hypertonic saline through a mouthpiece, the subject coughs and expectorates the sputum into a sterile container or in special conditions; sputum can be suctioned. The induced sputum method with hypertonic saline has been shown to effectively and safely recruit the mucus from the alveoli of patients. Each inhalation is followed by spirometry to check for any FEV_1 reduction. However, if a 20% reduction from the baseline value of FEV_1 occurs after salbutamol, sputum induction should be discontinued. This method allows the examination of inflammatory events and can also be applied to assess the effects of inhaled toxic gases or particles in the airways and lungs in both normal subjects and patients with disease [20, 21]. However, this method is relatively difficult to perform in the routine evaluation of children and adolescents [15, 22] and it is time-consuming [13]. Interestingly, studies have raised the possibility to trace metals, such as zinc, manganese, and copper, in induced sputum as biomarkers of inflammation in lung diseases [23].

Exhaled Breath

The presence of NO in exhaled air, FeNO, of human and animals was first described in 1991. FeNO is the most extensively studied exhaled biomarker in respiratory diseases (fig. 2). Measurements of FeNO can be performed online and offline, with similar application in epidemiology. However, influence of ambient NO on FeNO should be carefully examined [24]. NO is a simple gaseous molecule composed of a single nitrogen atom and one of oxygen atom, but it is a highly reactive chemical agent that has a short half-life when diluted (<10 s) due to its rapid oxidation. NO is a messenger of physiological process that stimulates the synthesis of cyclic GMP and promotes the relaxation of bronchial smooth muscle. NO is constitutively expressed in bronchial epithelium and alveolar epithelial type II cells are also found in human pulmonary blood vessels and all types of arteries, particularly in the radial artery. The NO generated by NO synthase is responsible for maintaining low vascular tone and preventing the adhesion of leukocytes and platelets in the vascular wall. On the contrary, it can also lead to vasodilatation in the arterioles, leading to plasma extravasation and edema. NO produced from induced NO synthase may have cytostatic and cytotoxic effects. NO has pro- and antioxidant effects, depending on location and concentration. At low concentrations, NO has protective actions, including neuromodulation, smooth muscle relaxation and reduction of bronchial hyperresponsiveness caused by bronchoconstrictor stimuli. However, in high concentrations, as observed in several pathological conditions, NO has deleterious effects, such as proinflammatory activity with increased gland secretion into the airways, activation and recruitment of numerous inflammatory cells, apoptosis and necrosis. Significantly increased values of FeNO are observed in patients with asthma, COPD patients with sputum eosinophilia, and cystic fibrosis [25, 26]. However, FeNO measurement in COPD is of limited value due to the smoking effect and the results are dependent of exhalation rates. Recently, Saraiva-Romanholo et al. [27] have reported a similar pattern to asthma of increased FeNO in non-asthmatic patients during bronchospasm episodes in the surgical room. The concentration of FeNO has also been used to measure human response to air pollutants. Increased levels of FeNO can be found in non-smoking subjects exposed to air pollution showing that airways inflammation is present with no clinical presentation [7].

Exhaled Breath Condensate

EBC is a promising biological fluid that can be easily and quickly obtained by cooling exhaled air under condition of spontaneous breathing. Participants are asked to breathe tidally through the mouthpiece connected to the tube during 10–15 min to collect approximately 2–3 ml of EBC, which is aliquoted and frozen to –70°C. [28]. The analysis of EBC is increasingly studied as a non-invasive research method of sampling the lungs, as a real-time assessment of pulmonary pathobiology. Fluid pH and several biochemical components can be analyzed in EBC. EBC analysis is a simple, easy, safe, and non-invasive method to investigate the oxidative stress in many respiratory diseases and other conditions, also due to medication evaluation and air pollution exposure. Recently, in adult patients with mild and moderate asthma, McCreanor et al. [8] showed that breathing polluted air during a 2-hour walk on Oxford Street in London, where only diesel-powered vehicles are allowed, resulted in lung function reduction accompanied by respiratory inflammatory activity. They found airway acidification (a twofold increase in hydrogen ions after 2 h of exposure) in EBC samples, increased levels of myeloperoxidase and interleukin-8 in sputum samples and higher fraction of NO in exhaled breath. The endogenous airway acidification assessed by pH of EBC represents a biomarker associated with oxidative stress and sputum neutrophilia. There is evidence that oxidative stress may have an important role in exacerbating COPD. The concentration of hydrogen peroxide and 8-isoprostane are increased during COPD exacerbations. Many mechanisms are raised to enhance inflammation and proteolytic injury, such as the activation of transcription factor nuclear factor-κB [29]. Recently, Salvi and Barnes [30] reported evidence in the literature for the association of COPD with biomass fuel, occupational exposure to dusts and gases, and outdoor air pollution. EBC has limitations, such as considerable variability due to the sample collection and analysis [31]. The EBC sample from tidal breathing is obtained with the use of an apparatus ('breath condensate collector'). According to Koczulla et al. [32], there are no differences between EBC devices in healthy controls, asthmatics and COPD patients for pH measurements. An example of the modified apparatus is showed in figure 2B. Another point is the exact site of origin of substances measured in EBC. Jackson et al. [33] showed in a very elegant work that biomarkers of inflammation and oxidative stress are easily

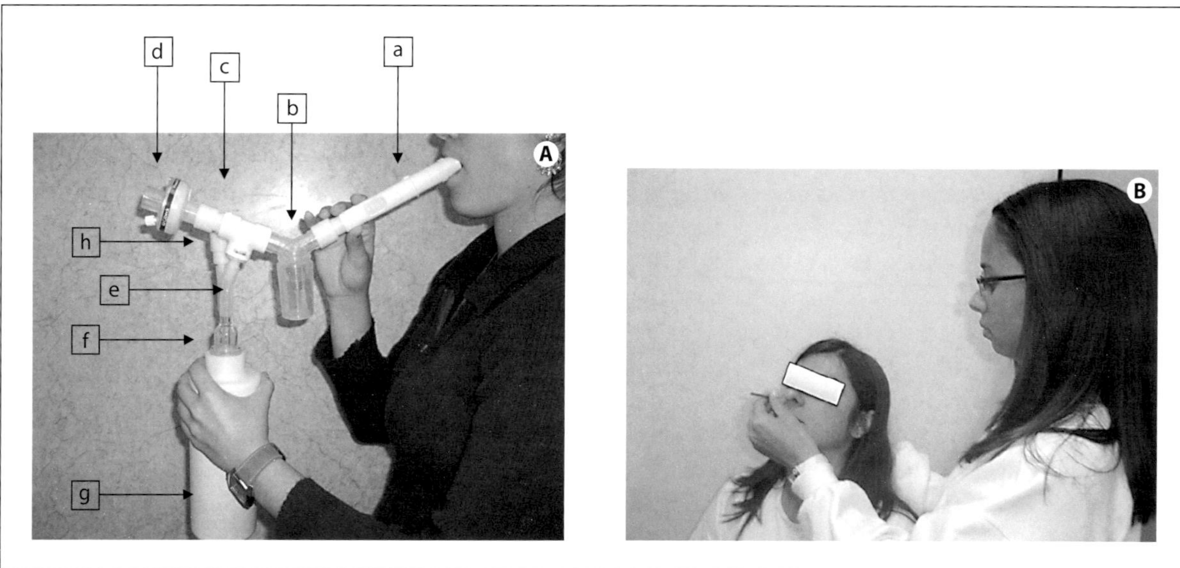

Fig. 3. The exhaled breath condensator modified apparatus (**A**): (a) buccal, (b) saliva collector, (c) T-piece with unidirectional valve, (d) filter (humid vent filter compact S, Louis Gibeck AB, Upplands Väsby, Sweden), (e) EBC tube connector, (f) EBC tube collector, (g) condenser reservoir, and (h) expiratory unidirectional valve. This apparatus was developed by Dr. Paulo Hilário Nascimento Saldiva, Dr. Naomi Kondo Nakagawa, Simão Bacht, and Dr. Idágene Cestari, and built by Bioengeering Division of Heart Institute (InCor) University of São Paulo Medical School; STT test (**B**).

detectable and measurable in EBC. However, comparing EBC with bronchoalveolar lavage, the biomarkers do not correlate (8-isoprostane, nitrogen oxides, total phospholipid and pH were higher in EBC than in bronchoalveolar lavage, total protein was lower in EBC compared with bronchoalveolar lavage, and hydrogen peroxide and keratin were similar).

Nasal Lavage

NL is a well-established, safe, well-tolerated and low-cost technique that has been used to study the acute inflammatory response in the upper respiratory tract for more than 20 years. It was first described by Naclerio et al. [34]. NL is performed by sitting the subject with the nasopharynx closed while tilting the neck back 45° from the vertical position. Five milliliters of warm (37°C) normal saline is instilled into each nostril by a syringe. After 10 s, the subject brings the head forward and expels the liquid into a sterile plastic receptacle [34–36]. The lavage fluid from both nostrils is pooled in the same receptacle and kept on ice until processed. Each lavage sample is vigorously shaken to break up clumps of mucus and then centrifuged (1,000 *g* at 4°C during 10 min). Cell counts are determined from the resuspended pellet and differential cell counts are performed using the cytospin preparation at 450 rpm for 6 min [35]. Many cell types found in the lining of the nasopharygeal region are similar to cells of the tracheal and bronchial lining. Therefore, it has been suggested that the cellular responses in the nose to toxicants are likely to be similar to the lower airway at the same dose of the agent. If these pollutants are respiratory irritants, capable of causing cellular damage, effects may therefore be detected in the nasal passage.

However, a number of studies have reported controversial findings in NL of workers and subjects exposed to several inhaled substances [37, 38]. Blaski et al. [37] did not find a relationship between NL cellularity and respiratory symptoms, airflow obstruction, and levels of short-term dust exposure in a cross-sectional field study of workers exposed to organic dusts. However, they found increased cellularity in NL in workers exposed to high levels of ambient organic dusts compared with low levels. On the other hand, Barraza-Vilarreal et al. [38] showed in a cohort study of 158 asthmatics and 50 non-asthmatic school-age children significant associations of increased inflammatory marker (interleukin-8) in NL, reduced pH of EBC and decreased FEV_1 and FVC after a short-term air pollutant exposure. FeNO and FEV_1 were inversely correlated in asthmatic children.

Saccharin Transit Time Test

STT test is a simple, inexpensive, repeatable and non-invasive method for some purposes: (a) in vivo evaluation of the abnormal mucociliary clearance in several conditions, (b) identification of subjects that other assessment studies should be carried out, such as mucus properties analysis, ciliary motility and structure, and (c) assessment of clinical and surgical interventions. The STT test was first described by Andersen et al. [39] and modified by Rutland and Cole [40]. To perform the STT test (fig. 2A), a 5-mg particle of saccharine is placed 2 cm inside the non-obstructed nostril, on the inferior turbinate under visual control while the subject is quiet and seated. A timer is displayed to measure the transit time. STT is the elapsed time from the placement of the particle into the nasal mucosa until the subject reports the sweet taste of saccharine. Subjects are allowed to swallow freely, and oriented to maintain normal ventilation, avoiding deep breaths, talking, sniffing, sneezing, eating, or coughing. The normal mean value reported for this assay is 11–12 min in young healthy adults [40–44]. However, despite its widespread use, there are factors that may affect STT. On the one hand, age and smoking prolong STT, and on the other hand, exercise and acute rhinitis accelerate STT.

Conclusions

Air pollutants may induce inflammation in the respiratory system. Inflammation is a fundamental process in the pathophysiological cascade leading to respiratory disorders, including asthma, COPD or interstitial lung disease. Several safe, repeatable, and non-invasive techniques of inflammatory monitoring, and assessment of a disease's severity or host response to treatments are available. The efficiency of these techniques depends on the standardization and implementation of the procedures and technology, and adequate interpretation of the results. Considering the adverse effects of air pollution, there is a special interest for biomarkers that reflect or induce oxidative stress, and inflammatory elements and processes.

Acknowledgments

The authors would like to thank S. Fidalgo, T.M. Lima, and A.S. Santos for providing the photographs shown of figures 1A, 3A, and 3B, respectively. The EBC-modified apparatus was developed by Dr. Paulo Hilário Nascimento Saldiva, Dr. Naomi Kondo Nakagawa, Simão Bacht, and Dr. Idágene Cestari, and built by Bioengeering Division of Heart Institute (InCor) University of São Paulo Medical School.

References

1 Pellegrino R, Viegi G, Brusasco V, et al: Interpretative strategies for lung function tests. Eur Respir J 2005;26:948–968.
2 Miller MR, Crapo R, Hankinson J, et al: General consideration for lung function testing. Eur Respir J 2005;26:153–161.
3 Global Initiative for Chronic Obstructive Lung Disease (GOLD), American Thoracic Society 2006. Spirometry for healthcare providers (http://www.goldcopd.com/OtherResourcesItem.asp?l1=2&l2=2&intId=1836).
4 American Thoracic Society: Standardization of spirometry. Am J Respir Crit Care Med 1995;152:1107–1136.
5 Liu L, Poon R, Chen L, et al: Acute effects of air pollution on pulmonary function, airway inflammation, and oxidative stress in asthmatic children. Environ Health Perspect 2009;117:668–674.
6 Steinvil A, Fireman E, Kordova-Biezuner L, et al: Environmental air pollution has decremental effects on pulmonary function test parameters up to one week after exposure. Am J Med Sci 2009;338:273–279.
7 Guarnieri G, Lodde V, Ferrazzoni S, et al: Acute effects of environmental pollution on the urban vigilants airways. G Ital Med Lav Ergon 2007;29:838–840.
8 McCreanor J, Cullinan P, Nieuwenhuijsen MJ, et al: Respiratory effects of exposure to diesel traffic in persons with asthma. N Engl J Med 2007;357:2348–2358.
9 Ackerman-Liebrih U, Leuenberger P, Shwartz J, et al: Lung function and long-term exposure to air pollutants in Switzerland. Study on air pollution and lung diseases in adults (SAPALDIA) team. Am J Respir Crit Care Med 1009;155:122–129.
10 Canova C, Torresan S, Simonato L, et al: Carbon monoxide pollution is associated with decreased lung function in asthmatic adults. Eur Respir J 2009;35:266–272.
11 Pizzichini E, Pizzichini MMM, Kidney JC, et al: Induced sputum, bronchoalveolar lavage and blood from mild asthmatics: inflammatory cells lymphocyte subsets and soluble markers compared. Eur Respir J 1998;11:828–834.
12 Drews AC, Pizzichini MM, Pizzichini E, et al: Neutrophilic airway inflammation is a main feature of induced sputum in nonatopic asthmatic children. Allergy 2009;64:1597–1601.
13 Saraiva-Romanholo BM, Barnabé V, Carvalho AL, Martins MA, Saldiva PH, Nunes MP: Comparison of three methods for differential cell count in induced sputum. Chest 2003;124:1060–1066.
14 Fireman E: Induced sputum as a diagnostic tactic in pulmonary diseases. Isr Med Assoc J 2003;5:524–527.
15 Gagliardo R, La Grutta S, Chanez P, et al: Non-invasive markers of airway inflammation and remodeling in childhood asthma. Pediatr Allergy Immunol 2009;20:780–790.
16 Fireman E, Gilberto D, Marmor S: Angiogenic cytokines in induced sputum of patients with sarcoidosis. Respirology 2009;14:117–123.
17 Fireman E, Kraiem Z, Sade O, et al: Induced sputum-retrieved matrix metalloproteinase-9 and tissue metalloproteinase inhibitor-1 in granulomatous diseases. Clin Exp Immunol 2002;130:331–337.
18 Murray MP, Pentland JL, Turnbull K, et al: Sputum colour: a useful clinical tool in non-cystic fibrosis bronchiectasis. Eur Respir J 2009;34:361–364.
19 Albertini-Yagi CS, Oliveira RC, Vieira JE, et al: Sputum induction as a research tool for the study of human respiratory mucus. Respir Physiol Neurobiol 2005;145:101–110.
20 Hogg JC, van Eeden S: Pulmonary and systemic response to atmospheric pollution. Respirology 2009;14:336–346.
21 Mussafi H, Fireman EM, Mei-Zahav M, et al: Induced sputum in the very young. Chest 2008;133:176–182.
22 Paro-Heitor ML, Bussamra MH, Saraiva-Romanholo BM, et al: Exhaled nitric oxide for monitoring childhood asthma inflammation compared to sputum analysis, serum interleukins and pulmonary function. Pediatr Pulmonol 2008;43:134–141.
23 Gray RD, Duncan A, Noble D, et al: Sputum trace metals are biomarkers of inflammatory and suppurative lung disease. Chest 2010;37:635–641.
24 Linn WS, Berhane KT, Rappaport EB, et al: Relationships of online exhaled, offline exhaled, and ambient nitric oxide in an epidemiological survey of schoolchildren. J Expo Sci Environ Epidemiol 2009;19:674–681.
25 Baraldi E, Jongste JC: Measurement of exhaled nitric oxide in children, 2001. Eur Respir J 2002;20:1–15.
26 Ricciardolo FLM, Sterk PJ, Gaston B, et al: Nitric oxide in health and disease of the respiratory system. Physiol Rev 2004;84:731–765.
27 Saraiva-Romanholo BM, Machado FS, Almeida FM, et al: Non-asthmatic patients show increased exhaled nitric oxide concentrations. Clinics 2009;64:5–10.
28 Cepelak I, Dodig S: Exhaled breath condensate: a new method for lung disease diagnosis. Clin Chem Lab Med 2007;45:945–952.
29 Barnes PJ: Medical progress: chronic obstructive pulmonary disease. N Engl J Med 2000;343:269–280.
30 Salvi SS, Barnes PJ: Chronic obstructive pulmonary disease in non-smokers. Lancet 2009;374:733–743.
31 Leung TF, Li CY, Yung E, et al: Clinical and technical factors affecting pH and other biomarkers in exhaled breath condensate. Pediatr Pulmonol 2006;41:87–94.
32 Koczulla R, Dragonieri S, Schot R, et al: Comparison of exhaled breath condensate pH using two commercially available devices in healthy controls, asthma and COPD patients. Respir Res 2009;10:78.
33 Jackson AS, Sandrini A, Campbell C, et al: Comparison of biomarkers in exhaled breath condensate and bronchoalveolar lavage. Am J Crit Care Med 2007;175:222–227.
34 Naclerio RM, Meier HL, Kagey-Sobotka A, et al: Mediator release after nasal challenge with allergen. Am Rev Respir Dis 1983;128:597–602.
35 Diaz-Sanches D, Dotson AR, Takanaka H, et al. Diesel exhaust particles induce local IgE production in vivo and alter the pattern of IgE messenger RNA isoforms. J Clin Invest 1994;94:1417–1425.

36 Diaz-Sanches D, Id RR, Gong H: Challenge with environmental tobacco smoke exacerbates allergic airway disease in human beings. J Allergy Clin Immunol 2006;118:441–446.
37 Blaski CA, Watt JL, Quinn TJ, et al: Nasal lavage cellularity, grain dust, and airflow obstruction. Chest 1996;109:1086–1092.
38 Barraza-Villarreal A, Sunyer J, Hernandez-Cadena L, et al: Air pollution, airway inflammation, and lung function in a cohort study of Mexico City schoolchildren. Environ Health Perspect 2008;116:832–838.
39 Andersen I, Camner P, Jensen PL, et al: Nasal clearance in monozygotic twins. Am Rev Respir Dis 1974;110:301–305.
40 Rutland J, Cole PJ: Nasal mucociliary clearance and ciliary beat frequency in cystic fibrosis compared with sinusitis and bronchiectasis. Thorax 1981;36:654–658.
41 Nakagawa NK, Franchini ML, Driusso P, et al: Mucociliary clearance is impaired in acutely ill patients. Chest 2005;128:2772–2777.
42 Persson C, Svensson C, Greiff L, et al: The use of the nose to study the inflammatory response of the respiratory tract. Thorax 1992;47:993–1000.
43 Stanley PJ, Wilson R, Greenstone MA, et al: Effect of cigarette smoking on nasal mucociliary clearance and ciliary beat frequency. Thorax 1986;41:519–523.
44 Goto DM, Torres GM, Seguro AC, Saldiva PHN, Lorenzi-Filho G, Nakagawa NK: Furosemide impairs nasal mucociliary clearance in humans. Respir Physiol Neurobiol 2010;170:246–252.

Naomi Kondo Nakagawa, BSc, PhD
Department of Physiotherapy, Communication Science and Disorders and Occupational Therapy
Laboratory of Medical Investigation 34, Faculdade de Medicina da Universidade de São Paulo
Av. Dr. Arnaldo 455, São Paulo 01246-903 (Brazil)
Tel. +55 11 3061 8529, Fax +55 11 3068 0072, E-Mail naomi.kondo@usp.br

Esquinas AM (ed): Applied Technologies in Pulmonary Medicine. Basel, Karger, 2011, pp 231–237

Air Pollution, Oxidative Stress and Pulmonary Defense

Mariangela Macchione[a] · Maria Lúcia Bueno Garcia[b]

[a]Department of Pathology, Laboratory of Experimental Air Pollution, Laboratory of Medical Investigation 05, and [b]Department of Internal Medicine, Laboratory of Experimental Therapeutics, Faculdade de Medicina da Universidade de São Paulo, Brazil

Abbreviations

ARE	Antioxidant response element
ERK	Extracellular signal-regulated protein kinases
JNK	Jun NH_2-terminal kinases
Keap1	Kelch-like ECH-associated protein
MAPK	Mitogen activation protein kinases
MAPKK	MAPK kinase
MAPKKK	MAPK kinase kinase
NF-κB	Nuclear factor-κB
Nrf2	Nuclear factor erythroid-2-related factor
PAH	Polycyclic aromatic hydrocarbons
PM	Particulate matter
ROS	Reactive oxygen species

Air Pollution and Oxidative Stress

Air pollutants affect different organs in mammalians and cause several health problems, including respiratory, cardiovascular, neurological, reproductive and developmental ailments and even cancer [1]. In addition, exposure to air pollutants is reported to alter immune response and enhance respiratory infection [1].

Respiratory epithelium cells are not a simple barrier between the body and the external environmental that protect against inhaled toxins, pathogens and particles. They also respond to attacks of air pollutants, ranging from responses of extracellular stimuli and stress by activating signaling pathways that lead to inflammation. Airway epithelial cells can produce a diverse array of proinflammatory mediators, growth factors and cytokines in response to environmental challenge, and are actively involved in different stages of epithelial repair. In vivo, the ability to generate oxidants correlates with the ability to produce inflammation [2]. In vitro, the acute inflammatory response to ambient particulate pollutants (PM) seems to reflect oxidative activation of fundamental cell signaling pathways [3].

Many air pollutants exert their major effects by causing oxidative stress in cells and tissues. Gaseous pollutants and PM are known to form ROS such as superoxide anion, hydrogen peroxide and hydroxyl radicals that may damage proteins, lipids and DNA directly, and form distinct products.

Exogenous Oxidants

Several air pollution components have been associated to particulate toxicity. An important determinant of the acute inflammatory response seems to be the dose of bioavailability of transition metals (copper, vanadium, chromium, nickel, cobalt and iron) as well as organic components (PAH) and biological fractions (endotoxins) [4].

Metals such as iron, copper, chromium, vanadium and cobalt are capable of redox cycling in which a single electron may be accepted or donated by the metal. This action catalyzes reactions that produce reactive radicals and can produce ROS. The most important reactions are probably Fenton's reaction and the Haber-Weiss reaction, in which hydroxyl radical is produced from the reduced iron and hydrogen peroxide.

Exposures to oxidant air pollutants can promote lipid peroxidation that is caused by a free radical reaction involving the polyunsaturated fatty acids of the membrane. This reaction can damage cell membrane leading to cell death and pathological consequences. In addition, one of these end-products, 4-hydroxy-2-noneal, causes in vitro depletion of intracellular glutathione and induction of peroxide production, airway remodeling through activation of the epidermal growth factor receptor, providing evidence for the hypothesis that secondary mediators generated by oxidant reactions with lipids, proteins and others biomolecules contribute to toxic effects of pollutants [5]. The oxidant air pollutants can also promote modification in the proteins, particularly those that have amino acid composition with cysteine and methionine residues, which are more susceptible to oxidation [6]. Studies also have shown that exposure to air pollutants can induce DNA damage, increasing the risk of lung cancer [7].

Air pollution is made up of several components constantly reacting to each other as particles and toxic gases. Both components are toxic to healthy. PM contains a carbonaceous core with adsorbed organic and inorganic materials as metals. Fine PM is within 2.5 μm of aerodynamic diameter (PM <10 μm) as they can reach the distal lung tissue and blood circulation. PM may alter the function of mitochondria, reduce nicotinamide adenine phosphate oxidase, activate inflammatory cells capable of generating ROS and reactive nitrogen species as well as DNA damage [8]. Exposures to diesel exhaust particles, which contains polyaromatic hydrocarbons, quinones and redox-active metals adsorbed to it, has shown to increase IL-6 and IL-8 in bronchial alveolar lavage in humans and upregulate endothelial adhesion molecules P-selectin and vascular cell adhesion molecule-1 [9].

In concern to toxic gaseous, ozone is a very reactive gas that forms secondary ROS directly by ozonization of the tract lining fluid lipids, inducing lipid peroxidation as well as activation of transcription factors such as NF-κB and increased expression of several proinflammatory cytokines and adhesion genes [10]. Nitrogen dioxide, like ozone, reacts with substrates present in the lung lining fluid compartment where the signaling cascade of inflammatory cells into the lung occurs [11].

PAH air pollution originates mainly due to the incomplete combustion of wood or fuel used for residential heating, industrial or motor vehicle exhaust. A number of studies have considered DNA damage as the endpoint or the effects of pollution in particular 'bulky' DNA adducts and also protein adducts which are related to exposure to aromatic compounds including PAH [12]. Select PAH as quinones can also induce oxidative stress in cells and decrease the GSH concentration through electrophilic reaction [13]. Kikuno et al. [14] showed that 1,2-naphthoquinone, a PM quinone, may cause tyrosine kinase, phosphorylation by activating phospholipase A_2/lipoxygenase/vanilloid receptor 1, signaling and increasing calcium levels which, in turn, resulted in contraction of tracheal smooth muscle.

Oxidant-Induced Cell Signaling

Oxidant pollutants through ROS may activate signalization pathways that lead to cellular responses which can trigger pathological responses in the

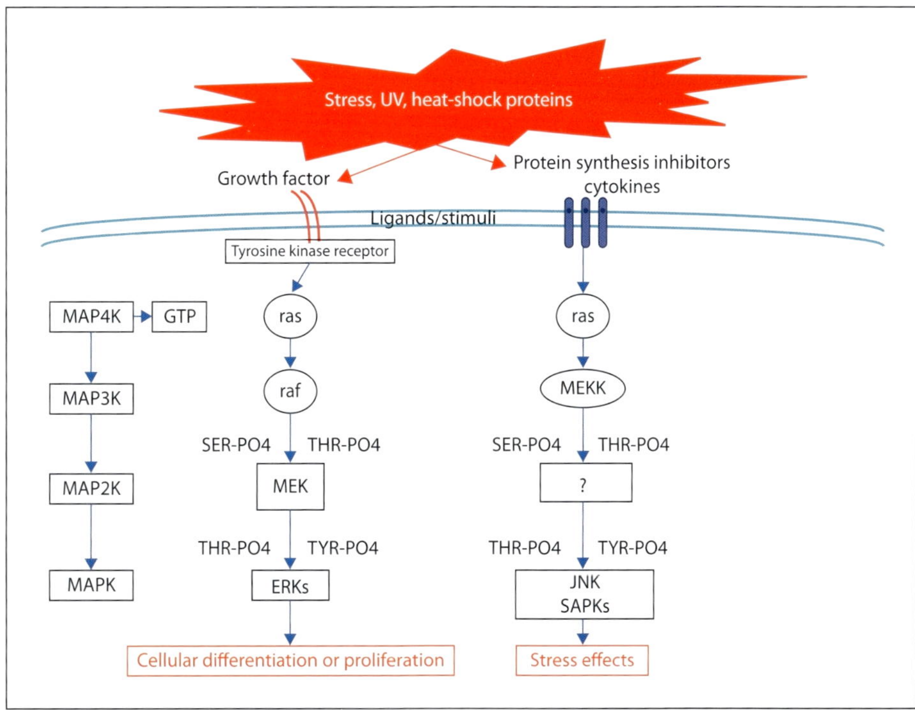

Fig. 1. MAPK cascades. Illustration of the three-tiered MAPK cascades for ERK and JNK family members.

lung. The main types of signal transduction pathways in eukaryotic cells are protein kinase cascades that culminate in activation of a family of protein kinases known as MAPK [15]. They are a group of 38–110 kDA Ser/Thr that translate signals which lead to diverse cellular responses. There are three major MAPK pathways which includes a Ser/Thr MAPK that is phosphorylated by a Thr/Tyr MAPKK which is itself phosphorylated by a Ser/Thr kinase known as a MAPKKK (fig. 1). There are three subtypes of MAPK: one is activated through ERK that mediates cell proliferation, while the other two subtypes are p38 MAPK and p46 to p54 MAPK (JNK) that mediate signals in response to environmental stress and cytokines which results in the phosphorylation-dependent activation of a variety of transcription factors (e.g. Elk1, c-Jun, ATF-2). They also mediate the specific response to the stimulus [16]. Other studies have demonstrated the ability of air pollutants to activate NF-κB through of the epidermal growth factor receptor activation and the MAPK signaling pathway, which is involved in the stress response [17].

Endogenous Oxidants

Endogenous sources of ROS may have an indirect role in the toxicity induced by exposure to air pollutants. The cells that produce ROS in the lung are neutrophils, eosinophils, alveolar macrophages, epithelial cells and endothelial cells. These cells are recruited when air pollutants induce lung inflammation and release ROS, enhancing inflammation with tissue damage and other pathological

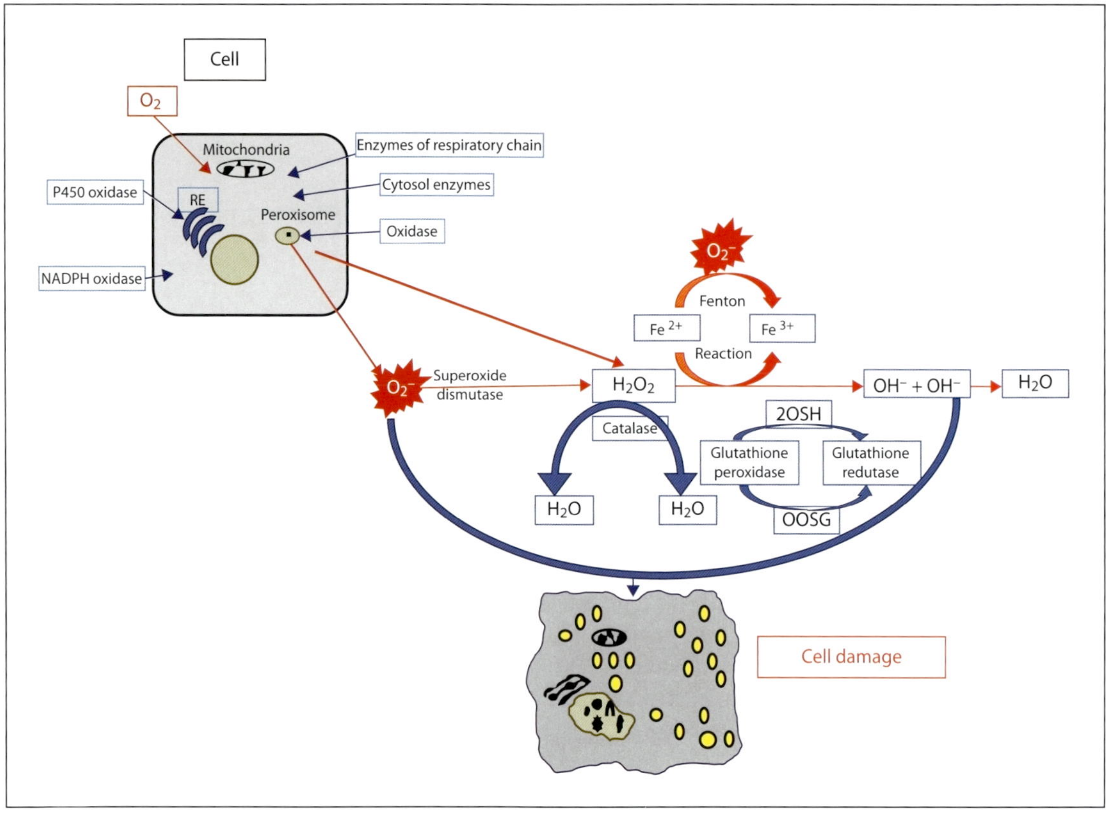

Fig. 2. Glutathione peroxidase and oxidative stress.

effects. Inflammatory cells produce mainly superoxide and hydrogen peroxide that can react with a number of substrates and biomolecules that generate radicals. ROS is also involved with reactions of the electron transport chain within the mitochondria and enzyme reactions involving cyclooxygenases, lipoxygenases, peroxygenases and cytochrome P450. Alteration in these processes or decrement in the antioxidants that offset the production of ROS may also lead to tissue damage and other pathological consequences [18].

Peroxynitrite is another potential oxidant that is formed by the reaction of nitric oxide and superoxide, inducing lipid peroxidation, DNA damage and protein oxidation. These studies demonstrate how endogenous sources of ROS can contribute to air pollutant-induced toxicity through an enhancement of the oxidative burden within the lung.

Pulmonary Antioxidants

There are several enzymatic and non-enzymatic systems that contribute to the inactivation of free radicals. Most of them are in the airways, the main and first barrier to external aggressors.

The non-enzymatic antioxidant system blocks the beginning of free radicals formation as well as their inactivation by scavengers and the final cellular and tissue damage. Some examples of this category are vitamins: vitamin E (α-tocopherol)

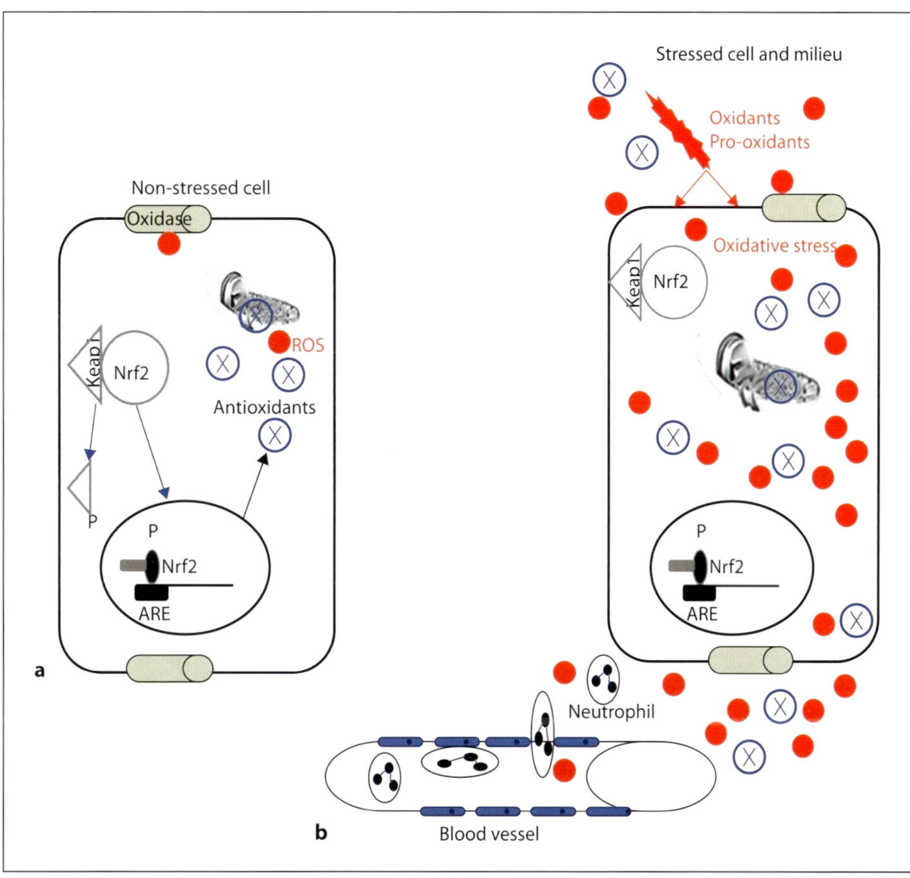

Fig. 3. Nrf2-antioxidant defense system in airway cells. **a** In normal physiologic conditions, a balance between antioxidants and oxidants maintains cellular redox equilibrium. **b** Under stressed conditions, oxidative stimuli could accelerate ROS production, directly or indirectly, and activate Nrf2 for production of ARE-driven antioxidants, while overwhelming ROS over antioxidant capacity may cause oxidative injury leading to pulmonary pathologic symptoms.

is secreted by type II pneumocyte with the surfactant, it is located in intra- and extracellular fluids, blocking the membrane lipid peroxidation by the peroxyl radicals clearance; vitamin A (and its precursors β-carotene) and vitamin C (ascorbic acid) induce endothelial stabilization and trigger vitamin E increment; uric acid, found in the nasal mucus and in the respiratory epithelium, clears oxidants in the mucus and superoxides; metallothionine, albumin and ceruloplasmin are extracellular metal-binding proteins able of clearing some radicals produced by the protein-copper or iron complex, associated with iron compartmentalization and homeostasis which facilitate the metal disponibility to interact with transferrin by the ceruloplasmin-ferroxidase activity.

Several other enzymes are included as enzymatic antioxidant systems which clear free radicals and lyse hydrogen peroxide and superoxide anion. These enzymes are the following: catalase located in the peroxisomes, decomposes H_2O_2 to $O_2 + H_2O$, enabling the membrane lipid peroxidation through peroxyl radicals clearance; superoxide dismutase group (MnSOD-SOD manganese in the mitochondria and copper-zinc-SOD in the cytosol) is able to turn the superoxide into H_2O_2 by blocking transition metals; glutathione peroxidase catalyzes and lyses free radicals (fig. 2) and the oxidized/reduced glutathione intracellular ratio reflects the oxidative state of the cell and is a key element in the cellular detoxification ability of ROS; heme oxygenase, ferritin, transferrin and lactoferrin catalyze the heme degradation into biliverdin and may be induced by several stimuli as hyperoxia, hypoxia, LPS and oxidative stress, modulated by NF-κB and activator protein-1; transferrin, ferritin, lactoferrin and ceruloplasmin are metal protein ligands, diminish transition metals storage levels and thus decrease the $OH^{\bullet}$ production; use of chelating agents as EDTA, DPTA, deferoxamine and D-penicilamine (cuprimine). The metal chelation also improves the heme oxygenase and ferritin effects.

Response to Oxidative Stress – Nrf2

Responsible for the procedure of the antioxidant molecules is the promoter of the genes for phase II detoxifying enzymes and antioxidants that contain a *cis*-acting element called ARE [19]. ARE is activated by phenolic antioxidants, hydroperoxides, quinones, heavy metals and other diverse inducers that bind Nrf2 with ARE sequence and activate the transcription of target genes. Under homeostatic conditions, Nrf2 is in the cytoplasm of the cell attached to an actin-binding cytosolic protein named Keap1 [20]. These proteins are uncoupled when Nrf2-Keap1 is exposed to electrophiles and ROS, leading to the translocation of Nrf2 to the nucleus where it can dimerize with other transcription factors binding to the ARE, which causes the transcriptional activation of phase II detoxifying enzymes and antioxidants (fig. 3).

Conclusion

Oxidative stress caused by air pollution may induce several inflammatory signs in the lung including exudates, cellular proliferation and influx, matrix accumulation and airway obstruction. Progress has been made to understand the mechanisms through which oxidants initiate and trigger cell and tissue toxicity, however critical questions still remain to be addressed.

References

1 Rubio V, Valverde M, Rojas E: Effects of atmospheric pollutants on the Nrf2 survival pathway. Environ Sci Pollut Res Int 2010;17:369–382.

2 Schaumann F, Borm PJ, Herbrich A, et al: Metal-rich ambient particles (particulate matter 2.5) cause airway inflammation in healthy subjects. Am J Respir Crit Care Med 2004;170:898–903.

3 Churg A, Xie C, Wang X, et al: Air pollution particles activate NF-κB on contact with airway epithelial cell surfaces. Toxicol Appl Pharmacol 2005;208:37–45.

4 Soukup JM, Becker S: Human alveolar macrophage responses to air pollution particulates are associated with insoluble components of coarse material, including particulate endotoxin. Toxicol Appl Pharmacol 2001;171:20–26.

5 Ciencewicki J, Trivedi S, Kleeberger SR: Oxidants and the pathogenesis of lung diseases. J Allergy Clin Immunol 2008;122:456–468.

6 Kelly FJ, Mudway IS: Protein oxidation at the air-lung interface. Amino Acids 2003;25:375–396.

7 Prahalad AK, Inmon J, Ghio AJ, et al: Enhancement of 2′-deoxyguanosine hydroxylation and DNA damage by coal and oil fly ash in relation to particulate metal content and availability. Chem Res Toxicol 2000;13:1011–1019.

8 González-Flecha B: Oxidant mechanisms in response to ambient air particles. Mol Aspects Med 2004;25:169–182.

9 Stenfors N, Nordenhäll C, Salvi SS, et al: Different airway inflammatory responses in asthmatic and healthy humans exposed to diesel. Eur Respir J 2004;23:82–86.

10 Kelly FJ: Oxidative stress: its role in air pollution and adverse health effects. Occup Environ Med 2003;60:612–616.
11 Janssen-Heininger YM, Persinger RL, Korn SH, et al: Reactive nitrogen species and cell signaling: implications for death or survival of lung epithelium. Am J Respir Crit Care Med 2002;166:S9–S16.
12 Peluso M, Merlo F, Munnia A, et al: ^{32}P-post-labeling detection of aromatic adducts in the white blood cell DNA of nonsmoking police officers. Cancer Epidemiol Biomarkers Prev 1998;7:3–11.
13 Bolton JL, Trush MA, Penning TM, et al: Role of quinones in toxicology. Chem Res Toxicol 2000;13:135–160.
14 Kikuno S, Taguchi K, Iwamoto N, Yamano S, et al: 1,2-Naphthoquinone activates vanilloid receptor-1 through increased protein tyrosine phosphorylation, leading to contraction of guinea pig trachea. Toxicol Appl Pharmacol 2006;210:47–54.
15 Wu W, Graves LM, Jaspers I, et al: Activation of the EGF receptor signaling pathway in human airway epithelial cells exposed to metals. Am J Physiol 1999;277:L924–931.
16 Treisman R: Regulation of transcription by MAP kinase cascades. Curr Opin Cell Biol 1996;8:205–215.
17 Dagher Z, Garçon G, Billet S, et al: Role of nuclear factor-κB activation in the adverse effects induced by air pollution particulate matter (PM2.5) in human epithelial lung cells (L132) in culture. Appl Toxicol 2007;27:284–290.
18 Lee OH, Jain AK, Papusha V, et al: An autoregulatory loop between stress sensors INrf2 and Nrf2 controls their cellular abundance. J Biol Chem 2007;282:36412–36420.
19 Ciencewicki J, Trivedi S, Kleeberger SR: Oxidants and the pathogenesis of lung diseases. J Allergy Clin Immunol 2008;122:456–468.
20 Lee JM, Li J, Johnson DA, et al: Nrf2, a multi-organ protector? FASEB J 2005;19:1061–1066.

Mariangela Macchione, PhD
Department of Pathology, Laboratory of Experimental Air Pollution, Laboratory of Medical Investigation 05
Faculdade de Medicina da Universidade de São Paulo
Av. Dr. Arnaldo 455, São Paulo 01246-903 (Brazil)
Tel./Fax +55 11 3068 0072, E-Mail mmacchione@lim05.fm.usp.br

Esquinas AM (ed): Applied Technologies in Pulmonary Medicine. Basel, Karger, 2011, pp 238–245

Mechanical Ventilation in Disaster Management

Richard Branson[a] · Thomas C. Blakeman[a] · Dario Rodriquez[b]

[a]Division of Trauma and Critical Care, University of Cincinnati, and [b]Cincinnati CSTARS, United States Air Force, University Hospital, Cincinnati, Ohio, USA

Abbreviations

AARC	American Association for Respiratory Care
ARDS	Adult respiratory distress syndrome
CMV	Continuous mandatory ventilation
FiO_2	Inspired oxygen concentration
HMEs	Heat and moisture exchangers
MCRF	Mass casualty respiratory failure
PEEP	Positive end-expiratory pressure
PPE	Personal protective equipment
SARS	Severe acute respiratory syndrome

Recent history provides compelling tales of natural disasters, the threat of terrorism, and outbreaks of severe febrile respiratory illness including H1N1 influenza and SARS. These threats have focused healthcare planners, hospitals, and communities on how to care for large numbers of critically ill patients. Planning requires not only space for the care of patients, but equipment and staff [1]. MCRF is defined as an event resulting in patients requiring mechanical ventilation in excess of the space to care for them and devices to provide ventilatory support [2–4].

The work is solely that of the authors and does not reflect the official position of the US Air Force, Department of Defense or US Government.

History

History's most instructive presentation of MCRF occurred in the 1950s during the European poliomyelitis epidemic. During the summer of 1952 the hospital owned five ventilators, while treating 100 patients requiring mechanical ventilation. This 'surge' of patients, relative to available ventilators, has not been seen since. Lassen and colleagues [5] devised a clever solution to their problem. Instead of negative pressure ventilation they performed tracheostomy and enlisted medical students to perform manual ventilation in 4-hour shifts. Using a non-self-inflating bag and carbon dioxide absorber, they were able to use very low flows of oxygen to sustain ventilation and oxygenation. Interestingly, manual ventilation was also used following Hurricane Katrina, when electricity failed at Charity Hospital in New Orleans [6].

In 2009, while the world awaited an anticipated H5N1 (avian flu) outbreak, a novel H1N1 virus originated in Mexico. The resulting pandemic taxed ICUs around the world with severe respiratory failure in pediatrics, obese, and obstetric patients. The H1N1 epidemic is a lesson in the unpredictability of viruses. The severity of ARDS associated with H1N1 spurred a renewed interest in rescue therapies for refractory hypoxemia [7].

The Threat

In the USA, the Department of Homeland Security National Planning Guidelines are intended to coordinate and prioritize emergency preparedness efforts at all response levels. Contained within the Guidelines are 15 National Planning Scenarios, and at least two-thirds of these may result in MCRF [8]. The relevant scenarios are reviewed below.

Traumatic Injury

Traumatic injury may result on a local level from fire, explosion, or terrorist attack typically resulting in <100 casualties. The experience from Israel with public explosions suggests that most incidents result in 20–30 casualties with half being hospitalized, half admitted to an ICU and the majority of those for life-saving mechanical ventilation [8].

Expected Number of Victims. In a local explosion or fire, typically <100 victims require hospitalization and fewer require mechanical ventilation. In the instance of an earthquake or flood, many more victims may be expected, although the severity of injury is likely to be lower.

Time from Injury to Need for Mechanical Ventilation. The severity of trauma may require immediate airway management and ventilation while others only require ventilation after operative repair.

Pathophysiology. Traumatic injuries resulting in a need for mechanical ventilation include closed head injury, hemothorax, pneumothorax, pulmonary contusion, flail chest, traumatic amputation, blood loss, and blast injury.

Area Affected. In an explosion or fire, the affected area is usually finite and managed locally. A larger natural event may affect greater numbers of patients and result in damage to hospitals and transportation systems. In these instances, critically ill victims at the scene are likely to expire.

Chemical Weapons

Injuries following chemical weapons exposure vary with the agent. Chemical agents are classified as lung-damaging agents, blood agents, blister agents and nerve agents. These agents include chlorine, phosgene, and ammonia, all of which are commonly used in industrial processes and readily available. Mustard gas is perhaps the best known blister agent and cyanide the most likely blood agent.

Expected Number of Victims. Under the appropriate environmental conditions, population density, and dispersion, chemical agents may result in thousands of victims. Despite this prediction however, to date the number of victims has been in the hundreds and the number of victims requiring mechanical ventilation has been less than a dozen.

Time from Injury to Need for Mechanical Ventilation. The time until respiratory failure requires mechanical ventilation varies with the agent and exposure. Pulmonary agents can cause sudden death as a result of laryngeal obstruction and severe respiratory failure days after exposure. Nerve agents causing paralysis may require ventilation at the scene.

Pathophysiology. Chemical weapons enter the body through the respiratory system and skin. Blistering agents and choking agents result in bronchospasm and over time ARDS. Cyanide poisons mitochondria and prevents cellular respiration resulting in death from cellular hypoxia. Nerve agents result in flaccid paralysis and apnea, but also produce significant bronchorrhea and bronchospasm. So while patients exposed to nerve agents may have normal lung compliance, airway resistance may be elevated.

Area Affected. Optimum effectiveness of these agents as a weapon includes exposure of a large number of victims in a closed space. As such, these exposures are limited to a well-defined area.

Epidemics and Febrile Respiratory Illness

Epidemics and febrile illness may result from both natural and man-made causes. SARS and pandemic flu are good examples resulting in illness around the world in a short time frame. Anthrax and botulism exposure are most likely the result of bioterrorism although botulism poisoning can occur from improperly preserved foods. Anthrax, caused by *Bacillus anthracis*, has been used in the USA as a weapon, infecting 22 people and killing 5. Anthrax is however not contagious.

Expected Number of Victims. Epidemics can infect people from all over the world affecting tens of thousands of people. Weaponized botulism and anthrax have the ability to infect large numbers of patients as well, but to date this has not occurred.

Time from Injury to Need for Mechanical Ventilation. Epidemics are likely to result in the greatest number of casualties and typically the time from exposure until respiratory failure develops is prolonged (days to weeks). In these cases, patients may seek relief of early symptoms prior to progression to respiratory failure.

Pathophysiology. Pandemic flu and SARS have caused severe ARDS requiring rescue therapies for refractory hypoxemia. Botulism results in neuromuscular ventilatory failure from paralysis and may require prolonged support. Anthrax results in hemorrhagic mediastinitis, hemoptysis, sepsis, profound hypoxemia, and acute respiratory failure.

Area Affected. Natural epidemics and bioterrorism agents in this class have the ability to infect entire regions depending on the length of the incubation period and the continued presence of the contagion. In the case of pandemic flu, entire portions of a country may be affected.

Planning for Mass Casualty Respiratory Failure

Staffing. Any MCRF scenario will result in an exponential need for mechanical ventilation and will dramatically increase the need for ICU nurses, respiratory therapists, and physicians. Each hospital and public health agency should have a plan for support of healthcare workers and a disaster plan. Equipment is of no use if skilled caregivers are not available to operate it [9–11].

Personal Protective Equipment. Several of the febrile respiratory illnesses associated with MCRF are highly contagious. PPE is a critical component of mass casualty care in this setting. Availability of PPE is important, as it allows caregivers to feel safe during patient interactions. In the absence of sufficient PPE, concerns about personal health may lead to employees avoiding the workplace. Training caregivers in the use of PPE is also critical. The risk of secondary transmission is likely greater in the ICU as a result of the number of interventions causing aerosolization of infectious material. Procedures such as endotracheal intubation, open-circuit suctioning, and bronchoscopy are associated with increased risk of transmission. The use of filters in the ventilator circuit on the inspired and/or expired side or inside an HME may make sense but there is not data to support this practice. If filters are used, increased resistance may result in overdistension. Ventilators that compress room air should have a filter on the inspiratory inlet.

Oxygen. Liquid oxygen is readily available at most hospitals. Under normal circumstances, a hospital has reserves to operate for 3 weeks. A typical liquid system has 6,000–9,000 gallons of liquid oxygen which evaporates to nearly 30,000,000 gaseous liters of oxygen. Ritz and Privitera [12] estimated that their 500-bed hospital used 1.5 million liters of oxygen per day. During a disaster, oxygen conservation can be helpful. This includes use of reservoir or pendant cannulas, turning off flow to manual resuscitators, switching from heated aerosols to HMEs, and accepting lower levels of oxygen saturation in patients.

Disposables. A frequently overlooked aspect of MCRF are disposables. Ventilators require circuits, HMEs or humidifiers, and suction catheters. Oxygen requires delivery tubing, cannulas, masks, and other appliances. In keeping with cost containment, these devices are commonly kept at a level sufficient for several weeks of supply. In MCRF, most experts suspect that the disposables will be among the first supplies to run out. Re-use of circuits has been suggested, but this should only be considered as a last resort.

Ventilators

Ventilators may be needed following a disaster in three distinct environments. In the field to move patients from the scene of an accident to definitive care, between facilities (decompressing a localized event), and in-hospital care of critically ill and injured patients. The following discussion reviews the requirements of mechanical ventilators used for surge capacity in hospitals for definitive care.

Evidence-based management of the patient with ARDS is based on the results of the ARDSnet trial. The principles of ARDS management are straightforward: (a) low tidal volume (6–8 ml/kg of predicted body weight based on height); (b) ability to give a constant tidal volume; (c) plateau pressure ≤30 cm H_2O; (d) stable FiO_2 from 0.21 to 1.0; (e) CMV – maintain minute ventilation; (f) PEEP to prevent alveolar collapse and lung injury.

On day 1 of the ARDSnet trial, patients received a PEEP of 6–13 cm H_2O, an FiO_2 of 0.35–0.75, and a minute ventilation of 10–16 l/min. These data provide some standard requirements for the functional performance of ventilators for use in MCRF. We could suggest that ventilators for MCRF should be capable of setting PEEP from 6 to 13 cm H_2O, FiO_2 from 0.35 to 0.75, and a minute ventilation of 10–18 l/min. Assuming predicted body weights of 62–90 kg, tidal volumes of 375 up to 540 ml (6 ml/kg) should be capable of being set. These would be minimum requirements. Clearly some patients will require PEEP up to or >20 cm H_2O. Ventilators which are unable to produce these settings at a minimum *are not suitable* for in hospital MCRF.

Ventilator Performance Characteristics. Operational characteristics of ventilators for MCRF have been published by the AARC [13]. Some explanation and clarification of these characteristics are in order [14, 15]. Table 1 lists the desirable characteristics of ventilators for MCRF. The optimal ranges for operation remain to be determined. Characteristics of ventilators for MCRF which are more difficult to quantify are clearly just as important. A ventilator for MCRF should be rugged, portable, withstand shock and vibration, and continue operation if dropped. Portability is important and ideally devices would be well 'portable'. A weight of <10 kg is often a goal. In our minds, a portable device is one that a caregiver can pick up with one hand and move it without difficulty.

A ventilator for MCRF should have a low gas consumption. Equally important is battery life. Battery life is affected by age of the battery, temperature, and charging history regardless of the ventilator. Ventilator characteristics which decrease battery life include the mode of ventilation, the FiO_2, and PEEP. Patient characteristics can also affect battery life, the greater the load the shorter the duration of operation.

The ventilator should be easy to trigger and have an acceptable work of breathing. Most current-generation portable ventilators meet this requirement. Cost should be less than USD 10,000. The ventilator should be intuitive and easy to use.

Table 1. Suggested performance characteristics of ventilators for MCRF

Characteristic	Rationale	Characteristics	
		mandatory	desirable
FDA-approved for adults and pediatrics	Natural disasters, pandemics, and chemical/bioterrorism will also affect children	Ventilate 10-kg patient	Ventilate 5-kg patient
Ability to operate without 50 psig compressed gas	The redundancy for electrical power in hospitals far exceeds oxygen stores and redundancy In the absence of high-pressure oxygen, low flow oxygen from a flowmeter can be used to increase FiO_2	Operate without 50 psig input FiO_2 from 0.21 to 1.0	Operate with or without 50 psig input alone
Battery life of 4 h of greater	Allow for transport from facility to facility Provide continuous support during intermittent power failure	4 h of operation at nominal settings	>4 h operation at nominal settings
Constant volume delivery	Meet guidelines for tidal volume delivery as dictated by ARDSnet protocol Reduce potential for ventilator-induced lung injury Provide age-appropriate settings	Volume control ventilation (350–600 ml)	Pressure control and volume control ventilation
Mode: CMV	Meet ARDSnet guidelines Assure minimum ventilation in a situation of multiple patients and a shortage of caregivers	CMV	CMV, intermittent mandatory ventilation, and pressure support
PEEP	Meet ARDSnet guidelines Prevent ventilator-induced lung injury Reverse hypoxemia	Adjustable from 5 to 15 cm H_2O	Adjustable from 5 to 20 cm H_2O
Separate controls for respiratory rate and tidal volume	Meet ARDSnet guidelines Assure minute ventilation in apneic patients	Respiratory rate from 6 to 35 breaths/min	Respiratory rate from 6 to 75 breaths/min (for pediatrics)
Monitor airway pressures and tidal volume	Meet ARDSnet guidelines Provide assessment of patient's lung compliance Patient safety – prevent overdistension	Monitor peak inspiratory pressure and delivered tidal volume	Monitor plateau pressure and patient tidal volumes
Appropriate alarms	Patient safety Improve ability to monitor large numbers of patients with reduced staff	Alarms for circuit disconnect High airway pressure Low airway pressure (leak) Loss of electric power Loss of high pressure source gas	Alarms for high tidal volume in pressure modes Low minute ventilation Remote alarms

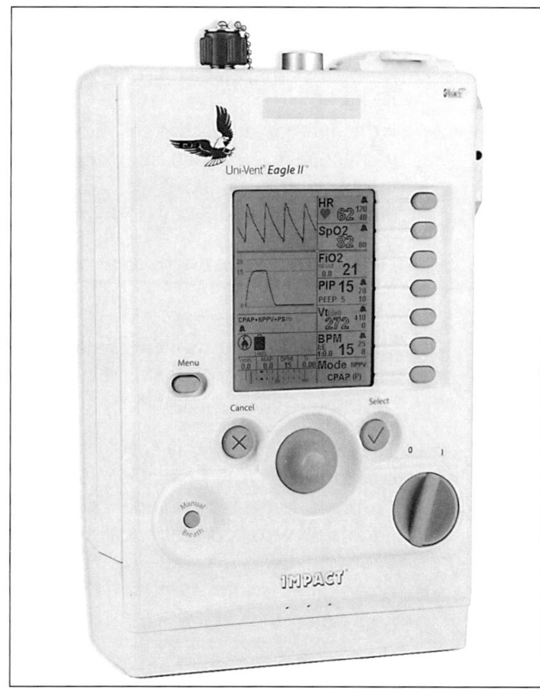

Fig. 1. A sophisticated portable ventilator capable of ventilating critically ill patients. This device has an internal air source (compressor) and a suite of monitoring and alarms allowing it to be used in a number of situations.

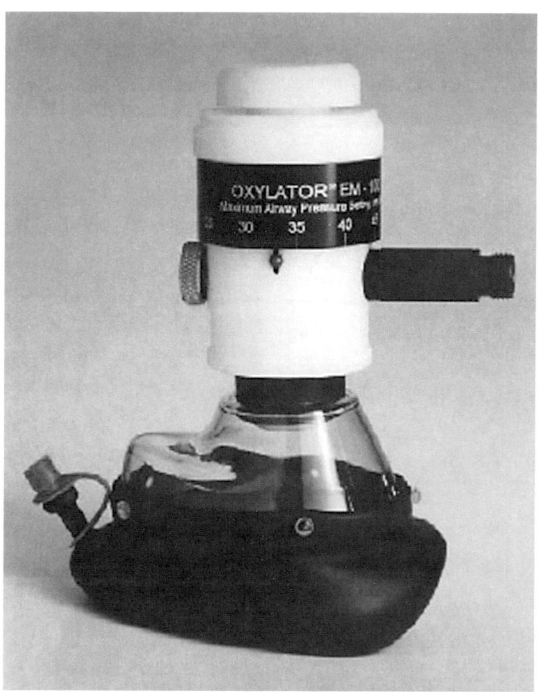

Fig. 2. Automatic resuscitator with limited capability. These devices must be used with a caregiver present at each patient.

Ventilators. Classification of mechanical ventilators is a complex task. For the purposes of describing ventilators for MCRF, operation and application leads to description of types of ventilators which might be used based on characteristics. This description includes automatic resuscitators, EMS ventilators, pneumatically-powered portable ventilators, electrically-powered portable ventilators, and full-feature ICU ventilators.

Automatic Resuscitators. An automatic resuscitator is designed to replace the need for hand-bagging. These devices are predominantly pneumatically-powered and pressure-cycled. Automatic resuscitators have few to no alarms, cannot provide a constant tidal volume, cannot set rate and tidal volume separately, and commonly provide 100% source gas or a lower concentration with the use of a Venturi. These devices are inexpensive, but fail to meet the demands of the patient with ARDS and are not suitable for stockpiling to treat MCRF. The best that can be said is that these devices are better than no support at all. An example of an automatic resuscitator is shown in figure 1.

EMS Portable Ventilators. An EMS portable ventilator is used in patient transport, typically in emergency care via ambulance. These devices are more reliable, rugged, and have greater functionality than automatic resuscitators. The functionality and cost in this group is variable. Some devices set tidal volume and respiratory rate via a single control. Others have separate controls for both settings. PEEP is usually supplied by an external

Table 2. Sources of additional ventilators for a MCRF scenario

Affected hospital	Cancel elective surgeries Repurpose anesthesia workstations as mechanical ventilators and ICU monitoring (during non-trauma disasters)	Number of anesthesia machines is limited If the duration of mechanical ventilation is prolonged, anesthesia machines will be needed when surgeries and other procedures are reinitiated
Unaffected hospital	Redistribution of available equipment from unaffected hospitals to those in need	There are few extra available ventilators at most hospitals even during usual conditions Delayed situational awareness may reduce willingness of 'unaffected' hospitals to share equipment
Mechanical ventilator rental services	Provision of additional ventilators by a rental company	The same company may have contracts with a number of affected hospitals, so the total number of additional ventilators may be limited Logistical delays may be encountered when sending ventilators from distant geographic areas
Strategic National Stockpile	Deployment of mechanical ventilators to states or cities in need	Delay in distribution since most states still have limited capacity to distribute equipment from the Strategic National Stockpile Unclear how distribution will be prioritized when multiple hospitals are requesting ventilators at the same time

valve. FiO_2 is commonly 100% source gas or a single lower concentration with use of an air entrainment system. Monitoring and alarms are limited.

Sophisticated Portable Ventilators (Pneumatically-Powered). Sophisticated pneumatically-powered, portable ventilators have the ability to provide CMV and intermittent mandatory ventilation, set PEEP, have a low work of breathing, and allow separate control of tidal volume and respiratory rate. These devices meet most of the performance characteristics for MCRF. The limitations of these devices surround the pneumatic power source. These devices cannot operate in the absence of a 50-psig gas source. FiO_2 is typically limited to 100% source gas which wastes oxygen. Few alarms are also a weakness.

Sophisticated Portable Ventilators (Electronically-Powered). These devices are often used in homecare and for in-hospital transport. Electronically-powered, sophisticated portable ventilators meet the performance characteristics required of a ventilator for MCRF. There is some significant difference in weight of these devices (5–15 kg). Battery life and gas consumption vary depending on the driving system of the ventilator. Figure 2 depicts a commonly used portable ventilator.

Critical Care Ventilators. Critical care ventilators are capable of managing all types of respiratory failure. These devices have not been recommended for MCRF due to the large size, cost (USD 30,000+), and complexity.

Non-Invasive Ventilators. Non-invasive ventilation is a standard of care for respiratory failure in the patient with chronic obstructive pulmonary disease, under normal circumstances. The use of non-invasive ventilation in MCRF however has significant limitations. In a MCRF situation, we suggest the repurposing of non-invasive ventilators for use as invasive ventilators. Table 2 lists the possible sources of additional ventilators during MCRF.

Triage. No discussion of MCRF is complete without mentioning triage of ventilators. This is an ethical dilemma which the modern world has not yet had to face. In MCRF, all patients will receive care based on the likelihood of survival. These systems are being developed by national societies to allow the most good to be done for the most patients with the best possible outcome. All patients receive care in a mass casualty situation, even if it is comfort care.

Conclusion

MCRF represents a significant concern for healthcare systems and governments around the world. The best solution is thoughtful planning and cooperation between all the shareholders. Despite our inability to predict when an event may occur and how many patients will require mechanical ventilation, we must plan using best evidence. Ventilators purchased for MCRF must meet the demands of the patient and the skills of the operator.

References

1 Hotchkin DL, Rubinson L: Modified critical care and treatment space consideration for mass casualty critical illness and injury. Respir Care 2008;53:67–74.
2 Rubinson L, Nuzzo JB, Talmor DS, O'Toole T, Kramer BR, Inglesby TV: Augmentation of hospital critical care capacity after bioterrorist attacks or epidemics: recommendations of the Working Group on Emergency Mass Critical Care. Crit Care Med 2005;33:2393–2403.
3 Rubinson L, O'Toole T: Critical care during epidemics. Crit Care 2005;9:311–313.
4 Rubinson L, Branson RD, Pesik N, Talmor D: Positive-pressure ventilation equipment for mass casualty respiratory failure. Biosecur Bioterror 2006;4:183–194.
5 Lassen HCA: Management of Life-Threatening Poliomyelitis. Copenhagen, 1952–1956, with a Survey of Autopsy Findings in 115 cases. Edinburgh, Livingstone, 1956.
6 DeBoisblanc BP: Black Hawk, please come down: reflections on a hospital's struggle to survive in the wake of Hurricane Katrina. Am J Respir Crit Care Med 2005;172:1239–1240.
7 Tang JW, Shetty N, Lam TT: Features of the new pandemic influenza A/H1N1/2009 virus: virology, epidemiology, clinical and public health aspects. Curr Opin Pulm Med 2010;16:235–241.
8 Homeland Security: National Preparedness Guidelines, October 2007. Accessed April 24, 2010 (http://www.dhs.gov/xlibrary/assets/National_Preparedness_Guidelines.pdf).
9 Muskat P: Mass casualty chemical exposure and implications for respiratory failure. Respir Care 2008;53:58–63.
10 Hanley ME, Bogdan GM: Mechanical ventilation in mass casualty scenarios. Augmenting staff: project XTREME. Respir Care 2008;53:176–188.
11 Daugherty E, Branson RD, Desai A, Rubinson L: Infection control in mass respiratory failure: preparing to respond to H1N1. Crit Care Med 2010;38(suppl):e103–e109.
12 Ritz RH, Privitera JE: Oxygen supplies during a mass casualty situation. Respir Care 2008;53:215–224.
13 AARC Guidelines for Acquisition of Ventilators to Meet Demands for Pandemic Flu and Mass Casualty Incidents American Association Accessed April 14, 2008 (http://www.aarc.org/headlines/ventilator_acquisitions/vent_guidelines.pdf).
14 Branson RD, Johannigman JA, Daugherty EL, Rubinson L: Surge capacity mechanical ventilation. Respir Care 2008;53:78–90.
15 Daugherty EL, Branson RD, Rubinson L: Mass casualty respiratory failure. Curr Opin Crit Care 2007;13:51–56.

Richard Branson, MS, RRT
Division of Trauma and Critical Care, University of Cincinnati
231 Albert Sabin Way, Cincinnati, OH 45267-0558 (USA)
Tel. +1 513 558 6785, Fax +1 513 558 3747
E-Mail Richard.branson@uc.edu

Esquinas AM (ed): Applied Technologies in Pulmonary Medicine. Basel, Karger, 2011, pp 246–249

Postoperative Intensive and Intermediate Care?

Charles Weissman

Department of Anesthesiology and Critical Care Medicine, Hadassah-Hebrew University Medical Center, Hebrew University-Hadassah School of Medicine, Jerusalem, Israel

Contemporary hospital medicine must cope with increasing numbers and proportions of very ill patients requiring greater nursing and medical care than afforded on regular hospital floors. To care for such patients requires clinical areas with increased nurse:patient ratios and specialized medical personnel. Therefore, hospitals require increasing numbers of ICUs (intensive therapy units), intermediate care units (high dependency units) and postoperative recovery rooms (post-anesthesia care units). This situation has placed hospitals in the perpetual quandary of how many and what proportion of beds should be intensive care, intermediate care and regular beds [1].

Analysis of Main Topics

Increasingly complex surgery is being performed on patients suffering from preexisting chronic diseases and who are elderly. Such patients frequently require enhanced care after surgery to monitor, prevent and, if necessary, treat life-threatening complications as soon as they appear. In the UK, surgical patients make up 60–70% of the ICU workload [2]. The British National Confidential Enquiry into Perioperative Deaths for 1992/1993 recommended that surgery not be performed on physiologically compromised patients without adequate facilities for postoperative care [3]. This situation requires provisions for graduated levels of care (intensive, intermediate, routine floor care). The importance of graduated care was emphasized in a report from hospitals without intermediate care units so that postoperative intermediate care patients were sent to regular wards. The greater care requirements of such patients adversely affected the care of less ill patients [4]. The advantages of postoperative intermediate care was demonstrated by comparing major abdominal surgery patients who were cared for on a general surgical ward because the hospital lacked an intermediate unit with those who were initially managed in an intermediate unit. Intermediate care resulted in fewer cardiorespiratory complications, without differences in mortality, but with a trend towards shorter hospital stays [5, 6]. Alternately, the introduction of a 4-bed intermediate unit in a teaching hospital failed to reduce postoperative serious events or mortality, nor did it decrease the mean duration of hospitalization [7].

Graduated postoperative care requires that specific criteria be established for equipping, staffing and admissions to each type of unit. Surgical ICUs generally care for four types of patients: (1) Those after extensive elective surgery (e.g. open abdominal aneurysm repairs, anterior-posterior spine fusion) and those with severe preexisting diseases undergoing major to moderate elective surgery [8]. (2) Emergency surgery patients who have cardiopulmonary instability following surgery. (3) Surgical patients who have cardiopulmonary, septic or hemorrhagic deteriorations on surgical floors or intermediate care units. (4) Trauma victims admitted for non-operative management (e.g. observation of splenic, renal or hepatic lacerations). Many institutions have subspecialty ICUs to care for high volumes of specific patients. The leading example is the cardiothoracic surgical ICU which specializes in caring for postoperative cardiac and thoracic surgery patients. Such ICUs are unifocused and thus can optimize protocol and care plans for such patients. Neurosurgical and burn ICUs serve much the same purpose. Specialized units offload routine elective cardiac surgery and neurosurgery patients from the main surgical ICU allowing it to focus on caring for the remaining heterogeneous population of critically ill surgical patients many of whom require extensive physiological monitoring, multiple diagnostic and therapeutic procedures and much medical and nursing care.

Intermediate care units differ from ICUs by caring for lower acuity patients. They, thus, have higher nurse:patient ratios (ICU 1:1–1:2 vs. intermediate 1:4) and lower intensity of physician coverage. Surgical intermediate care units take a number of forms: (1) *Postoperative/post-procedure units* monitor (24–48 h) hemodynamically stable patients after complex surgeries, patients with underlying cardiopulmonary disorders after moderate surgery and those receiving peripheral arterial thrombolytic therapy [1, 9]. (2) *Step-down units* admit patients who no longer need ICU care but require more intense nursing care than provided on the surgical floors. (3) *Mechanical ventilator units* care for patients requiring long-term mechanical ventilation. Alternately, the post-anesthesia care unit can be used as a postoperative/post-procedure intermediate unit for patients needing up to 24 h of such care. The rationale is that post-anesthesia care units are equipped with physiological monitors and staffed by specially trained nurses but are not fully occupied during the evening and night. Among the disadvantages of this arrangement is the need to discharge these overnight patients early enough in the morning so as not to interfere with the elective surgical schedule.

Discussion

The types of patients admitted to each kind of unit is institution-specific, i.e. depends on the patient population, number and types of ICU and intermediate units, the number of such beds, the monitoring, nursing and medical capabilities of each unit, the nursing capabilities on regular floors (i.e. nurse:patient ratio) and institutional administrative and medical policies. For example, in our institution, 12% of postoperative patients were admitted directly to an ICU or intermediate unit [10].

A recent prospective observational study of 1,233 adult postoperative patients transferred after a short recovery room stay to a floor bed or the ambulatory surgery unit and 1,883 patients admitted to intermediate and ICU areas, examined the effects of pre- and intraoperative factors on receipt of postoperative ICU or intermediate care. There were distinct differences between the preoperative (preexisting systemic disease) and intraoperative characteristics (complexity of surgery and intraoperative care intensity) of postoperative ICU/intermediate care patients and those receiving routine floor care [11]. Moreover, there were differences between elective and emergency surgery. Most patients undergoing elective operations of the highest complexity (e.g. craniotomy, cardiac surgery) received intermediate or ICU care including those without preexisting systemic illness (ASA class 1). Classic examples were healthy teenagers undergoing elective orthognathic jaw surgery and anterior-posterior spine fusion for scoliosis. The former because they remained tracheally intubated overnight because of upper airway edema and the latter because they were monitored for hemorrhage. Another example was elective neurosurgery patients with minimal (ASA class 2) underlying systemic diseases who underwent craniotomies for brain tumor excision. Alternately, patients undergoing less complex major elective surgery often tended to receive intermediate or ICU care if they had significant preexisting systemic disorders (ASA classes 3 and 4).

Emergency surgery patients differed substantially from elective surgery ones with a greater proportion receiving ICU rather than intermediate care. ASA class was not significantly associated with receipt of ICU rather than intermediate care. This was true even when trauma patients, many of whom were ASA classes 1 and 2, were removed from the analysis. Like the elective surgery patients, high intraoperative care intensity and postoperative mechanical ventilation were associated with the receipt of ICU rather than intermediate care. This is in contrast to the elective patients were ASA class, operative complexity and age were also so associated. This suggests that the intensity of non-surgical care received during emergency surgery and the decision to leave the patient mechanically ventilated after surgery resulted in ICU rather than intermediate admission. Therefore, the severity of the acute illness or trauma dictates the need for significant interventions during surgery (e.g. blood products, hemodynamic monitoring) resulting in a decision to leave the patient mechanically ventilated after surgery.

Interestingly, 10% of the elective surgery patients unexpectedly received ICU or intermediate care because of unanticipated intraoperative or immediate postoperative issues, such as upper airway problems or unexpected hemorrhage. Similar observations have been made by others, who consider unexpected admissions a quality indicator [12].

Recommendations

- Modern in-patient surgical care systems require graduated levels of care (intensive, intermediate and floor care).
- Postoperative patients are major consumers of ICU and intermediate care as surgery is increasingly performed on the elderly and on patients with significant preexisting illness.
- Receipt of postoperative intermediate and intensive care is associated with distinct patterns of both preoperative and intraoperative factors.
- Postoperative mechanically ventilation is the major indication for ICU rather than intermediate care.
- The ASA class and complexity of the surgery are important factors determining postoperative intensive/intermediate care after elective surgery. After emergency surgery the intensity of intraoperative interventions, and not surgical complexity, is a major determining factor.

References

1 Heller J, Murch P: Development in service provision. Making major elective surgery happen. The development of a postoperative surgical unit. Nurs Crit Care 2008;13:97–104.

2 Cuthbertson BH, Webster NR: The role of the intensive care unit in the management of the critically ill surgical patient. J R Coll Surg Edinb 1999;44: 294–300.

3 Campling EA, Devlin HB, Hoile RW, et al: The report of the National Confidential Enquiry into Perioperative Deaths 1992/1993. London, NCEPOD, 1995.

4 Coggins RP: Delivery of surgical care in a district general hospital without high dependency unit facilities. Postgrad Med J 2000;76:223–226.
5 Jones HJ, Coggins R, Lafuente J, et al: Value of a surgical high-dependency unit. Br J Surg 1999;86:1578–1582.
6 Armstrong K, Young J, Hayburn A, et al: Evaluating the impact of a new high dependency unit. Int J Nurs Pract 2003; 9:285–293.
7 Bellomo R, Goldsmith D, Uchino S, et al: A before and after trial of the effect of a high-dependency unit on post-operative morbidity and mortality. Crit Care Resusc 2005;7:16–21.
8 Cavaliere F, Conti G, Costa R, et al: Intensive care after elective surgery: a survey on 30-day postoperative mortality and morbidity. Minerva Anestesiol 2008;74:459–468.
9 Angel D, Sieunarine K, Finn J, et al: Comparison of short-term clinical postoperative outcomes in patients who underwent carotid endarterectomy: intensive care unit versus the ward high-dependency unit. J Vasc Nurs 2004;22:85–90.
10 Weissman C, Klein N: The importance of differentiating between elective and emergency postoperative critical care patients. J Crit Care 2008;23:308–316.
11 Weissman C, Klein N: Who receives postoperative intensive and intermediate care? J Clin Anesth 2008;20:263–270.
12 Haller G, Myles PS, Langley M, et al: Assessment of an unplanned admission to the intensive care unit as a global safety indicator in surgical patients. Anaesth Intensive Care 2008;36:190–200.

Charles Weissman, MD
Department of Anesthesiology and Critical Care Medicine
Hadassah-Hebrew University Medical Center, Hebrew University-Hadassah School of Medicine
Jerusalem 91120 (Israel)
Tel. +972 2 677 7269, Fax +972 2 642 9392, E-Mail Charles@hadassah.org.il

Author Index

Subject Index

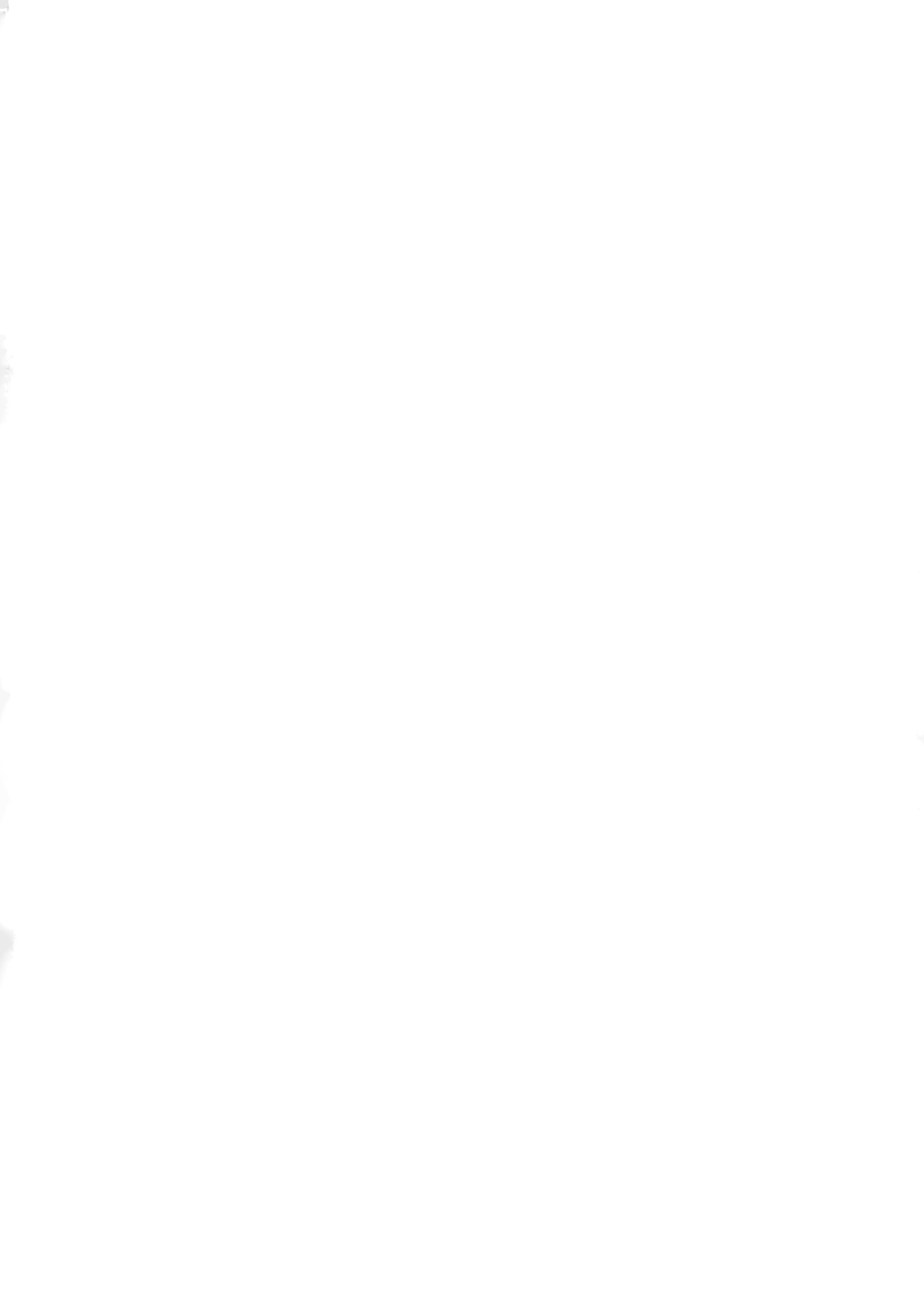